Functional Biomaterials

With the emergence of additive manufacturing, mass customization of biomaterials for complex tissue regeneration and targeted drug delivery applications is possible. This book emphasizes the fundamental concepts of biomaterials science, their structure–property relationships and processing methods, and biological responses in biomedical engineering. It focuses on recent advancements in biomedical applications, such as tissue engineering, wound healing, drug delivery, cancer treatments, bioimaging, and theranostics.

This book

- Discusses design chemistry, modification, and processing of biomaterials.
- Describes the efficacy of biomaterials at various scales for biological response and drug delivery.
- Demonstrates technological advances from conventional to additive manufacturing.
- Covers future of biofabrication and customized medical devices.

This volume serves as a go-to reference on functional biomaterials and is ideal for multi-disciplinary communities such as students and research professionals in materials science, biomedical engineering, healthcare, and medical fields.

Emerging Materials and Technologies

Series Editor:
Boris I. Kharissov

The *Emerging Materials and Technologies* series is devoted to highlighting publications centered on emerging advanced materials and novel technologies. Attention is paid to those newly discovered or applied materials with potential to solve pressing societal problems and improve quality of life, corresponding to environmental protection, medicine, communications, energy, transportation, advanced manufacturing, and related areas.

The series takes into account that, under present strong demands for energy, material, and cost savings, as well as heavy contamination problems and worldwide pandemic conditions, the area of emerging materials and related scalable technologies is a highly interdisciplinary field, with the need for researchers, professionals, and academics across the spectrum of engineering and technological disciplines. The main objective of this book series is to attract more attention to these materials and technologies and invite conversation among the international R&D community.

PUBLISHED TITLES

Two-Dimensional Nanomaterials for Fire-Safe Polymers
Yuan Hu and Xin Wang

3D Printing and Bioprinting for Pharmaceutical and Medical Applications
Edited by Jose Luis Pedraz Muñoz, Laura Saenz del Burgo Martínez, Gustavo Puras Ochoa, and Jon Zarate Sesma

Wastewater Treatment with the Fenton Process
Principles and Applications
Dominika Bury, Piotr Marcinowski, Jan Bogacki, Michal Jakubczak, and Agnieszka Maria Jastrzebska

For more information about this series, please visit: www.routledge.com/Emerging-Materials-and-Technologies/book-series/CRCEMT

Functional Biomaterials

Advances in Design and Biomedical Applications

Edited By
Anuj Kumar, Durgalakshmi Dhinasekaran,
Irina N. Savina and Sung Soo Han

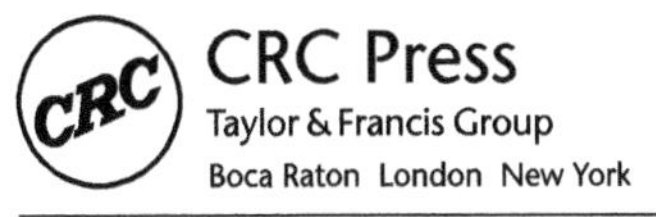

CRC Press is an imprint of the
Taylor & Francis Group, an **informa** business

First edition published 2024
by CRC Press
2385 Executive Center Drive, Suite 320, Boca Raton, FL 33431

and by CRC Press
4 Park Square, Milton Park, Abingdon, Oxon, OX14 4RN

CRC Press is an imprint of Taylor & Francis Group, LLC

ISBN: 978-1-032-17089-3 (hbk)
ISBN: 978-1-032-17090-9 (pbk)
ISBN: 978-1-003-25176-7 (ebk)

DOI: 10.1201/9781003251767

Typeset in Times
by codeMantra

Contents

Preface vii
About the Authors ix
Contributors xi

Chapter 1 Stimuli-Responsive Hydrogels for Tissue Engineering and Drug Delivery Applications 1

Remziye Aysun Kepekçi

Chapter 2 3D Printing of Hydrogels for Cartilage Tissue Engineering Applications 19

Sena Su Torun, Ecem Dogan, Nazmi Ekren, Cem Bulent Ustundag, and Oguzhan Gunduz

Chapter 3 Advances in 3D Hydrogel Matrix and Their Role in Neural Tissue Engineering 37

Sumeyye Cesur, Tuba Bedir, Nazmi Ekren, Oguzhan Gunduz, and Cem Bulent Ustundag

Chapter 4 Evolution of Biogenic Synthesized Scaffolds for Tissue Engineering Applications 77

Deepa Suhag and Yogita Basnal

Chapter 5 3D Bioprinting of Hydrogels for Bones and Skin Tissue Regeneration 99

Sümeyra Ayan, Rıdvan Yıldırım, Nazmi Ekren, Oguzhan Gunduz, and Cem Bulent Ustundag

Chapter 6 Design and Development of Biopolymers-Based Gene Delivery Applications 131

S. Sajeesh, A.K. Dipin Das, and M.R. Rekha

Chapter 7 Stimuli-Responsive Microgels as Drug Carriers and Theranostics 151

Aastha Gupta, Ankita Dhiman, Sangram K. Samal, and Garima Agrawal

Chapter 8 Bioactive Glasses: Multifunctional Delivery Systems for Cancer Theranostic Applications 175

Saeid Kargozar, Sara Gorgani, Sahar Mollazadeh, Farzad Kermani, and Francesco Baino

Chapter 9 Cryogels, Macroporous Hydrogels, as Promising Materials for Tissue Engineering and Drug Delivery 193

I. N. Savina

Chapter 10 Constructing Three-Dimensional Microenvironments Using Engineered Biomaterials for Bone and Cartilage Tissue Regeneration 213

Ketki Holkar, Isha Behere, and Ganesh Ingavle

Chapter 11 Collagen-Based Functionalized Nanocomposite for Bone Tissue Regeneration 237

Sougata Ghosh, Sirikanjana Thongmee, Hisao Haniu, and Ebrahim Mostafavi

Chapter 12 Composite Hydrogels for Adipose Tissue Engineering 255

P.N. Blessy Rebecca, D. Durgalakshmi, and R. Ajay Rakkesh

Chapter 13 Recent Progress in Organic-Inorganic Hybrids for Bone Tissue Reconstruction 275

Toshiki Miyazaki

Chapter 14 Biomaterials and Microfluidics Systems Used for Modeling Pathological Tissues 289

Baeckkyoung Sung

Index 309

Preface

Over the past decades, functional biomaterials have been evolved to improve the functionality of the living systems in the healthcare, especially in tissue engineering and delivery of bioactive molecules or theranostics. A biomaterial is commonly characterized as the substance, manufactured into various forms (single or as component of a complex structure), that adapts various therapeutic or diagnostic progressions by governing interactions with the components of native living tissues. There has been extensive research in the functionality of different classes of biomaterials for diverse biomedical applications over the past few decades and they are designed to function as anticipated by demonstrating superior aptitudes to elucidate various challenges related to human health. The designing and development of a wide range of innovative functional biomaterials is a promising aspect in diverse biomedical areas for their successful clinical translation. In the design of functional biomaterials, it is not focused only on manufacturing bioinert systems but rather on systems that can respond to the cellular 3D micro-/nanoenvironment around them to enhance biomaterial integration and tissue regeneration. However, the precise manufacturing of biomaterials to bestow them with functions at the anticipated scales or through multiple scales for targeted tissue or delivery of bioactive molecules is a long-researched sub-area of the biomedical field, and yet there are various challenges to be overcome. A better understanding of the science of biomaterials is imperative to engineering sophisticated functional biomaterials for diverse biomedical applications.

The prime purpose of this book is to provide information on a broad range of biomaterial-based structures, design approaches, processing, properties, and their particular utilizations in different biomedical areas such as tissue engineering, drug delivery carriers and theranostics, gene delivery, or modeling pathological tissues. Individual chapters focus on the materials utilized in functional biomaterials, their properties and applications, such as biogenic synthesized scaffolds, composite hydrogels, stimuli-responsive hydrogels and microgels, 3D printing of hydrogel-systems, cryogels, biopolymers, collagen, bioactive glasses, organic–inorganic hybrids, and the utility of biomaterials and microfluidic systems for modeling pathological tissues. Moreover, the key issues and challenges associated with the design of complex functional biomaterials are also discussed in each chapter. Therefore, an updated collection of biomaterial research will be a useful reference text for undergraduate/postgraduate students and essential reading for professors, scientists, engineers, and clinicians working on biomaterials in diverse biomedical areas.

At last, but most notably, we would like to thank and acknowledge the authors who contributed to this book. Furthermore, we thank all the reviewers for giving their valuable time and providing timely constructive comments and suggestions to improve the quality of this book.

Varanasi, India; Anuj Kumar
Chennai, India; Durgalakshmi Dhinasekaran
Brighton, UK; Irina N. Savina
Gyeongsan, South Korea; Sung Soo Han

About the Authors

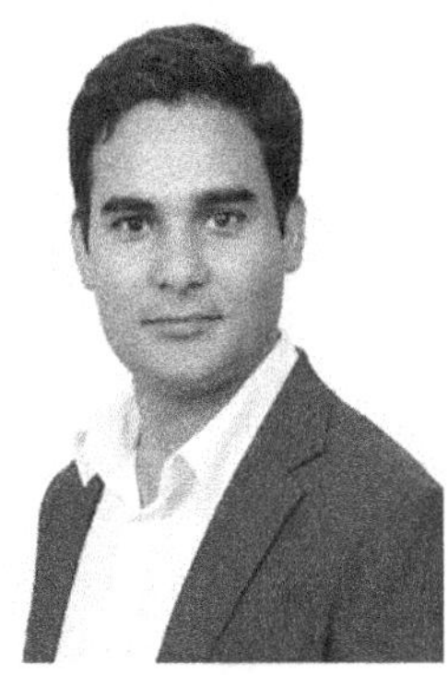

Anuj Kumar is a DBT-Ramalingaswami Faculty (Assistant Professor) at the School of Materials Science and Technology, Indian Institute of Technology (Banaras Hindu University), Varanasi, India. Prior to this position, he was an Assistant Professor (Polymers and Biomaterials) in the School of Chemical Engineering at Yeungnam University (YU) in Gyeongsan, South Korea. He has been awarded 3 sponsored research projects *(including the Indo-Korea joint research project as Co-PI)*, DBT-Ramalingaswami Re-entry Fellowship, and BK21 participating professorship. He was Postdoctoral Research Associate in YU (South Korea) and Assistant Professor (Chemistry) at DIT University (India). He received his PhD (Polymer Science and Engineering), MTech (Fibre Science and Technology), and MSc (Organic Chemistry) from IIT Roorkee, IIT Delhi, and CCSU Meerut, India, respectively. His research interests are focused on polymer chemistry, lignocellulosic biomass, nanocellulose, biomaterials, 3D bioprinting, microfluidics, tissue engineering, cultured meat production, drug delivery, cancer therapy, wearable bioelectronics, etc.

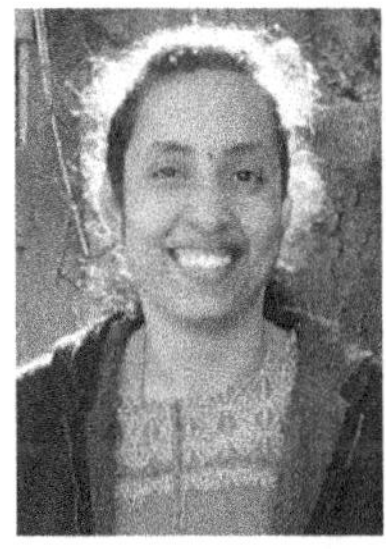

Durgalakshmi Dhinasekaran received her Bachelor's degree in Physics from Thiruvalluvar University and Master's degree in Physics from Bharathidasan University. She did her Master of Philosophy in Physics-Material Science from the University of Madras. She completed her Ph.D. degree in the field of "Physics-Nano-Biomaterials" from the National Centre for Nanoscience and Nanotechnology, University of Madras, India. For her doctoral work, *she also awarded Lady Tata Junior and senior fellowship, a prestigious fellowship from Tata Memorial Trust*, a prestigious award given for the students doing medicinal research. For her PhD thesis, she was awarded the best thesis of the year 2016 *in the area of Material Science by Material Research Society of India for this she also got the G.C. Jain Memorial prize award.* Now, she is working as an Assistant Professor in the Department of Medical Physics, Anna University, Chennai. Prior to this position, she also worked as an Assistant Professor at Ethiraj College for Woment and DST-INPSIRE faculty in the Department of Medical Physics, Anna University, Chennai. She has nearly 75 research publications, 16 book chapters, and edited one book for Springer International Publication. Her research focuses on nanostructured materials for energy, environmental, and biomedical applications.

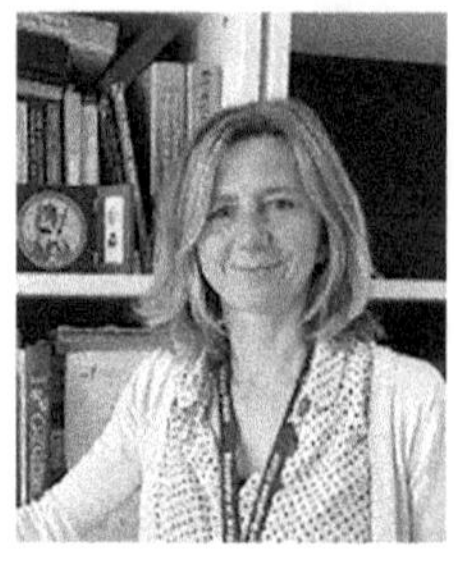

Irina N. Savina graduated from the Ryazan State Pedagogical University, Russia, with the qualification of Teacher of Biology and Chemistry. She did her PhD at the A.N. Nesmeyanov Institute of Organoelement Compounds, Russian Academy of Sciences, Moscow, Russia. She did her postdoctoral studies at the University of Gent in Belgium and at Lund University in Sweden. In May 2007, Dr. Irina Savina joined the University of Brighton and is currently working as a Senior Lecturer at the School of Applied Sciences. Dr. Savina's research work is diverse and multi-disciplinary, with the core subject being the synthesis of novel polymer materials. Her interests cover polymer synthesis, physical chemistry of polymer gels, macroporous polymer materials, organic/inorganic hybrid materials, nanocomposites, polymer graft polymerization, and polymer surface modification, with a special emphasis on designing novel hydrogel materials for biotechnology, biomedical, and environmental applications. She is an expert in cryogel (macroporous hydrogel) production. Dr. Savina is actively participating in national and international industry-focused research (UK Department of Trade and Industry, National Science Foundation, British Council, European Commission). She has been awarded two prestigious (MC) individual fellowships (IEF and CIG), as recognition of her excellence in science. Dr. Savina has published more than 60 papers in international peer reviewed journals, nine book chapters, and two patents. She is a member of the Engineering and Physical Science Research Council (UK), the National Center of Science and Technology Evaluation of Republic of Kazakhstan and European Commission expert panels. She is a member of the Editorial Board of Toxicology, Pollution and the Environment within the journal *Frontiers in Environmental Science*, a Guest Editor of two special issues of Molecules (MDPI) and a Guest Editor of RSC Advances themed collection titled 'Nanomaterials in Drug Delivery' (RSC).

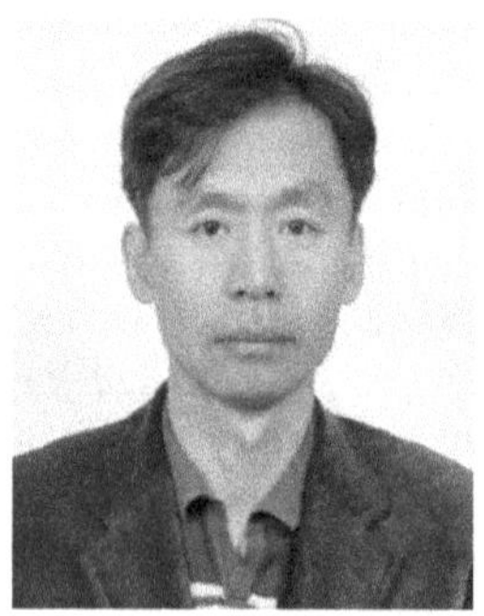

Sung Soo Han is a Professor at the School of Chemical Engineering at Yeungnam University (YU) in Gyeongsan, South Korea. He received his PhD, MS, and BS degrees from the Department of Polymer and Textile Engineering, Seoul National University (SNU), Seoul, South Korea. He has published several research and review articles in internationally reputed journals. His research interests are focused on biomaterials, nanomaterials, tissue engineering, drug delivery, cancer therapy, bioprocess engineering, and artificial meat culture.

Contributors

Garima Agrawal
School of Chemical Sciences
Indian Institute of Technology Mandi
Himachal Pradesh, India

Sümeyra Ayan
Department of Bioengineering
Yildiz Technical University
Istanbul, Turkey
and
Materials Institute, Marmara Research Center
TUBITAK
İzmit, Turkey

Francesco Baino
Institute of Materials Physics and Engineering, Applied Science and Technology Department
Politecnico di Torino
Torino, Italy

Yogita Basnal
Amity Centre for Nanotechnology
Amity University Haryana
Manesar, India

Tuba Bedir
Center for Nanotechnology & Biomaterials Application and Research (NBUAM)
Marmara University
Istanbul, Turkey
and
Department of Metallurgical and Materials Engineering, Faculty of Technology
Marmara University
Istanbul, Turkey

Isha Behere
Symbiosis Centre for Stem Cell Research (SCSCR)
Symbiosis International (Deemed University)
Pune, India

Sumeyye Cesur
Center for Nanotechnology & Biomaterials Application and Research (NBUAM)
Marmara University
Istanbul, Turkey

A.K. Dipin Das
Division of Biosurface Technology, Biomedical Technology Wing
SCTIMST
Thiruvananthapuram, India

Ankita Dhiman
School of Chemical Sciences
Indian Institute of Technology Mandi
Himachal Pradesh, India

Ecem Dogan
Department of Bioengineering, Faculty of Chemical and Metallurgical Engineering
Yildiz Technical University
Istanbul, Turkey
and
Center for Nanotechnology & Biomaterials Application and Research (NBUAM)
Marmara University
Istanbul, Turkey

D. Durgalakshmi
Department of Medical Physics
Anna University
Chennai, India
and
Department of Physics
Ethiraj College for Women
Chennai, India

Nazmi Ekren
Department of Bioengineering, Faculty of Chemical and Metallurgical Engineering
Yildiz Technical University
Istanbul, Turkey
and
Electrical and Electronics Engineering, Faculty of Technology
Marmara University
Istanbul, Turkey

Sougata Ghosh
Department of Physics, Faculty of Science
Kasetsart University
Bangkok, Thailand
and
Department of Microbiology, School of Science
RK University
Rajkot, India

Sara Gorgani
Tissue Engineering Research Group (TERG), Department of Anatomy and Cell Biology, School of Medicine
Mashhad University of Medical Sciences
Mashhad, Iran

Oguzhan Gunduz
Center for Nanotechnology & Biomaterials Application and Research (NBUAM)
Marmara University
Istanbul, Turkey
and
Department of Metallurgical and Materials Engineering, Faculty of Technology
Marmara University
Istanbul, Turkey

Aastha Gupta
School of Chemical Sciences
Indian Institute of Technology Mandi
Himachal Pradesh, India

Hisao Haniu
Institute for Biomedical Sciences, Interdisciplinary Cluster for Cutting Edge Research
Shinshu University
Asahi, Japan

Ketki Holkar
Symbiosis Centre for Stem Cell Research (SCSCR)
Symbiosis International (Deemed University)
Pune, India

Ganesh Ingavle
Symbiosis Centre for Stem Cell Research (SCSCR)
Symbiosis International (Deemed University)
Pune, India

Saeid Kargozar
UT Southwestern Medical Center, USA
Tissue Engineering Research Group (TERG), Department of Anatomy and Cell Biology, School of Medicine
Mashhad University of Medical Sciences
Mashhad, Iran

Remziye Aysun Kepekçi
Department of Biology
Gaziantep University
Gaziantep, Turkey

Farzad Kermani
Tissue Engineering Research Group (TERG), Department of Anatomy and Cell Biology, School of Medicine
Mashhad University of Medical Sciences
Mashhad, Iran

Toshiki Miyazaki
Graduate School of Life Science and Systems Engineering
Kyushu Institute of Technology
Kitakyushu, Japan

Sahar Mollazadeh
Department of Materials Engineering, Faculty of Engineering
Ferdowsi University of Mashhad (FUM)
Mashhad, Iran

Ebrahim Mostafavi
Stanford Cardiovascular Institute
and
Department of Medicine
Stanford University School of Medicine
Stanford, California

R. Ajay Rakkesh
Department of Physics and Nanotechnology
SRM Institute of Science and Technology
Kattankulathur, India

P.N. Blessy Rebecca
Department of Physics and Nanotechnology
SRM Institute of Science and Technology
Kattankulathur, India

M.R. Rekha
Division of Biosurface Technology, Biomedical Technology Wing
SCTIMST
Thiruvananthapuram, India

S. Sajeesh
Department of Bioengineering
Lehigh University
Bethlehem, Pennsylvania

Sangram K. Samal
Materials Research Centre
Indian Institute of Science
Bangalore, India

I. N. Savina
School of Applied Sciences
University of Brighton
Brighton, United Kingdom

Deepa Suhag
Amity Centre for Nanotechnology
Amity University Haryana
Manesar, India

Baeckkyoung Sung
Biosensor Group
KIST Europe Forschungsgesellschaft mbH
Saarbrücken, Germany
and
Division of Energy & Environment Technology
University of Science & Technology
Daejeon, Republic of Korea

Sirikanjana Thongmee
Department of Physics, Faculty of Science
Kasetsart University
Bangkok, Thailand

Sena Su Torun
Department of Bioengineering, Faculty of Chemical and Metallurgical Engineering
Yildiz Technical University
Istanbul, Turkey
and
Center for Nanotechnology & Biomaterials Application and Research (NBUAM)
Marmara University
Istanbul, Turkey
and
Nanortopedi Technology Industry and Trade Inc.
Marmara University Technopark
Istanbul, Turkey

Cem Bulent Ustundag
Department of Bioengineering, Faculty of Chemical and Metallurgical Engineering
Yildiz Technical University
Istanbul, Turkey

Rıdvan Yıldırım
Department of Bioengineering
Yildiz Technical University
Istanbul, Turkey
and
Center for Nanotechnology & Biomaterials Application and Research (NBUAM)
Marmara University
Istanbul, Turkey

1 Stimuli-Responsive Hydrogels for Tissue Engineering and Drug Delivery Applications

Remziye Aysun Kepekçi
Gaziantep University

CONTENTS

1.1 Introduction: Hydrogels as Smart Biomaterials 1
 1.1.1 Physical Stimuli-Responsive Hydrogels 2
 1.1.2 Chemical-Responsive Hydrogels 5
 1.1.3 Biological-Responsive Hydrogels 7
1.2 Applications of Stimuli-Responsive Hydrogels in Drug Delivery 8
1.3 Applications of Stimuli-Responsive Hydrogels in Tissue Engineering 10
1.4 Current Challenges and Future Prospects 11
References 11

1.1 INTRODUCTION: HYDROGELS AS SMART BIOMATERIALS

Biomaterials can be defined as "materials of natural or synthetic origin that come in contact with tissue, blood or biological fluids, and intended for use in diagnostic, prosthetic, therapeutic or storage application" (Kulinets 2015).

Biomaterial science has undergone a revolutionary advancement in the past few years thanks to the advancements in nanobiotechnology and bioengineering. Biomaterials have evolved from conventional static biomaterials lacking many functionalities to "smart" responsive biomaterials. These new-generation innovative biomaterials are distinguished from conventional biomaterials by their ability to change their physical properties as a result of their interaction with one or more stimuli. This ability gives them meticulous control over the desired cellular response (Amukarimi, Ramakrishna, and Mozafari 2021).

Owing to their outstanding characteristics, hydrogels have gained priority as smart biomaterials among other biomaterials (El-Husseiny et al. 2022). Among these features, there is no doubt that their high biocompatibility makes them preferred over other biomaterials (Mathew et al. 2018; Murdan 2003). Like ECM, hydrogels are

DOI: 10.1201/9781003251767-1

composed of crosslinked polymeric networks with high hydrophilicity (Mantha et al. 2019). This unique structure can simulate living tissues and maintain an appropriate microenvironment for cell growth (Hoffman 2012).

Hydrogels can serve as potent delivery matrices for therapeutic compounds due to their porous structure. Upon exposure to stimuli, stimuli-responsive hydrogels can transform their network structure as a response. As a consequence of this transformation, their mechanical strength and permeability change (Amukarimi et al. 2021). This property provides controlled release of the bioactive molecule from porous structure as needed.

The human body presents a diverse environment for physical, biological and chemical stimuli, allowing hydrogel properties to be controlled in response to external conditions at different sites throughout the body (Singh, Laverty, and Donnelly 2018). Hydrogels can be formulated to swell or deswell in response to any stimulus. They can change their volume dramatically in response to several environmental signals. Thus, stimuli-responsive hydrogels can behave as an "on–off" switch for various purposes. They are mainly categorized as physical, chemical, and biological stimulus-responsive hydrogels.

1.1.1 Physical Stimuli-Responsive Hydrogels

Temperature/Thermo-responsive hydrogels: Thermo-sensitive hydrogels are the most examined type of stimuli-responsive hydrogels. Being easily controllable and variable in the native environment provided temperature to be used extensively as physical stimuli. Thermo-responsive hydrogels can change their volume according to temperature differences in their surroundings (El-Husseiny et al. 2022; Li, Guo, and Zhang 2021). The hydrophobic and hydrophilic subunits interact with water differently at distinct temperatures, and this brings out the thermal response.

The hydrophobic groups like propyl, ethyl, and methyl moieties in the crosslinked network of these hydrogels show temperature-sensitive transitions. Thermo-responsive hydrogels can be classified as "negative" or "positive temperature-responsive hydrogels" (Figure 1.1).

The term "Critical Solution Temperature" (CST) is determinative in this classification. CST is "the temperature at which a mixture of two liquids, immiscible at ordinary temperatures, ceases to separate into two phases." Temperature-sensitive hydrogels have shown great promise for engineering various types of tissues, including cardiac (Li et al. 2014), dermal (Zhang, Lv, et al. 2021), corneal (Lin et al. 2017), osseous (Deng et al. 2020; Li, Guo, and Zhang 2021), tendinous (Huang et al. 2022), cartilaginous (Zhang et al. 2022) and meniscal (Chen et al. 2020) tissues. Additionally, many types of thermo-sensitive hydrogels were formulated to deliver various drugs such as Docetaxel, Doxorubicin, Ketoprofen, Diclofenac Sodium, luteolin and Dexamethasone (Huang et al. 2019; García-Couce et al. 2022).

Light/photo-responsive hydrogels: Light-responsive hydrogels that recognize light signal arouse broad attention. To develop light-responsive hydrogels, light-sensitive groups have to be inserted into gel polymers (Li, Zhou, et al. 2021).

The photo-responsive groups can be situated in different locations. These locations are listed by Li et al. (2019) as "in the crosslinking points, along the polymer or

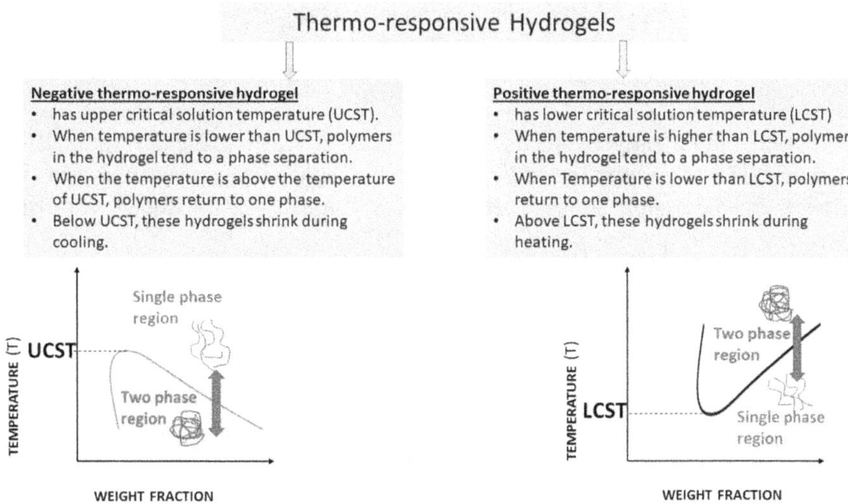

Thermo-responsive Hydrogels
Negative thermo-responsive hydrogel
has upper critical solution temperature (UCST).
When temperature is lower than UCST, polymers in the hydrogel tend to a phase separation.
When the temperature is above the temperature of UCST, polymers return to one phase.
Below UCST, these hydrogels shrink during cooling.
Positive thermo-responsive hydrogel
has lower critical solution temperature (LCST)
When temperature is higher than LCST, polymers in the hydrogel tend to a phase separation.
When Temperature is lower than LCST, polymers return to one phase.
Above LCST, these hydrogels shrink during heating.
Single phase region
UCST
Two phase region
TEMPERATURE (T)
WEIGHT FRACTION
Two phase region
LCST
Single phase region
TEMPERATURE (T)
WEIGHT FRACTION

FIGURE 1.1 Classification of thermo-responsive hydrogels as positive and negative thermo-responsive hydrogels and their shrinking behavior according to the temperature of surrounding medium.

supramolecular backbone, along the side chains, or dissolved in the aqueous medium of hydrogels." The location and type of photo-responsive subunit determine the photoresponse of hydrogel. This response may appear as follows: shrinking, partial de-crosslinking, complete de-crosslinking, photothermal excitation, activation/deactivation of the reactive site and release of the target molecule (Li, Scheiger, and Levkin 2019). Light-responsive hydrogels have been employed for the engineering of various tissue types like neural (Dong et al. 2020; Peng et al. 2022), cartilage (Giammanco et al. 2016) and dermal (Wei, Wang, et al. 2022), as well as for controlled drug release (Li, Scheiger, and Levkin 2019).

Electric/magnetic (electro-magnetic)-responsive hydrogels: Hydrogels composed of polyelectrolytes can respond to electrical stimuli. The magnitude of the response changes according to some factors. These factors are reported by Koetting et al. (2015) as "the charge density of the hydrogel, the degree of crosslinking in the hydrogel, the magnitude of the applied voltage, the dielectric properties of the surrounding medium, and the pH and ionic strength of the surrounding medium" (Koetting et al. 2015). In order to synthesize electro-responsive hydrogels, electro-conductive materials like conductive polymers and carbon-based nanoparticles are commonly encoded in the structure of hydrogels (El-Husseiny et al. 2022). Electro-induced gel deswelling, gel deswelling and gel erosion can be regarded as possible responses of electro-sensitive hydrogels to electrical signals (Murdan 2003). This type of hydrogel systems have been employed in electrically active tissues like nerves and cardiac tissue in tissue engineering (Xu et al. 2018). Upon exposure to an electrical field, they respond by supporting the contraction–relaxation of these tissues, which could cause hydrogel disruption. They hold great promise in regenerative medicine for restoring the lost function of impaired tissues by modulating cell proliferation and differentiation. They also have the potential to deliver drugs as a response to electrical stimuli (Carayon et al. 2020).

Magnetic-responsive hydrogels: Magnetic-responsive hydrogels are generated by connecting hydrogel systems with additives that can respond to magnetic fields, while other stimulus-responsive hydrogels are derived from only the hydrogel networks themselves. Generally, various magnetic materials at the nanoscale can be incorporated into hydrogel systems (Messing et al. 2011; Hermenegildo et al. 2019; Liu et al. 2010) as additives in order to generate magnetic-responsive hydrogels for various biomedical applications (Chen et al. 2019; Zhou et al. 2018; Zhang et al. 2015; Huang et al. 2020; Wu et al. 2017; Tang et al. 2017; Silva et al. 2018). Magnetic hydrogels give various responses such as locomotion, deformation and thermogenesis as a result of an external magnetic stimulus (Noh et al. 2017; Wu et al. 2018). Magnetic nanoparticles (MNPs) are able to convert magnetic energy into other types of energy under various densities of magnetic fields. They can convert magnetic energy into mechanical energy at low frequencies, while they can transform magnetic energy into thermal energy at high frequencies. MNPs in hydrogels can be magnetized rapidly by a magnetic field. Ion channels in cells can be activated by oscillations generated by magnetized MNPs (Li, Li, et al. 2021).

Magnetic-responsive hydrogels come into prominence due to their specialities such as rapid reply, temporospatial control, noninvasive nature, and ability to activate remotely. Additionally, different smart hydrogels can be combined with magnetic subunits to provide responsiveness to more than one stimulus. This expands the applicability of magnetic hydrogels (Li, Li, et al. 2021).

Pressure/strain-responsive hydrogels: The piezoresistive effect describes the change in the electrical resistivity of a substance as the mechanical strain on it changes. A piezoresistive pressure sensor converts mechanical signals into current signals (Yang et al. 2021). Pressure-responsive hydrogels respond to extrinsic mechanical stimuli by swelling–deswelling and/or extension–shrinkage (El-Husseiny et al. 2022).

Currently, hydrogel-based wearable strain sensors have gained significant momentum since they conquer the limitations of elastomer-based sensors, such as inadequate biocompatibility, brittle structure, and complex production stages. Their electrical conductivity, suitable mechanical properties and high biocompatibility put forward their usage in wearables and healthcare materials (Rahmani and Shojaei 2021) to deliver many drugs for control of various diseases (El-Husseiny et al. 2022).

Ultrasound-responsive hydrogels: Ultrasound (US) is a mechanical sound wave with high frequencies (≥20 kHz). The sounds with these frequencies are outside the upper audible limit of human hearing (Mitragotri 2005). US-responsive hydrogels respond to US stimuli through one of the following mechanisms: induction by temperature, stimulation by mechanical forces or gas vaporization through bubbles (Zardad et al. 2016). Easy of penetration of US into the tissue and its noninvasive nature have favored the usage of US-responsive hydrogels as drug carriers, especially in cancer treatment (Norris et al. 2005).

Ultrasonic waves enhance drug penetration into the target side of the body through biological barriers, which is a key challenge in drug delivery. When the polymers in the hydrogel network are activated by ultrasonic waves, microbubbles that are filled with air generate a transitory porous structure in the membrane. US-responsive hydrogel can behave as an on/off switch for delivering target molecules at the required time and place (Gholamali 2019; Wei, Cornel, and Du 2021).

1.1.2 Chemical-Responsive Hydrogels

pH-responsive hydrogels: Polymers in this type of hydrogel can take or discharge protons in response to alterations in the pH values of their surrounding medium. Hydrogels respond to variations in the pH of their environment by either swelling or deswelling (Gholamali 2019; Singh, Laverty, and Donnelly 2018). Changes in the hydrophobic–hydrophilic nature of the chains, inter- and intramolecular complexation by hydrogen bonding and electrostatic repulsion are the key mechanisms controlling the swelling behavior of hydrogels (Gholamali 2019).

Considering the pendant molecules in the polymer backbone, pH-responsive hydrogels are classified as anionic and cationic hydrogels (Figure 1.2).

These groups show variations in the ionization of pendant groups and the ensuing swelling attitude (Koetting et al. 2015). The ionized structure provides an increment in the electrostatic repulsion between chains and the hydrophilicity of the polymer network. Consequently, hydrogels can absorb large amounts of water (Gholamali 2019). Owing to the fact that several parts within the human body display a broad range of pH values during either physiological or pathological states, many pH-responsive hydrogels have been developed to deliver various drugs to different sites in the body, such as the gastrointestinal tract, tumor microenvironment and wounds and also to induce tissue regeneration (Anirudhan, Mohan, and Rajeev 2022; He et al. 2021; Zhang, Zhou, et al. 2021; Wu et al. 2020; Sahoo et al. 2017).

Glucose-responsive hydrogels: Particularly, glucose-responsive hydrogels have been designed to deliver insulin. Glucose sensing and responding to glucose presence are the two main functions that glucose-responsive hydrogels should perform. Glucose-responsive hydrogels can be divided into three groups depending on their mode of glucose sensing. The first category of glucose-responsive hydrogels is glucose oxidase hydrogels. These hydrogels utilize glucose oxidase as a glucose-detecting

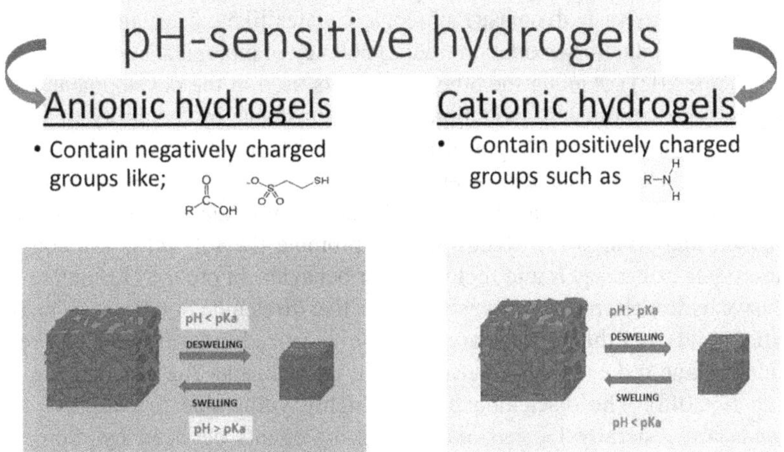

FIGURE 1.2 Classification of pH-responsive hydrogels as anionic and cationic hydrogels and their swelling /deswelling behavior according to pH of surrounding medium and their pKa (the negative log base ten of the Ka (acid dissociation constant)) value.

enzyme that is entrapped in their structure. When glucose is available, oxidation of glucose into gluconic acid causes pH to decrease. Indeed, the actual response is pH dependent since upon a decrease in pH, the hydrogel swells and insulin is released from the hydrogel. The main pathway for the second category of glucose-responsive hydrogels relies on the immobilization of concanavalin A (Con A), a lectin (carbohydrate-binding protein) originally extracted from the jack bean (*Canavalia ensiformis*), within the hydrogel system. Binding of Con A with glycosylated moieties of the polymer backbone provides a firmly complexed hydrogel matrix with a small pore size. In this way, insulin can be ensnared within the hydrogel. The affinity of Con A for glucose is higher than for the glycosylated components. When glucose is available in the surrounding environment, Con A will bind with glucose, causing the hydrogel to decompose and to release insulin. The last category of glucose-responsive hydrogels is phenylboronic (PBA) acid gels. These glucose-responsive systems are dependent on boronic acid–diol complexation. Polymers having phenylboronic groups build up a gel through interaction between the pendant phenyl borate and hydroxyl groups. PBA binds covalently to saccharides and forms complexes with diols (Hisamitsu et al. 1997). Commonly, there is an equilibrium between uncharged and cationically charged forms of the phenyl borate group in aqueous environments (Koetting et al. 2015). Glucose only reacts in a cationically charged form, resulting in another cationic product. When glucose enters the hydrogel matrix, PBA reversibly binds with glucose, leading to a shift of equilibrium toward cationically charged boron residual groups. The increase in charge enhances ionic repulsion and enables hydrogels to become more hydrophilic. Consequently, swelling behavior of hydrogel appears. Among the three classes of glucose-responsive hydrogels, PBA hydrogels are the most promising candidates for clinical usage (Koetting et al. 2015). The synthetic nature of PBA hydrogels overcomes the drawback of protein-based hydrogels, which are susceptible to denaturation under nonbiological conditions (Roy, Cambre, and Sumerlin 2010). Besides, they offer sensitive glucose responsiveness (Koetting et al. 2015).

Redox-responsive hydrogels: Pathological states like cancer and inflammation can change the reduction–oxidation (redox) potency of biological systems (Lennicke and Cochemé 2021). Among the other stimulants used in the development of smart hydrogels, redox (reduction–oxidation) is distinguishable by its ability to simulataneously alter the charge and spin of a molecule. Their suitability to be integrated into present electronic devices also gives them priority to be used in industry. Redox stimuli can be generated through the action of oxidants/reductants (Fukino, Yamagishi, and Aida 2017). Redox stimuli promote the sol–gel phase conversion of these types of hydrogels and regulate their behavior. In order to formulate redox-responsive hydrogels, redox-responsive agents like diselenide bonds, disulfide bonds, thioether bonds and thiol groups are commonly utilized to target sites that respond to oxidation and reduction. (Mollazadeh, Mackiewicz, and Yazdimamaghani 2021; Guo et al. 2018). The diselenide bond is highly vulnerable to oxidative agents. Se bonds are generally located as crosslinking agents between hydrophilic and hydrophobic segments (Choi et al. 2021). Besides the anticancer activity of Se, the responsiveness of Se bonds to the redox environment puts forward the utilization of redox-responsive hydrogel in drug delivery systems (Varlamova et al. 2021; Gebrie et al. 2021; Monteiro et al. 2021). Reduction of the disulfide bond to the thiol group occurs when a reducing agent is present in the environment. Oxidative agents can regenerate the disulfide bond. Thus, this bond can be utilized as a redox-responsive linkage. Intracellular glutathione (GSH) behaves as a reducing agent for S–S bonds. Tumor sites contain higher levels (at least four times) of GSH in the cytoplasm as compared to normal tissues (Cui et al. 2012; Cheng et al. 2011). In the tumor microenvironment containing high levels of GSH, reduction of the disulfide bond, which is stable in the structure of hydrogel in a medium with low reducing potential, to the mercaptan group occurs. This provides the breach of the hydrogel and the release of the target molecule (Zong et al. 2022). Thus, redox-sensitive disulfide bonds, which can be cleaved under high GSH concentrations, can be used as effective agents, especially to release drugs precisely at tumor sites and minimize the invasive damage to healthy tissues (Zhao et al. 2015; Li et al. 2015; Guo et al. 2018). Disulfide bonds are vulnerable to oxidation and reduction, while thioether bonds are responsive to oxidizing agents. Oxidation of the thioether bond to a hydrophilic sulfoxide or sulphone by an oxidizing agent occurs. Redox-responsive hydrogels can also be generated to recognize reactive oxygen species (ROS), including hydrogen peroxide, superoxide, hydroxyl radical, peroxynitrite, and hypochlorite. ROS play essential roles in normal cell metabolism and are significantly increased in many diseases (Xu, He, Xiao, et al. 2016). Thus, ROS have aroused much interest since ROS have been documented as highly related to pathological conditions. ROS-responsive hydrogels have shown encouraging potential, especially for anticancer drug delivery systems (Zhou et al. 2021; Zong et al. 2022) and inflammation-related diseases (Zhao et al. 2020, 2022; Saw et al. 2021), as well as cell protection against excess oxidation (Li, Zhu, et al. 2021; Xu, He, Ren, et al. 2016; Gupta et al. 2014). Mostly, this type of hydrogel is based on ROS-triggered degradation and bioactive compound release.

1.1.3 Biological-Responsive Hydrogels

Enzyme-responsive hydrogels: Hydrogels can be generated to respond to the target enzyme. In the native environment of cells, mostly enzymes control many stimulus-responsive mechanisms, and many pathological disorders are associated with altered enzyme levels. Thus, enzymes can be utilized as biological triggers to provide controlled releases of biomolecules at desired sites (Chandrawati 2016). Enzymatic regulation of hydrogels enables responsiveness to the body's own signals, which are highly selective and comprise catalytic augmentation to provide a fast reply (Abul-Haija and Ulijn 2014). This property gives them priority among other stimulus-responsive hydrogels.

Hydrogels may be designed to render them degradable, which may involve detaching chemical crosslinks (polymeric hydrogels) or controlled disassembly (supramolecular hydrogels) (Abul-Haija and Ulijn 2014). Enzyme-responsive hydrogels can be formulated by using peptide chains as linkers, either as crosslinks within the hydrogel or as links between the polymer backbone and drug molecules. These peptide chains, as short sequences, can be digested, especially by certain enzymes. So, the hydrogel degrades when the target enzyme is present. In the case of incorporation of peptides into hydrogels as the chemical crosslinker rather than as a pendant linker, gel–sol degradation of the hydrogel occurs upon digestion by the target enzyme (Koetting et al. 2015). Enzymatic degradation is selective, can in principle be tightly regulated and is therefore a highly attractive option in stimuli-responsive hydrogels. Matrix metalloproteinases (MMPs), extracellular proteinases that can degrade proteins in the ECM, are involved in tumor invasion and tissue remodeling. MMP-responsive hydrogels come at the forefront of other enzyme-responsive hydrogels, especially in tissue engineering applications (Purcell et al. 2014; Fan et al. 2019; Wei, Chen, et al. 2022; Zhou et al. 2022).

Antigen/antibody-responsive hydrogels: "Antigen–antibody interaction" is utilized in the production of this type of hydrogel. These hydrogels are prepared by implanting the antigen and corresponding antibody into the polymer structure. In this way, the crosslinks in the hydrogel network are formed. Binding of the free antigen competitively to the hydrogel structure decomposes the hydrogel network (Miyata, Asami, and Uragami 1999). The antigens/antibodies may also be captured in the hydrogel structure in different ways. They can be chemically conjugated in the hydrogel or their binding part, and the hydrogel can be copolymerized (El-Husseiny et al. 2022).

1.2 APPLICATIONS OF STIMULI-RESPONSIVE HYDROGELS IN DRUG DELIVERY

Conventional drug administration methods can cause side effects and harm healthy tissues since drugs usually need large amounts or persistent applications to be efficacious. In addition to this drawback, especially for hydrophobic drugs, the loading/release potential of traditional drug delivery systems are still inadequate. To address these issues, research in drug delivery has therefore focused on achieving controlled and local drug delivery for both hydrophobic and hydrophilic drugs (Dreiss 2020).

Outstanding features of hydrogels have given them superiority among other drug delivery agents. The aqueous nature of hydrogels diminishes the probability of drug degradation and accumulation upon exposure to any solvent. Not only can hydrogels be loaded with high amounts of water-soluble drugs, but they can also encapsulate water-insoluble drugs (Li and Mooney 2016). Hydrogels as drug delivery agents can be used for oral, rectal, ocular, epidermal and subcutaneous applications. Many hydrogel-based products were approved by the FDA (Table 1.1) and became available commercially (Gayatri and Dalwadi 2013).

TABLE 1.1

Some Commercial Hydrogel-Based Products

Product	Hydrogel Type	Application
Lupron depot™	conventional	treatment of prostate cancer
Sandostatin™	conventional	treatment of Acromegaly
Infuse™	conventional	bone regeneration
Azasite™	conventional	treatment of bacterial conjunctivitis
BST-Gel™	thermo sensitive hydrogel	cartilage repair
OnkoGel™	thermo sensitive hydrogel	treatment of tumors
LeGoo™	thermo sensitive hydrogel	treatment of vascular injury
sQZ gel™	pH sensitive hydrogel	treatment of hypertension

Poor controllability and limited responsiveness of traditional hydrogels often overshadow their admirable properties (Wei, Cornel, and Du 2021). Currently, a better understanding of chronopharmacokinetics and the influence of circadian rhythm on diseases has aroused a great interest in designing innovative drug carriers that can target the molecular clock and release the drug at the peak time of the disease (Choudhary et al. 2021). Especially, stimuli-responsive hydrogels as smart drug delivery agents stand at the forefront of other biomaterials due to their versatility and biocompatibility. They are distinguished as more talented among others thanks to their remotely controllable drug release profile and drug loading capacity (Dreiss 2020). Exposure of stimuli-responsive hydrogels to stimuli maintains accurately targeted delivery of drugs/biomolecules that are loaded in their structure at the required time and place (Soppimath et al. 2002). Unique properties of stimuli-responsive hydrogels enable their function to protect, target and locally deliver drugs in a controllable way. There is enough research on the delivery of drug molecules to a desired site as a response to an external signal such as temperature, pH, glucose or light (Koetting et al. 2015; Gholamali 2019; Hoffman 2012; Li and Mooney 2016; Qiu and Park 2001). Many patents and papers about potential applications of stimuli-responsive hydrogels in drug delivery have been published. However, many significant obstacles remain to be overcome, including low drug load, inadequate release rate, a narrow range of appropriate drugs, and translation from laboratory to industrial scale (Zhu et al. 2022; Mantha et al. 2019).

The drug release profile is highly influenced by the interaction between the drug and polymer molecules in hydrogel. Covalent conjugation, electrostatic interaction and hydrophobic association are types of interactions between the drug and polymers of hydrogel. These chemical interactions mediate drug release. Controlled drug release can occur through network degradation, swelling or mechanical deformation Thus, selection of hydrogel formulation considering physicochemical characteristics of the polymeric compounds in the hydrogel network is crucial for achieving the desired performance *in vivo*. Although many investigations have reported the basic mechanisms of drug release in different stimuli-responsive hydrogel networks, theoretical modeling of drug release profiles remains unrevealed (Li and Mooney 2016). In terms of modeling the *in vivo* release profiles of stimuli-responsive hydrogels, a lot of research is also required to translate them to clinical trials.

Currently, multiple stimuli-responsive hydrogels as safer and more targeted drug delivery systems than those with one stimulus have become the subject of many investigations (Palmese et al. 2020; Yang et al. 2022; Fu et al. 2018). Drug delivery systems that can respond to multiple stimuli have become a popular strategy for much research, especially for cancer treatment (Jo et al. 2022; Jahanban-Esfahlan et al. 2021). Cancer microenvironments containing high levels of GSH are slightly acidic. Thus, hydrogels that are vulnerable to local pH and reduction conditions may contribute to drug delivery applications as carriers for anticancer drugs in the cancer microenvironment (Mazidi et al. 2022). However, the difficulty of introducing multi-stimuli-responsive functions and degradability at the same time in a biological microenvironment limits their application. Additionally, the preparation of these hydrogels generally requires multi-step reactions and is rather complicated (Komatsu et al. 2021). The chemical crosslinker used in the synthesis of the hydrogels may be toxic. To overcome the mentioned issue, the physically crosslinked hydrogel preparation method can be used. However, the physically crosslinked hydrogels exhibit mechanical instability in some cases (MohanKumar et al. 2021). These drawbacks represent barriers to the clinical use of smart hydrogels. Although smart hydrogels as drug delivery agents are highly promising, many challenges need to be addressed for their translation into clinical applications.

Recently, advances in bioelectronics have broadened the range of hydrogels designed for controlled drug delivery. Hydrogels possess a unique set of properties (including high stretchability, transparency and conductivity to ionic currents) to bridge the gap between biology and electronics, holding great promise for bioelectronics applications (Yuk, Lu, and Zhao 2019). Especially microelectronics could be integrated with smart hydrogel drug delivery systems to develop next-generation bioelectronics with healing effects (Li and Mooney 2016). However, this technology is still in an early stage of development.

1.3 APPLICATIONS OF STIMULI-RESPONSIVE HYDROGELS IN TISSUE ENGINEERING

Scaffold matrices play an essential role in the applications of tissue engineering. They facilitate the generation of new tissues by supporting cell proliferation, migration, and differentiation. A proper scaffold must have the ability to repair body tissues by permitting oxygen and nutrient passage and mimicking the natural structure of the tissue for required cell growth, vascularization and proliferation. Besides, an ideal scaffold should be degraded naturally during or shortly after the healing process without any toxic effects. Lack of these properties can cause cell necrosis and defective tissues (Mantha et al. 2019). Among other polymeric scaffolds, hydrogel-based scaffolds have attracted great interest among researchers since they mimic the dynamic structure of ECM, which plays crucial roles in many physiological events of cells, including cell proliferation, differentiation, migration and apoptosis (Peng et al. 2022). Hydrogels are regarded as bioinspired networks with biomimetic and bioactive properties (Li, Zhou, et al. 2021). Their porous structure allows the penetration of cell metabolites and the removal of cell waste (Mantha et al. 2019). Furthermore, the flexibility and firmness of hydrogels can maintain the required stability for cell proliferation (Li, Li, et al. 2021).

Specific body tissues, such as cartilage and meniscus, are incapable of healing in the case of damage since they have limited or no blood supply. Stem cells and growth factors can be encapsulated in hydrogel systems to promote tissue regeneration (Mantha et al. 2019). Hydrogels loaded with repair cells or drugs may encourage tissue repair and regeneration in injured areas. The potential of smart hydrogels has been investigated for application in the engineering of various types of tissues, including cardiac, neural, dermal, corneal, osseous, cartilaginous, tendinous, meniscal and intervertebral disc (Chen et al. 2020; Mantha et al. 2019; Zhang, Zhou, et al. 2021; El-Husseiny et al. 2022; Dong et al. 2020). The alluring outcomes of these stimuli-responsive hydrogel systems in tissue regeneration hold great promise for their usage in tissue engineering and clinical practice. Additionally, the possibility of their injectability makes them superior to other biomaterials. Especially biotherapeutic molecules like stem cells can be delivered by injectable hydrogels to hard-to-reach parts of the body, such as the joints, the back of the eye or the sinuses (Mathew et al. 2018; Gaffey et al. 2015).

Developments in biomaterial science and bioprinting have expanded the boundaries of additive manufacturing technology. Recently, four-dimensional (4D) bioprinting has emerged as the next-generation biofabrication technology. This technique aims to fabricate dynamic three-dimensional (3D)-patterned biological structures that can change their shapes and behavior as a response to different stimulants (Amukarimi and Mozafari 2021; Li et al. 2016). Stimuli-responsive hydrogels hold great promise as bioprintable materials, which are known as bioinks (Mobaraki et al. 2020; Ramiah et al. 2020; Kumar, Voicu, and Thakur 2021). Studies on 4D bioprinting are still in the early stages of progress. Obviously, the development of this cutting-edge technology would lead to the emergence of novel bioprinted smart hydrogels as commercial products in the biomaterial market for applications in tissue engineering and drug delivery.

1.4 CURRENT CHALLENGES AND FUTURE PROSPECTS

Conventional hydrogels are widely present in many products, while smart hydrogels as commercial products in tissue engineering and drug delivery are still limited. Many responsive hydrogel-based drug delivery agents and scaffolds for tissue engineering applications have been formulated, examined and patented. However, very few have reached the market. Some commercial stimuli-responsive hydrogel-based products are shown in Table 1.1. The limited number of hydrogel-based commercial products in drug delivery and tissue engineering can be attributed to some drawbacks, such as high production costs, nonbiodegradable structure of some synthetic hydrogels, difficulty in sterilization, handling and loading due to the fragile structure of hydrogels, inhomogeneous crosslink density distribution (spatial inhomogeneity), which reduces the strength of hydrogels, and the probability of toxicity in the case of long-term usage of synthetic hydrogels. Further analyses are needed to overcome these existing limitations. The efficiency and biocompatibility of smart hydrogels should be confirmed by well-designed clinical trials and pharmacological and toxicological evaluations. Commercialization of smart hydrogels requires extensive research and outstanding collaboration between clinicians and researchers. The biomaterial market for tissue engineering and drug delivery applications represents a multibillion-dollar market potential worldwide. In the foreseen future, thanks to advancements in cutting-edge technologies like 4D bioprinting, nanotechnology and bioelectronics, smart hydrogels as next-generation biomaterials will dominate the market.

REFERENCES

Abul-Haija, Yousef M., and Rein V. Ulijn. 2014. Enzyme-responsive hydrogels for biomedical applications. *Hydrogels in Cell-Based Therapies*; Royal Society of Chemistry. doi: 10.1039/9781782622055-00112.

Amukarimi, Shukufe, and Masoud Mozafari. 2021. "4D bioprinting of tissues and organs." *Bioprinting* 23; e00161. Doi: 10.1016/j.bprint.2021.e00161.

Amukarimi, Shukufe, Seeram Ramakrishna, and Masoud Mozafari. 2021. "Smart biomaterials-A proposed definition and overview of the field." *Current Opinion in Biomedical Engineering*; 100311. doi: 10.1016/j.cobme.2021.100311.

Anirudhan, T.S., Maneesh Mohan, and M.R. Rajeev. 2022. "Chitosan-hyaluronic acid-based hydrogel for the pH-responsive Co-delivery of cisplatin and doxorubicin." *International Journal of Biological Macromolecules*. doi: 10.1016/j.ijbiomac.2022.01.022.

Carayon, Iga, Alexandra Gaubert, Yannick Mousli, and Barthélémy Philippe. 2020. "Electro-responsive hydrogels; Macromolecular and supramolecular approaches in the biomedical field." *Biomaterials Science* 8(20); 5589–5600. doi: 10.1039/d0bm01268h.

Chandrawati, Rona. 2016. "Enzyme-responsive polymer hydrogels for therapeutic delivery." *Experimental Biology Medicine* 241(9); 972–979. doi: 10.1177/1535370216647186.

Chen, Chen, Jialin Song, Jiayu Qiu, and Jinzhong Zhao. 2020. "Repair of a meniscal defect in a rabbit model through use of a thermosensitive, injectable, in situ cross-linked hydrogel with encapsulated bone mesenchymal stromal cells and transforming growth factor β1." *The American Journal of Sports Medicine* 48(4); 884–894. doi: 10.1177/0363546519898519.

Chen, Xueyun, Ming Fan, Huaping Tan, Bowen Ren, Guoliang Yuan, Yang Jia, Jianliang Li, Dangsheng Xiong, Xiaodong Xing, and Xiaohong Niu. 2019. "Magnetic and self-healing chitosan-alginate hydrogel encapsulated gelatin microspheres via covalent cross-linking for drug delivery." *Materials Science Engineering C* 101; 619–629. doi: 10.1016/j.msec.2019.04.012.

Cheng, Ru, Fang Feng, Fenghua Meng, Chao Deng, Jan Feijen, and Zhiyuan Zhong. 2011. "Glutathione-responsive nano-vehicles as a promising platform for targeted intracellular drug and gene delivery." *Journal of Controlled Release* 152(1); 2–12. doi: 10.1016/j.jconrel.2011.01.030.

Choi, Yeon Su, Kang Moo Huh, Min Suk Shim, In Suh Park, Yong-Yeon Cho, Joo Young Lee, Hye Suk Lee, and Han Chang Kang. 2021. "Disrupting the redox balance with a diselenide drug delivery system; Synergistic or antagonistic?" *Advanced Functional Materials* 31(6); 2007275. doi: 10.1002/adfm.202007275.

Choudhary, Devendra, Hanmant Goykar, Kuldeep Rajpoot, and Rakesh Kumar Tekade. 2021. "Chronopharmacokinetics." In Rakesh Tekade (ed.) *Biopharmaceutics and Pharmacokinetics Considerations*, 163–194. Elsevier, Amsterdam.

Cui, Yanna, Haiqing Dong, Xiaojun Cai, Deping Wang, and Yongyong Li. 2012. "Mesoporous silica nanoparticles capped with disulfide-linked PEG gatekeepers for glutathione-mediated controlled release." *ACS Applied Materials Interfaces* 4(6); 3177–3183. doi: 10.1021/am3005225.

Deng, Jiajia, Jie Pan, Xinxin Han, Liming Yu, Jing Chen, Weihua Zhang, Luying Zhu, Wei Huang, Shangfeng Liu, and Zhengwei You. 2020. "PDGFBB-modified stem cells from apical papilla and thermosensitive hydrogel scaffolds induced bone regeneration." *Chemico-Biological Interactions* 316; 108931. doi: 10.1016/j.cbi.2019.108931.

Dong, Mei, Bo Shi, Dun Liu, Jia-Hao Liu, Di Zhao, Zheng-Hang Yu, Xiao-Quan Shen, Jia-Min Gan, Ben-Long Shi, and Yong Qiu. 2020. "Conductive hydrogel for a photothermal-responsive stretchable artificial nerve and coalescing with a damaged peripheral nerve." *ACS Nano* 14(12); 16565–16575. doi: 10.1021/acsnano.0c05197.

Dreiss, Cécile A. 2020. "Hydrogel design strategies for drug delivery." *Current Opinion in Colloid Interface Science* 48; 1–17. doi: 10.1016/j.cocis.2020.02.001.

El-Husseiny, Hussein M., Eman A. Mady, Lina Hamabe, Amira Abugomaa, Kazumi Shimada, Tomohiko Yoshida, Takashi Tanaka, Aimi Yokoi, Mohamed Elbadawy, and Ryou Tanaka. 2022. "Smart/stimuli-responsive hydrogels; Cutting-edge platforms for tissue engineering and other biomedical applications." *Materials Today Bio* 13; 100186. doi; 10.1016/j.mtbio.2021.100186.

Fan, Caixia, Jiajia Shi, Yan Zhuang, Lulu Zhang, Lei Huang, Wen Yang, Bing Chen, Yanyan Chen, Zhifeng Xiao, and He Shen. 2019. "Myocardial-infarction-responsive smart hydrogels targeting matrix metalloproteinase for on-demand growth factor delivery." *Advanced Materials* 31(40); 1902900. doi: 10.1002/adma.201902900.

Fu, Xiao, Leticia Hosta-Rigau, Rona Chandrawati, and Jiwei Cui. 2018. "Multi-stimuli-responsive polymer particles, films, and hydrogels for drug delivery." *Chem* 4(9); 2084–2107. doi: 10.1016/j.chempr.2018.07.002.

Fukino, Takahiro, Hiroshi Yamagishi, and Takuzo Aida. 2017. "Redox-responsive molecular systems and materials." *Advanced Materials* 29(25); 1603888. doi: 10.1002/adma.201603888.

Gaffey, Ann C., Minna H. Chen, Chantel M. Venkataraman, Alen Trubelja, Christopher B. Rodell, Patrick V. Dinh, George Hung, John W. MacArthur, Renganaden V. Soopan, and Jason A. Burdick. 2015. "Injectable shear-thinning hydrogels used to deliver endothelial progenitor cells, enhance cell engraftment, and improve ischemic myocardium." *The Journal of Thoracic Cardiovascular Surgery* 150(5); 1268–1277. doi: 10.1016/j.jtcvs.2015.07.035.

García-Couce, Jomarien, Miriela Tomás, Gastón Fuentes, Ivo Que, Amisel Almirall, and Luis J. Cruz. 2022. "Chitosan/Pluronic F127 thermosensitive hydrogel as an injectable dexamethasone delivery carrier." *Gels* 8(1); 44. doi: 10.3390/gels8010044.

Gayatri, C. Patel and Chintan A. Dalwadi. 2013. "Recent patents on stimuli responsive hydrogel drug delivery system." *Recent Patents on Drug Delivery Formulation* 7(3); 206–215.

Gebrie, Hailemichael Tegenu, Kefyalew Dagnew Addisu, Haile Fentahun Darge, Tefera Worku Mekonnen, and Hsieh-Chih Tsai. 2021. "Development of thermo/redox-responsive diselenide linked methoxy poly (ethylene glycol)-block-poly (ε-caprolactone-co-p-dioxanone) hydrogel for localized control drug release." *Journal of Polymer Research* 28(11); 1–13. doi: 10.1007/s10965-021-02776-8.

Gholamali, Iman 2019. "Stimuli-responsive polysaccharide hydrogels for biomedical applications: A review." *Regenerative Engineering Translational Medicine*; 1–24. doi: 10.1007/s40883-019-00134-1.

Giammanco, Giuseppe E., Bita Carrion, Rhima M. Coleman, Alexis D. Ostrowski, and interfaces. 2016. "Photoresponsive polysaccharide-based hydrogels with tunable mechanical properties for cartilage tissue engineering." *ACS Applied Materials* 8(23); 14423–14429. doi: 10.1021/acsami.6b03834.

Guo, Xiaoshuang, Yuan Cheng, Xiaotian Zhao, Yanli Luo, Jianjun Chen, and Wei-En Yuan. 2018. "Advances in redox-responsive drug delivery systems of tumor microenvironment." *Journal of Nanobiotechnology* 16(1); 1–10. doi: 10.1186/s12951-018-0398-2.

Gupta, Mukesh K., John R. Martin, Thomas A. Werfel, Tianwei Shen, Jonathan M. Page, and Craig L. Duvall. 2014. "Cell protective, ABC triblock polymer-based thermoresponsive hydrogels with ROS-triggered degradation and drug release." *Journal of the American Chemical Society* 136(42); 14896–14902. doi: 10.1021/ja507626y.

He, Jiahui, Zixi Zhang, Yutong Yang, Fenggang Ren, Jipeng Li, Shaojun Zhu, Feng Ma, Rongqian Wu, Yi Lv, and Gang He. 2021. "Injectable self-healing adhesive pH-responsive hydrogels accelerate gastric hemostasis and wound healing." *Nano-micro Letters* 13(1); 1–17. doi: 10.1007/s40820-020-00585-0.

Hermenegildo, B., Clarisse Ribeiro, L. Pérez-Álvarez, José L. Vilas, David A. Learmonth, Rui A. Sousa, P. Martins, and S. Lanceros-Méndez. 2019. "Hydrogel-based magnetoelectric microenvironments for tissue stimulation." *Colloids Surfaces B; Biointerfaces* 181; 1041–1047. doi: 10.1016/j.colsurfb.2019.06.023.

Hisamitsu, Issei, Kazunori Kataoka, Teruo Okano, and Yasuhisa Sakurai. 1997. "Glucose-responsive gel from phenylborate polymer and poly (vinyl alcohol); prompt response at physiological pH through the interaction of borate with amino group in the gel." *Pharmaceutical Research* 14(3); 289–293. doi: 10.1023/A:1012033718302.

Hoffman, Allan S. 2012. "Hydrogels for biomedical applications." *Advanced Drug Delivery Reviews* 64; 18–23. doi: 10.1016/j.addr.2012.09.010.

Huang, Haiqin, Xiaole Qi, Yanhua Chen, and Zhenghong Wu. 2019. "Thermo-sensitive hydrogels for delivering biotherapeutic molecules: A review." *Saudi Pharmaceutical Journal* 27(7); 990–999. doi:10.1016/j.jsps.2019.08.001.

Huang, Jianghong, Zhaofeng Jia, Yujie Liang, Zhiwang Huang, Zhibin Rong, Jianyi Xiong, and Dapping Wang. 2020. "Pulse electromagnetic fields enhance the repair of rabbit articular cartilage defects with magnetic nano-hydrogel." *RSC Advances* 10(1); 541–550. doi: 10.1039/c9ra07874f.

Huang, K., J. Du, J. Xu, C. Wu, C. Chen, S. Chen, T. Zhu, J. Jiang, and J. Zhao. 2022. "Tendon-bone junction healing by injectable bioactive thermo-sensitive hydrogel based on inspiration of tendon-derived stem cells." *Materials Today Chemistry* 23; 100720. doi: 10.1016/j.mtchem.2021.100720.

Jahanban-Esfahlan, Rana, Khadijeh Soleimani, Hossein Derakhshankhah, Babak Haghshenas, Aram Rezaei, Bakhshali Massoumi, Amir Farnudiyan-Habibi, Hadi Samadian, and Mehdi Jaymand. 2021. "Multi-stimuli-responsive magnetic hydrogel based on Tragacanth gum as a de novo nanosystem for targeted chemo/hyperthermia treatment of cancer." *Journal of Materials Research* 36(4); 858–869. doi: 10.1557/s43578-021-00137-1.

Jo, Yi-Jun, Muhammad Gulfam, Sung-Han Jo, Yeong-Soon Gal, Chul-Woong Oh, Sang-Hyug Park, and Kwon Taek Lim. 2022. "Multi-stimuli responsive hydrogels derived from hyaluronic acid for cancer therapy application." *Carbohydrate Polymers*; 119303. doi: 10.1016/j.carbpol.2022.119303.

Koetting, Michael C., Jonathan T. Peters, Stephanie D. Steichen, and Nicholas A. Peppas. 2015. "Stimulus-responsive hydrogels; Theory, modern advances, and applications." *Materials Science Engineering; R; Reports* 93; 1–49. doi: 10.1016/j.mser.2015.04.001.

Komatsu, Syuuhei, Moeno Tago, Yu Ando, Taka-Aki Asoh, and Akihiko Kikuchi. 2021. "Facile preparation of multi-stimuli-responsive degradable hydrogels for protein loading and release." *Journal of Controlled Release* 331; 1–6. doi: 10.1016/j.jconrel.2021.01.011.

Kulinets, I. 2015. "Biomaterials and their applications in medicine." In *Regulatory Affairs for Biomaterials and Medical Devices*, 1–10. Elsevier. doi: 10.1533/9780857099204.1.

Kumar, Anuj, Stefan Ioan Voicu, and Vijay Kumar Thakur. 2021. *3D Printable Gel-inks for Tissue Engineering; Chemistry, Processing, and Applications*. Springer Nature, Berlin.

Lennicke, Claudia, and Helena M. Cochemé. 2021. "Redox metabolism; ROS as specific molecular regulators of cell signaling and function." *Molecular Cell* 81(18); 3691–3707. doi: 10.1016/j.molcel.2021.08.018.

Li, Jianyu, and David J. Mooney. 2016. "Designing hydrogels for controlled drug delivery." *Nature Reviews Materials* 1(12); 1–17. doi: 10.1038/natrevmats.2016.71.

Li, Lei, Johannes M. Scheiger, and Pavel A. Levkin. 2019. "Design and applications of photoresponsive hydrogels." *Advanced Materials* 31(26); 1807333. doi: 10.1002/adma.201807333.

Li, Na, Rui Guo, and Zhenyu Jason Zhang. 2021. "Bioink formulations for bone tissue regeneration." *Frontiers in Bioengineering and Biotechnology* 9; 630488. doi: 10.3389/fbioe.2021.630488.

Li, Xia, Jin Zhou, Zhiqiang Liu, Jun Chen, Shuanghong Lü, Hongyu Sun, Junjie Li, Qiuxia Lin, Boguang Yang, and Cuimi Duan. 2014. "A PNIPAAm-based thermosensitive hydrogel containing SWCNTs for stem cell transplantation in myocardial repair." *Biomaterials* 35(22); 5679–5688. doi: 10.1016/j.biomaterials.2014.03.067.

Li, Yi-Chen, Yu Shrike Zhang, Ali Akpek, Su Ryon Shin, and Ali Khademhosseini. 2016. "4D bioprinting; the next-generation technology for biofabrication enabled by stimuli-responsive materials." *Biofabrication* 9(1); 012001. doi: 10.1088/1758-5090/9/1/012001.

Li, Ze-Yong, Jing-Jing Hu, Qi Xu, Si Chen, Hui-Zhen Jia, Yun-Xia Sun, Ren-Xi Zhuo, and Xian-Zheng Zhang. 2015. "A redox-responsive drug delivery system based on RGD containing peptide-capped mesoporous silica nanoparticles." *Journal of Materials Chemistry B* 3(1); 39–44. doi: 10.1039/c4tb01533a.

Li, Zhenguang, Yingze Li, Chang Chen, and Yu Cheng. 2021. "Magnetic-responsive hydrogels: From strategic design to biomedical applications." *Journal of Controlled Release* 335; 541–556. doi: 10.1016/j.jconrel.2021.06.003.

Li, Zhenhua, Dashuai Zhu, Qi Hui, Jianing Bi, Bingjie Yu, Zhen Huang, Shiqi Hu, Zhenzhen Wang, Thomas Caranasos, and Joseph Rossi. 2021. "Injection of ROS-responsive hydrogel loaded with basic fibroblast growth factor into the pericardial cavity for heart repair." *Advanced Functional Materials* 31(15); 2004377. doi: 10.1002/adfm.202004377.

Li, Ziyuan, Yanzi Zhou, Tianyue Li, Junji Zhang, and He Tian. 2021. "Stimuli-responsive hydrogels; Fabrication and biomedical applications." *View* 3; 20200112. doi: 10.1002/Viw.20200112.

Lin, Yung-Kai, Ruchi Sharma, Hsu Ma Lin, Wen-Shyan Chen, and Chao-Ling Yao. 2017. "In situ polymerizable hydrogel incorporated with specific pathogen-free porcine platelet-rich plasma for the reconstruction of the corneal endothelium." *Journal of the Taiwan Institute of Chemical Engineers* 78; 65–74. doi: 10.1016/j.jtice.2017.06.006.

Liu, Hongxia, Chaoyang Wang, Quanxing Gao, Xinxing Liu, and Zhen Tong. 2010. "Magnetic hydrogels with supracolloidal structures prepared by suspension polymerization stabilized by Fe_2O_3 nanoparticles." *Acta Biomaterialia* 6(1); 275–281. doi: 10.1016/j.actbio.2009.06.018.

Mantha, Somasundar, Sangeeth Pillai, Parisa Khayambashi, Akshaya Upadhyay, Yuli Zhang, Owen Tao, Hieu M. Pham, and Simon D Tran. 2019. "Smart hydrogels in tissue engineering and regenerative medicine." *Materials Science* 12(20); 3323. doi: 10.3390/ma12203323.

Mathew, Ansuja Pulickal, Saji Uthaman, Ki-Hyun Cho, Chong-Su Cho, and In-Kyu Park. 2018. "Injectable hydrogels for delivering biotherapeutic molecules." *International Journal of Biological Macromolecules* 110; 17–29. doi: 10.1016/j.ijbiomac.2017.11.113.

Mazidi, Zahra, Sanaz Javanmardi, Seyed Morteza Naghib, and Zahra Mohammadpour. 2022. "Smart stimuli-responsive implantable drug delivery systems for programmed and on-demand cancer treatment; an overview on the emerging materials." *Chemical Engineering Journal*; 134569. doi: 10.1016/j.cej.2022.134569.

Messing, Renate, Natalia Frickel, Lhoussaine Belkoura, Reinhard Strey, Helene Rahn, Stefan Odenbach, and Annette M. Schmidt. 2011. "Cobalt ferrite nanoparticles as multifunctional cross-linkers in PAAm ferrohydrogels." *Macromolecules* 44(8); 2990–2999. doi: 10.1021/ma102708b.

Mitragotri, Samir. 2005. "Healing sound; the use of ultrasound in drug delivery and other therapeutic applications." *Nature Reviews Drug Discovery* 4(3); 255–260. doi: 10.1038/nrd1662.

Miyata, Takashi, Noriko Asami, and Tadashi Uragami. 1999. "A reversibly antigen-responsive hydrogel." *Nature* 399(6738); 766–769. doi: 10.1038/21619.

Mobaraki, Mohammadmahdi, Maryam Ghaffari, Abolfazl Yazdanpanah, Yangyang Luo, and D.K. Mills. 2020. "Bioinks and bioprinting: A focused review." *Bioprinting* 18; e00080. doi: 10.1016/j.bprint.2020.e00080.

MohanKumar, B.S., G. Priyanka, S. Rajalakshmi, Rakesh Sankar, Taj Sabreen, and Jayasree Ravindran. 2021. "Hydrogels; potential aid in tissue engineering—a review." *Polymer Bulletin*; 1–31. doi: 10.1007/s00289-021-03864-x.

Mollazadeh, Shirin, Marcin Mackiewicz, and Mostafa Yazdimamaghani. 2021. "Recent advances in the redox-responsive drug delivery nanoplatforms; A chemical structure and physical property perspective." *Materials Science Engineering: C* 118; 111536. doi: 10.1016/j.msec.2020.111536.

Monteiro, Patrícia F., Alessandra Travanut, Claudia Conte, and Cameron Alexander. 2021. "Reduction-responsive polymers for drug delivery in cancer therapy—Is there anything new to discover?" *Wiley Interdisciplinary Reviews: Nanomedicine Nanobiotechnology* 13(2); e1678. doi: 10.1002/wnan.1678.

Murdan, Sudaxshina. 2003. "Electro-responsive drug delivery from hydrogels." *Journal of Controlled Release* 92(1–2); 1–17. doi: 10.1016/s0168-3659(03)00303-1.

Noh, Seung-Hyun, Seung Ho Moon, Tae-Hyun Shin, Yongjun Lim, and Jinwoo Cheon. 2017. "Recent advances of magneto-thermal capabilities of nanoparticles: From design principles to biomedical applications." *Nano Today* 13; 61–76. doi: 10.1016/j.nantod.2017.02.006.

Norris, P., M. Noble, I. Francolini, A.M. Vinogradov, Philip S. Stewart, B.D. Ratner, J. William Costerton, and Paul Stoodley. 2005. "Ultrasonically controlled release of ciprofloxacin from self-assembled coatings on poly (2-hydroxyethyl methacrylate) hydrogels for Pseudomonas aeruginosa biofilm prevention." *Antimicrobial Agents Chemotherapy* 49(10); 4272–4279. doi: 10.1128/AAC.49.10.4272-4279.2005.

Palmese, Luisa L., Ming Fan, Rebecca A. Scott, Huaping Tan, and Kristi L. Kiick. 2020. "Multi-stimuli-responsive, liposome-crosslinked poly (ethylene glycol) hydrogels for drug delivery." *Journal of Biomaterials Science, Polymer Edition* 32(5); 635–656. doi: 10.1080/09205063.2020.1855392.

Peng, Ke, Lifei Zheng, Tieli Zhou, Chunwu Zhang, and Huaqiong Li. 2022. "Light manipulation for fabrication of hydrogels and their biological applications." *Acta Biomaterialia* 137; 20–43. doi: 10.1016/j.actbio.2021.10.003.

Purcell, Brendan P., David Lobb, Manoj B. Charati, Shauna M. Dorsey, Ryan J. Wade, Kia N. Zellars, Heather Doviak, Sara Pettaway, Christina B. Logdon, and James A. Shuman. 2014. "Injectable and bioresponsive hydrogels for on-demand matrix metalloproteinase inhibition." *Nature Materials* 13(6); 653–661. doi: 10.1038/nmat3922.

Qiu, Yong, and Kinam Park. 2001. "Environment-sensitive hydrogels for drug delivery." *Advanced Drug Delivery Reviews* 53(3); 321–339. doi: 10.1016/s0169-409x(01)00203-4.

Rahmani, Pooria, and Akbar Shojaei. 2021. "A review on the features, performance and potential applications of hydrogel-based wearable strain/pressure sensors." *Advances in Colloid Interface Science* 298; 102553. doi: 10.1016/j.cis.2021.102553.

Ramiah, Previn, Lisa C. Du Toit, Yahya E. Choonara, Pierre P.D. Kondiah, and Viness Pillay. 2020. "Hydrogel-based bioinks for 3D bioprinting in tissue regeneration." *Frontiers in Materials* 7; 76. doi: 10.3389/fmats.2020.00076.

Roy, Debashish, Jennifer N. Cambre, and Brent S. Sumerlin. 2010. "Future perspectives and recent advances in stimuli-responsive materials." *Progress in Polymer Science* 35(1–2); 278–301. doi: 10.1016/j.progpolymsci.2009.10.008.

Sahoo, Pratyusa, Kok Hoong Leong, Shaik Nyamathulla, Yoshinori Onuki, Kozo Takayama, and Lip Yong Chung. 2017. "Optimization of pH-responsive carboxymethylated iota-carrageenan/chitosan nanoparticles for oral insulin delivery using response surface methodology." *Reactive Functional Polymers* 119; 145–155. doi: 10.1016/j.reactfunctpolym.2017.08.014.

Saw, Phei Er, Zhen Zhang, Yangyang Chen, Senlin Li, Linzhuo Huang, Chi Zhang, Qianqian Zhao, Xiaoding Xu, and Qiuling Xiang. 2021. "ROS-scavenging hybrid hydrogel for genetically engineered stem cell delivery and limb ischemia therapy." *Chemical Engineering Journal* 425; 131504. doi: 10.1016/j.cej.2021.131504.

Silva, Elsa D., Pedro S. Babo, Raquel Costa-Almeida, Rui M.A. Domingues, Bárbara B. Mendes, Elvira Paz, Paulo Freitas, Márcia T. Rodrigues, Pedro L. Granja, and Manuela E. Gomes. 2018. "Multifunctional magnetic-responsive hydrogels to engineer tendon-to-bone interface." *Nanomedicine; Nanotechnology, Biology Medicine* 14(7); 2375–2385. doi: 10.1016/j.nano.2017.06.002.

Singh, Thakur Raghu Raj, Garry Laverty, and Ryan Donnelly. 2018. *Hydrogels; Design, Synthesis and Application in Drug Delivery and Regenerative Medicine*. CRC Press, Boca Raton, FL.

Soppimath, Kumaresh S., Tejraj M. Aminabhavi, Ashok M. Dave, Sangamesh G. Kumbar, and W.E. Rudzinski. 2002. "Stimulus-responsive "smart" hydrogels as novel drug delivery systems." *Drug Development Industrial Pharmacy* 28(8); 957–974. doi: 10.1081/Ddc-120006428.

Tang, Shijia, Ke Hu, Jianfei Sun, Yang Li, Zhaobin Guo, Mei Liu, Qi Liu, Feimin Zhang, and Ning Gu. 2017. "High quality multicellular tumor spheroid induction platform based on anisotropic magnetic hydrogel." *ACS Applied Materials Interfaces* 9(12); 10446–10452. doi: 10.1021/acsami.6b15918.

Varlamova, Elena G., Mikhail V. Goltyaev, Valentina N. Mal'tseva, Egor A. Turovsky, Ruslan M. Sarimov, Alexander V. Simakin, and Sergey V. Gudkov. 2021. "Mechanisms of the cytotoxic effect of selenium nanoparticles in different human cancer cell lines." *International Journal of Molecular Sciences* 22(15); 7798. doi: 10.3390/ijms22157798.

Wei, Ping, Erik Jan Cornel, and Jianzhong Du. 2021. "Ultrasound-responsive polymer-based drug delivery systems." *Drug Delivery Translational Research* 11(4); 1323–1339. doi: 10.1007/s13346-021-00963-0.

Wei, Qingcong, Yaxing Wang, Huan Wang, Li Qiao, Yuqin Jiang, Guanglei Ma, Weiwei Zhang, and Zhiguo Hu. 2022. "Photo-induced adhesive carboxymethyl chitosan-based hydrogels with antibacterial and antioxidant properties for accelerating wound healing." *Carbohydrate Polymers* 278; 119000. doi: 10.1016/j.carbpol.2021.119000.

Wei, Xiaojuan, Si Chen, Tian Xie, Hongchi Chen, Xin Jin, Jumin Yang, Shafaq Sahar, Huanlei Huang, Shuoji Zhu, and Nanbo Liu. 2022. "An MMP-degradable and conductive hydrogel to stabilize HIF-1α for recovering cardiac functions." *Theranostics* 12(1); 127. doi: 10.7150/thno.63481.

Wu, Congyu, Yajing Shen, Mengwei Chen, Kun Wang, Yongyong Li, and Yu Cheng. 2018. "Recent advances in magnetic-nanomaterial-based mechanotransduction for cell fate regulation." *Advanced Materials* 30(17); 1705673. doi: 10.1002/adma.201705673.

Wu, Haoan, Lina Song, Ling Chen, Yixin Huang, Yang Wu, Fengchao Zang, Yanli An, Hanbai Lyu, Ming Ma, and Jun Chen. 2017. "Injectable thermosensitive magnetic nanoemulsion hydrogel for multimodal-imaging-guided accurate thermoablative cancer therapy." *Nanoscale* 9(42); 16175–16182. doi: 10.1039/c7nr02858j.

Wu, Meng, Jingsi Chen, Weijuan Huang, Bin Yan, Qiongyao Peng, Jifang Liu, Lingyun Chen, and Hongbo Zeng. 2020. "Injectable and self-healing nanocomposite hydrogels with ultrasensitive pH-responsiveness and tunable mechanical properties: Implications for controlled drug delivery." *Biomacromolecules* 21(6); 2409–2420. doi: 10.1021/acs.biomac.0c00347.

Xu, Chao, Shui Guan, Shuping Wang, Weitao Gong, Tianqing Liu, Xuehu Ma, and Changkai Sun. 2018. "Biodegradable and electroconductive poly (3, 4-ethylenedioxythiophene)/carboxymethyl chitosan hydrogels for neural tissue engineering." *Materials Science Engineering: C* 84; 32–43. doi: 10.1016/j.msec.2017.11.032.

Xu, Qinghua, Chaoliang He, Kaixuan Ren, Chunsheng Xiao, and Xuesi Chen. 2016. "Thermosensitive polypeptide hydrogels as a platform for ROS-triggered cargo release with innate cytoprotective ability under oxidative stress." *Advanced Healthcare Materials* 5(15); 1979–1990. doi: 10.1002/adhm.201600292.

Xu, Qinghua, Chaoliang He, Chunsheng Xiao, and Xuesi Chen. 2016. "Reactive oxygen species (ROS) responsive polymers for biomedical applications." *Macromolecular Bioscience* 16(5); 635–646. doi: 10.1002/mabi.201500440.

Yang, Tao, Weili Deng, Xiang Chu, Xiao Wang, Yeting Hu, Xi Fan, Jia Song, Yuyu Gao, Binbin Zhang, and Guo Tian. 2021. "Hierarchically microstructure-bioinspired flexible piezoresistive bioelectronics." *ACS Nano* 15(7); 11555–11563. doi: 10.1021/acsnano.1c01606.

Yang, Xin, Changqing Zhang, Dawei Deng, Yueqing Gu, Huan Wang, and Qifeng Zhong. 2022. "Multiple stimuli-responsive mxene-based hydrogel as intelligent drug delivery carriers for deep chronic wound healing." *Small* 18(5); 2104368. doi: 10.1002/smll.202104368.

Yuk, Hyunwoo, Baoyang Lu, and Xuanhe Zhao. 2019. "Hydrogel bioelectronics." *Chemical Society Reviews* 48(6); 1642–1667. doi: 10.1039/c8cs00595h.

Zardad, Az-Zamakhshariy, Yahya Essop Choonara, Lisa Claire Du Toit, Pradeep Kumar, Mostafa Mabrouk, Pierre Pavan Demarco Kondiah, and Viness Pillay. 2016. "A review of thermo-and ultrasound-responsive polymeric systems for delivery of chemotherapeutic agents." *Polymers* 8(10); 359. doi: 10.3390/polym8100359.

Zhang, Keyan, Haijun Lv, Yuqi Zheng, Yueming Yao, Xiaoran Li, Jianyong Yu, and Bin Ding. 2021. "Nanofibrous hydrogels embedded with phase-change materials; temperature-responsive dressings for accelerating skin wound healing." *Composites Communications* 25; 100752. doi: 10.1016/j.coco.2021.100752.

Zhang, Li, Yuting Zhou, Dandan Su, Shangyan Wu, Juan Zhou, and Jinghua Chen. 2021. "Injectable, self-healing and pH responsive stem cell factor loaded collagen hydrogel as a dynamic bioadhesive dressing for diabetic wound repair." *Journal of Materials Chemistry B* 9(29); 5887–5897. doi: 10.1039/d1tb01163d.

Zhang, Naiyin, Jaclyn Lock, Amy Sallee, Huinan Liu, and Interfaces. 2015. "Magnetic nanocomposite hydrogel for potential cartilage tissue engineering; synthesis, characterization, and cytocompatibility with bone marrow derived mesenchymal stem cells." *ACS Applied Materials* 7(37); 20987–20998. doi: 10.1021/acsami.5b06939.

Zhang, Yu, Xiaowei Wang, Jian Chen, Dingfei Qian, Peng Gao, Tao Qin, Tao Jiang, Jiang Yi, Tao Xu, and Yifan Huang. 2022. "Exosomes derived from platelet-rich plasma administration in site mediate cartilage protection in subtalar osteoarthritis." *Journal of Nanobiotechnology* 20(1); 1–22. doi: 10.1186/s12951-022-01245-8.

Zhao, He, Jie Huang, Yan Li, Xinjing Lv, Huiting Zhou, Hairong Wang, Yunyun Xu, Chao Wang, Jian Wang, and Zhuang Liu. 2020. "ROS-scavenging hydrogel to promote healing of bacteria infected diabetic wounds." *Biomaterials* 258; 120286. doi: 10.1016/j.biomaterials.2020.120286.

Zhao, Qinfu, Jia Liu, Wenquan Zhu, Changshan Sun, Donghua Di, Ying Zhang, Pu Wang, Zhanyou Wang, and Siling Wang. 2015. "Dual-stimuli responsive hyaluronic acid-conjugated mesoporous silica for targeted delivery to CD44-overexpressing cancer cells." *Acta Biomaterialia* 23; 147–156. doi: 10.1016/j.actbio.2015.05.010.

Zhao, Xiaodan, Yuxuan Yang, Jing Yu, Rui Ding, Dandan Pei, Yanfeng Zhang, Gang He, Yilong Cheng, and Ang Li. 2022. "Injectable hydrogels with high drug loading through B–N coordination and ROS-triggered drug release for efficient treatment of chronic periodontitis in diabetic rats." *Biomaterials*; 121387. doi: 10.1016/j.biomaterials.2022.121387.

Zhou, Liangqin, Fan Chen, Zishuo Hou, Yuanwei Chen, and Xianglin Luo. 2021. "Injectable self-healing CuS nanoparticle complex hydrogels with antibacterial, anti-cancer, and wound healing properties." *Chemical Engineering Journal* 409; 128224. doi: 10.1016/j.cej.2020.128224.

Zhou, Wanyi, Zhiguang Duan, Jing Zhao, Rongzhan Fu, Chenhui Zhu, and Daidi Fan. 2022. "Glucose and MMP-9 dual-responsive hydrogel with temperature sensitive self-adaptive shape and controlled drug release accelerates diabetic wound healing." *Bioactive Materials*. doi; 10.1016/j.bioactmat.2022.01.004.

Zhou, Xiaohan, Longchen Wang, Yanjun Xu, Wenxian Du, Xiaojun Cai, Fengjuan Wang, Yi Ling, Hangrong Chen, Zhigang Wang, and Bing Hu. 2018. "A pH and magnetic dual-response hydrogel for synergistic chemo-magnetic hyperthermia tumor therapy." *RSC Advances* 8(18); 9812–9821. doi: 10.1039/c8ra00215k.

Zhu, Minze, Andrew K. Whittaker, Felicity Y. Han, and Maree T. Smith. 2022. "Journey to the market: The evolution of biodegradable drug delivery systems." *Applied Sciences* 12(2); 935. doi: 10.3390/app12020935.

Zong, Shiyu, Hankang Wen, Hui Lv, Tong Li, Ruilin Tang, Liujun Liu, Jianxin Jiang, Shengpeng Wang, and Jiufang Duan. 2022. "Intelligent hydrogel with both redox and thermo-response based on cellulose nanofiber for controlled drug delivery." *Carbohydrate Polymers* 278; 118943. doi: 10.1016/j.carbpol.2021.118943.

2 3D Printing of Hydrogels for Cartilage Tissue Engineering Applications

Sena Su Torun
Yildiz Technical University
Marmara University
Nanortopedi Technology Industry and Trade Inc

Ecem Dogan
Yildiz Technical University
Marmara University

Nazmi Ekren
Marmara University

Cem Bulent Ustundag
Yildiz Technical University

Oguzhan Gunduz
Marmara University

CONTENTS

2.1 Introduction 20
2.1.1 Cartilage 20
2.1.1.1 Composition and Function of the Cartilage 20
2.1.1.2 Degeneration and Current Treatment Techniques 21
2.1.1.3 Cartilage Tissue Engineering 22
2.1.2 Hydrogels for Cartilage Regeneration 22
2.1.2.1 Hydrogels with Natural Materials 22
2.1.2.2 Hydrogels with Synthetic Materials 24
2.2 Bioprinting Techniques 24
2.2.1 Extrusion-Based Bioprinting 25
2.2.2 Inkjet Bioprinting 26
2.2.3 Laser-Assisted Bioprinting 27
2.3 3D Printing of Hydrogels for Cartilage Tissue Engineering 29

DOI: 10.1201/9781003251767-2

2.4 3D Bioprinting of Cell-Laden Hydrogels for Cartilage Tissue Engineering 30
2.5 Conclusion 31
References 31

2.1 INTRODUCTION

2.1.1 Cartilage

Cartilage is a fibrous tissue that provides support and protection to soft tissues, acts as a sliding surface in joints, and aids both in the formation of long bones as well as the repair of bone fractures. There are three main types of cartilage: hyaline, elastic, and fibrocartilage. Hyaline cartilage is typically found in articulating joints and has a white, glassy appearance (Doran, 2015). Its ECM consists mostly of water, type II collagen, hyaluronate, and proteoglycans. It shows an excellent ability to soften the impact induced by the physical load during movement due to its high viscoelasticity. Elastic cartilage is distinguished among other types of cartilage by its high content of elastic fibers, which gives it flexibility. It is present at the places where maintaining a specific shape is critical to continuing its function, such as the external ear and the larynx (Jung, 2014). Fibrocartilage is a tough type of cartilage containing a larger amount of type I collagen and is found in areas that require great support or tensile strength, like intervertebral discs, the meniscus, and sites where ligaments and tendons are connected to bones (Benjamin & Ralphs, 2004). All three types of cartilage show limited self-repair and regeneration properties due to their low cell density, limited blood flow, and avascular structure.

2.1.1.1 Composition and Function of the Cartilage

Cartilage is composed of chondrocyte cells and extracellular matrix (ECM). Chondrocytes are metabolically active cells that synthesize ECM components like collagen, proteoglycans, glycoproteins, and hyaluronic acid (HA) to maintain and protect the cartilage (Akkiraju & Nohe, 2015).

Mesenchymal stem cells (MSCs) in the bone marrow initially become chondroblasts (immature cells) when they differentiate into cartilage cells. After insertion into the cartilage matrix, they are called chondrocytes (mature cells) and are located in the matrix spaces. They stop proliferation and begin to synthesize and accumulate more cartilage ECM and fibers (Kern, Eichler, Stoeve, Klüter, & Bieback, 2006).

The ECM of cartilage consists mainly of a collagen network and proteoglycans. The collagen network is related to the tensile strength of the cartilage tissue, and the proteoglycan structure is related to its swelling and elastic properties. Although there are more than 28 different types of collagen, type II collagen is the main type of collagen found in articular cartilage (Fratzl, 2008). Type II collagen forms a network-like structure by forming interlocking fibrils with Types IX and XI. This structure provides tensile strength as well as physically holding other macromolecules (Gartner, 2017).

Proteoglycans are large proteins consisting of a protein core with linked polysaccharide chains, which are glycosaminoglycans. The major glycosaminoglycans that bind to the proteoglycan central core protein are chondroitin/dermatan sulfate (CS), heparan sulfate (HS), and keratan sulfate (KS). Proteoglycans also have the ability to bind a wide array of growth factors and morphogens to their GAG side chains.

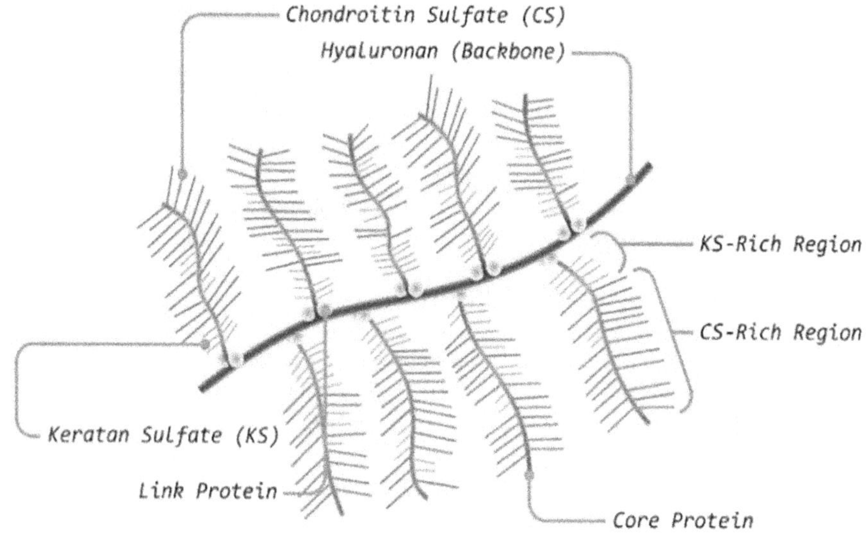

FIGURE 2.1 Schematic representation of the structure of aggrecan.

Aggregating proteoglycan (aggrecan) is the major proteoglycan form found in cartilage. Aggrecans have a specific HA binding site at the N-terminus of the molecule, which interacts ionically with HA. A glycoprotein known as the link protein mediates the connection between the HA binding site and HA. A schematic representation of the aggrecan structure is shown in Figure 2.1.

This organization is a stable structure in cartilage that attracts water molecules to hydrate the cartilage matrix and increases the resistance against compression (Tzanakakis, Kovalszky, Heldin, & Nikitovic, 2014). In hyalin cartilage, the proteoglycan's chondroitin sulfate side chains generate a cross-linked matrix by electrostatically binding to collagen fibrils.

HA, also called hyaluronan, is the simplest of the GAG groups and is composed of many thousands of repeating disaccharide units. HA-rich matrices facilitate the migration and condensation of mesenchymal cells during growth and development. In addition, HA is involved in the formation of the joint cavity and the growth of the longitudinal bone. HA binds to aggrecan in adult cartilage, thereby helping to maintain a high concentration of aggrecan, which is significant for tissue resistance to compression (Lin, Liu, Kampf, & Klein, 2020).

2.1.1.2 Degeneration and Current Treatment Techniques

Cartilage is a tissue with limited degeneration ability because there is no innervation or blood circulation. Microfracture and osteochondral autografting are the primary treatment techniques used for articular cartilage repair. In microfracture, holes are drilled into the subchondral bone underlying a cartilage defect to allow the release of MSCs from the bone marrow by inducing bleeding. After this procedure, fibrocartilage structure is mostly formed instead of natural cartilage, and this newly formed tissue is weaker than the natural tissue in terms of functional and biomechanical properties (Hurst, Steadman, O'Brien, Rodkey, & Briggs, 2010).

Osteochondral autografting is an autotransplantation procedure that involves harvesting osteochondral plugs from parts of the joint and implanting them into defects that have been prepared and sized (Hangody, Feczkó, Bartha, Bodó, & Kish, 2001). Although autografts have been found to have superior long-term clinical results than microfracture, they have a number of drawbacks, including donor site injury, prompting, scarring, and pain. Allograft and xenograft have more disadvantages compared to autograft, and they can also cause many complex problems such as disease transmission, infections, and transplant rejection (Tran, Park, Ching, Huynh, & Nguyen, 2020).

2.1.1.3 Cartilage Tissue Engineering

The tissue engineering approach involves building scaffolds in a 3D environment to support and guide cellular processes in immigration, proliferation, and differentiation into functional tissue. Chondrocytes and stem cells can be used in fabricating scaffolds; however, cell-free production of the scaffold is also often preferred since cell therapy can be more costly and challenging (Makris, Gomoll, Malizos, Hu, & Athanasiou, 2015). Biocompatibility, cellular functions, capability of waste and nutrient transport, and appropriate mechanical properties of equivalent strength to the original cartilage tissue should all be considered while producing bioscaffolds for cartilage engineering. A wide range of natural and synthetic biomaterials can be used for cartilage defects in various forms, such as fibrous mats, sponges, woven andnon-woven meshes, and hydrogels (Balakrishnan & Banerjee, 2011; Faust, Guo, & Elisseeff, 2019).

2.1.2 Hydrogels for Cartilage Regeneration

Hydrogels have been extensively studied in tissue engineering applications due to their superior properties such as biocompatibility, flexibility, and high water retention capacity. They can absorb water or biological fluids up to thousands of times their dry weight. Their structure simulates the ECM of original tissues, both physicochemically and biologically, and they can absorb fluids up to thousands of times their dry weight (Rey-Rico, Madry, & Cucchiarini, 2016).

Various natural and synthetic polymers such as collagen, HA, chitosan, fibrin, poly(ethylene glycol) (PEG), and poly(ethylene oxide) (PEO) can be used in the production of hydrogels. Due to the variety of chemical modifications and different cross-linking properties of hydrogels, they can be adjusted to the desired properties according to the targeted tissue (De Mori, Fernández, Blunn, Tozzi, & Roldo, 2018). Combining natural and synthetic polymers to construct ideal biomaterial scaffolds and induce new tissue formation is a promising strategy.

2.1.2.1 Hydrogels with Natural Materials

Natural hydrogels have properties like those of natural tissues, and natural hydrogel precursors occur naturally in most human bodies. Because of its high biocompatibility and bioactivity, it is often preferred by researchers in cartilage tissue engineering. Such materials promote cell attachment and stimulate ECM production. On the other hand, they have disadvantages such as being difficult to synthesize and process, having unstable material properties, and requiring rapid hydrolysis. Its low mechanical properties are also not sufficient to support cells, and therefore, scaffolds formed from natural hydrogels may be inadequate for tissue regeneration (Bao et al., 2020).

HA is an unsulfated glycosaminoglycan that is a crucial component of the ECM and has a function in cell signaling and wound healing. It is commonly produced by extraction from animal connective tissues such as rooster comb and by streptococcal fermentation (Prajapati & Maheriya, 2019). HA-based hydrogels are considered to be one of the most popular biomaterials for cartilage tissue engineering due to their unique properties. Studies have shown that HA has an inducing effect on chondrocyte production by type II collagen and proteoglycan (Akmal et al., 2005). Cross-linked HA hydrogels are used to provide better biocompatibility and controllable biodegradation.

Collagen, a protein found in approximately 30% of the mammalian body, is widely used as a hydrogel in medical fields. Collagen, a protein found in approximately 30% of the mammalian body, can be obtained from numerous sources, primarily the skin and bones of land animals (Silvipriya et al., 2015). It has the characteristic triple helical structure and thus can self-aggregate using covalent and hydrogen bonds. Hydrogels fabricated using collagen type I were shown to promote MSC adhesion, growth, proliferation, and cartilage differentiation in vitro in medical fields (Yang et al., 2019).

Gelatin is another natural polymer obtained by partial hydrolysis of collagen and used for cartilage regeneration. Gelatin-based hydrogels possess good biodegradability, biocompatibility, and cell/tissue affinity, making them one of the most studied polymers in this field. However, poor mechanical strength and low thermal stability are among its disadvantages (Han et al., 2017). Although there are various methods for the preparation of gelatin hydrogels, the most prominent method is the modification of gelatin with methacrylate anhydride. In this method, copolymerization is carried out by exposing the methacrylate gelatin (GelMA) solution to ultraviolet radiation under the influence of a photoinitiator. GelMA hydrogels considered a star product due to their advantages such as high biocompatibility and non-toxicity in tissue engineering, but pure GelMA hydrogels alone do not show sufficiently high mechanical properties in cartilage applications (Bao et al., 2020).

Alginate is an anionic biopolymer produced from seaweed and has been extensively researched and used in cartilage tissue engineering applications due to its biocompatibility, ease of preparation, and relatively low cost. Alginate is a linear copolymer of (1–4)-linked-β-d-mannuronic acid and R-l-guluronic acid. The most common method of preparing alginate hydrogel is to bind the alginate solution with various divalent metal ions such as calcium, magnesium, and barium. These ions bind to the guluronate blocks of alginate chains and form a porous hydrogel (Liu et al., 2017).

Fibrin is another natural biopolymer that forms naturally during blood coagulation and has an important function in hemostasis and tissue regeneration, promoting wound healing and implant engraftment. It has multiple important amino acid binding sequences, including two RGD sites that are involved in cell-integrin interactions. According to previous studies, fibrin gels are a good polymer gel for constructing new cartilage tissue and are capable of forming mechanical links between cartilage disks, resulting in healing and integration (Han et al., 2021).

Chitosan is a linear polysaccharide composed of 1,4-linked 2-amino-2-deoxy-d-glucose (GlcNH2) residues and randomly distributed *N*-acetyl-glucosamine (GlcNAc) groups and is the deacetylated derivative of chitin, which is commonly found in crab and shrimp shells (Iber, Kasan, Torsabo, & Omuwa, 2022). It is vital to improve cell adhesion by combining chitosan-based hydrogels with additional bioactive species that assist chondrocyte adhesion, proliferation, and chondrogenesis in order to generate chitosan-based hydrogels for cartilage tissue engineering. Poor wettability, a long degradation time, and a lack of cellular adhesion and interaction are among its disadvantages. In addition, it can cause adverse tissue reactions caused by its acidic degradation products. It is a suitable option to use with other natural biopolymers and bioactive agents to increase its biocompatibility and hydrophilicity when producing scaffolds for cartilage applications (Davachi et al., 2022).

2.1.2.2 Hydrogels with Synthetic Materials

Synthetic polymers are used in tissue engineering due to their wide availability, biocompatibility, controlled degradation, tailored mechanical properties, ease of processing, and ability to be modified to meet the specific needs of various applications. They are commonly used in cartilage regeneration because they can be easily processed into the desired shape and size and have relatively low toxicity, immunogenicity, and infection risks. The main disadvantage of synthetic polymers is the absence of biological factors that can promote cell adhesion and proliferation (Simionescu & Ivanov, 2016).

Some of the synthetic polymers used in hydrogel formulations for cartilage tissue engineering are mainly poly(d,l-lactic acid-co-glycolic acid) (PLGA), PEO, PEG, and polycaprolactone (PCL) (Faust et al., 2019).

PLGA, a copolymer of lactic and glycolic acids, is exclusively used in bone and cartilage tissue engineering due to its biocompatibility, tailorable biodegradation rate, good mechanical strength, and surface modification capability. The degradation rate of PLGA is strongly dependent on its crystallinity and the lactic/glycolic ratio. Monomers (lactic acid and glycolic acid) released in consequence of PLGA biodegradation do not cause adverse effects in the body as they are non-toxic natural byproducts of metabolic pathways (He et al., 2017).

PEG- and PEO-based hydrogels are promising materials for cartilage tissue engineering due to their photopolymerization ability and tunable mechanical properties. They are biodegradable and non-immunogenic, and it is easy to embed cells and growth factors into the gel matrix (Xiongfa, Hao, Liming, & Jun, 2018).

Polycaprolactone (PCL), which has received FDA approval for a variety of medical applications, is a biodegradable, hydrophobic semi-crystalline polyester. PCL is preferred for use in cartilage tissue regeneration because of its good processability, chemical diversity, and excellent mechanical properties. Poor wettability, a lack of cellular adhesion and interaction, and a long degradation rate are among its disadvantages. It is a suitable option to use with other biopolymers like PEG, chitosan, etc. to increase its biocompatibility and hydrophilicity for effective cartilage regeneration (Chang et al., 2018).

2.2 BIOPRINTING TECHNIQUES

The method of 3D bioprinting is employed in tissue engineering and regenerative medicine. 3D printers are also important to meet the increasing need for organ transplantation worldwide (Hacıoglu, Yılmazer, & Ustundag, 2018). 3D bioprinting is an emerging technique that can be used to manufacture tissue and organ structures to replace those that have been wounded or diseased.

Five centuries after the development of the printing industry, 3D printing technology was discovered and broke new ground in both industry and medicine. After the developments and advances, new scientific domains, for example "tissue engineering", have emerged (Papaioannou et al., 2019). In tissue engineering, cells are seeded onto scaffolds. These scaffolds can direct cell growth and differentiation into functional 3D tissues. Synthetic and natural polymers are used to produce different textures. To meet the challenges, materials must be biocompatible and biodegradable (Ozbolat & Yu, 2013). Artificial tissues and organs are produced by the 3D printing technique by combining cells, biomaterials, and growth factors. Organs and tissues can be produced by selecting the appropriate bioprinting technique and ink. With bioprinting technology, bioactive molecules, cells, biomaterials, or cell clusters are printed to produce a structure. With this technology, it is aimed at imitating tissues and organs by developing the desired complex structures (Mobaraki, Ghaffari, Yazdanpanah, Luo, & Mills, 2020).

Compared to conventional production methods, 3D printing allows for the design and fabrication of more complicated designs. With 3D printing, the prototyping process can be accelerated, and the stages can be completed quickly. Also, this technology saves resources and time.

A standard scaffold bioprinting process consists of several basic steps. It's the initial stage in making a tissue scaffold that can reflect tissue composition and organization in structural design. After this step, cells and biomaterials that can sustain their cellular and extracellular functions appropriately are synthesized. These materials must also be compatible with the bioprinting process. Following these steps, the extrusion-based bioprinting technique is used to produce tissue scaffolds that, depending on the structural design and material or cells selected, can be grown in vitro or inserted into a specific tissue location for in vivo applications (Harrison, St-Pierre, & Stevens, 2014).

The material of scaffolding is very important in 3D bioprinting. Cells are controlled by both the material composition of the scaffolds and the interior architectural features of the scaffolds, such as pores. In this section, extrusion-based, inkjet, and laser-assisted bioprinting techniques will be explained.

2.2.1 Extrusion-Based Bioprinting

Extrusion-based bioprinting can be defined as a technique that can form various tissue scaffolds from various biomaterials and cell types (Ning & Chen, 2017). A 3D structure is formed as a result of shaping thermoplastic polymers or polymer composites by extrusion from nozzles. The extrusion-based method has been used for many years to shape both metals and plastics (Abeykoon, Martin, Kelly, & Brown, 2012).

With extrusion-based bioprinting, bioprinting of cells, tissues, tissue structures, and organs has become possible (Almeida et al., 2014). Many different tissues, such as cartilage (W. Zhang et al., 2014), vascular system (Norotte, Marga, Niklason, & Forgacs, 2009), bone (Poldervaart et al., 2013), skin (Won, Patel, & Bull, 2014), liver (Godoy et al., 2013), and cardiac (Gaetani et al., 2012), have been produced with this

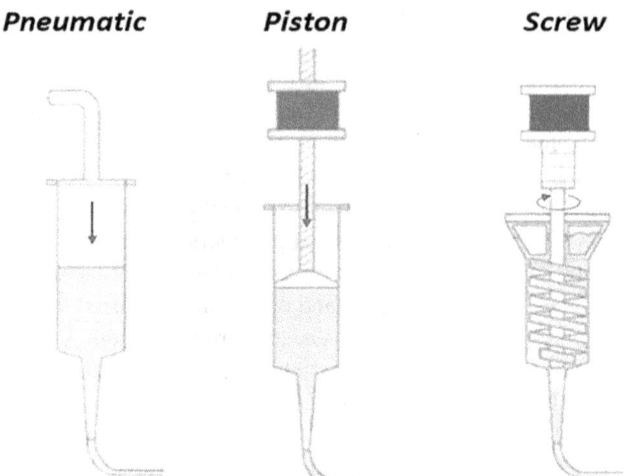

FIGURE 2.2 Types of extrusion bioprinting.

method. Factors such as thickness layer, nozzle advance speed, infill density, and printing pattern affect printing (Arslan, Ay, & Korkmaz, 2020). After the structural design and synthesis of cells and biomaterials, which are the main steps in the typical scaffold bioprinting process, the extrusion-based bioprinting technique is applied to the selected structural design and materials/cells to produce scaffolds that are cultured in vitro or implanted into localized tissue space for in vivo applications (Chang Yan, Nair, & Sun, 2010). A schematic representation of the types of extrusion bioprinting is shown in Figure 2.2.

2.2.2 Inkjet Bioprinting

Inkjet printing uses drops of ink non-contactly by receiving digital data from a computer and reproducing it on the substrate. Another name for the inkjet bioprinting method is drop-on-demand printers (Xu, Kincaid, Atala, & Yoo, 2008). In the inkjet bioprinting method, cells and/or biomaterials are used as bioink. In this way, living tissue or organs are printed on the substrates. The inkjet printing technique has several advantages, including great efficiency, low cost, and high sensitivity. Due to these superior features, it has been used in fields such as paper printing and has contributed to fields such as education and scientific research (Calvert, 2001; Dababneh & Ozbolat, 2014).

Hydrogels, powders, polymers, and small molecules are examples of biomaterials utilized in inkjet bioprinting. Hydrogels are a good choice for inkjet bioprinting since their viscosity can be regulated and the desired shape is easy to achieve. It also contributes positively to cell adhesion, proliferation, and migration due to its ability to mimic the microenvironment well (Kyle, Jessop, Al-Sabah, & Whitaker, 2017).

Polymers are preferred in biomedical areas due to features such as ease of processing, lightness, flexibility, high specific strength, good usability, and recyclability. By using inkjet bioprinting, the polymers PCL, polyurethanes (PUs), PLA, and PLGA have been used as scaffolds and drug delivery systems (Zhang, Wen, Vyavahare, & Boland, 2008; Scoutaris et al., 2016). In the bioprinting process, polymers are dissolved in organic solvents. It has been reported that the molecular weights of polymers and their printability are inversely proportional (De Gans, Duineveld, & Schubert, 2004). Since solvents such as acetic acid, ethanol, and dimethylformamide are used, the inkjet bioprinting process is done without cells. Therefore, solvents must be eliminated through dehydration or drying before cells are cultivated. High resolution, user-friendly, inexpensive, and sterilizable qualities are desirable in an inkjet bioprinter (Li et al., 2020). A schematic representation of the thermal, piezoelectric, and mechanical inkjet bioprinters is shown in Figure 2.3.

2.2.3 Laser-Assisted Bioprinting

Laser-assisted bioprinters (LAB) are a fast, precise, and accurate printing method. In laser-assisted bioprinting, cells print with a laser beam, and this beam vibrates at a controlled rate. Unlike the inkjet bioprinting method, materials with a wide viscosity range can be printed using this method (Hacıoglu et al., 2018).

Laser-assisted bioprinting method consists of three parts: a pulsed laser source, a strip and the receiving substrate (Guillemot, Souquet, Catros, & Guillotin, 2010). The laser part is used as an energy source to achieve energy accumulation. The ribbon portion is a multilayered component consisting of a thin layer of laser-absorbing metal like clear glass, gold, or titanium and a suspended bioink layer made up of cells, hydrogels, and bioactive substances. When the laser beam strip is focused, the metal layer on top of the hydrogel evaporates. Bioink droplets are sprayed onto the receiving substrate by the pressure bubble formed by this steam. The sprayed drops of acceptor substrate contain culture medium to promote growth. Printing the cells one after the other without stopping at the desired coordinates means resolution (Bishop et al., 2017).

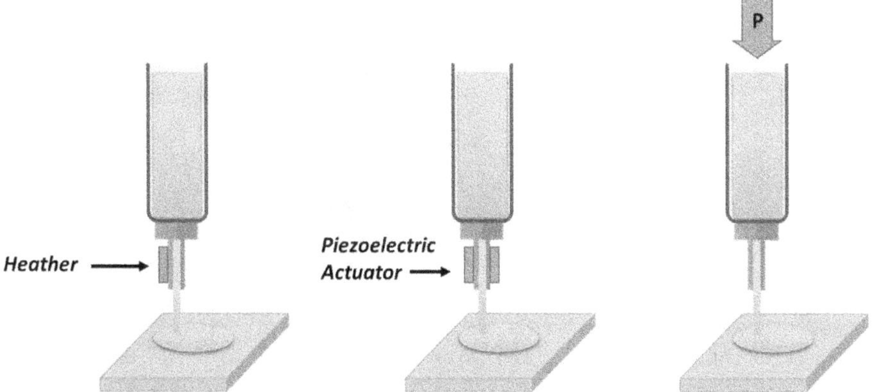

FIGURE 2.3 Thermal, piezoelectric, and mechanical inkjet bioprinters, respectively.

Structurally complex scaffolds can be produced with LAB technology. For this purpose, the necessary cells and various biomaterials are used. With this printing method, cell-scaffold interaction becomes easier, and tissues and organs that cannot be obtained with traditional scaffold manufacturing can be produced. In this method, artificial cell niches or architectures can be obtained without affecting the viability or material integrity of the cells (Ventura, 2021).

Stem cells are versatile cells and are preferred as a source of cells in 3D printing due to their ability to divide for cell renewal and proliferation. The materials to be used for bioprinting are expected to be biocompatible, suitable for biomimicry, and have sufficient mechanical and rheological qualities to endure bioprinting and degradation. The materials used as bioinks for the LAB process are polymers that resemble a natural ECM. These polymers support cell function and proliferation (Murphy & Atala, 2014). Especially when producing bioinks from synthetic polymers, it may be necessary to use organic solvents that can induce cell toxicity. These organic solvents must be well removed after producing the scaffold to provide biocompatibility (De Mori et al., 2018). Collagen, one of these polymers, is a very important component of the ECM. It can be used for cell growth and tissue regeneration (Zhang et al., 2021). A schematic representation of the laser-assisted bioprinting is shown in Figure 2.4.

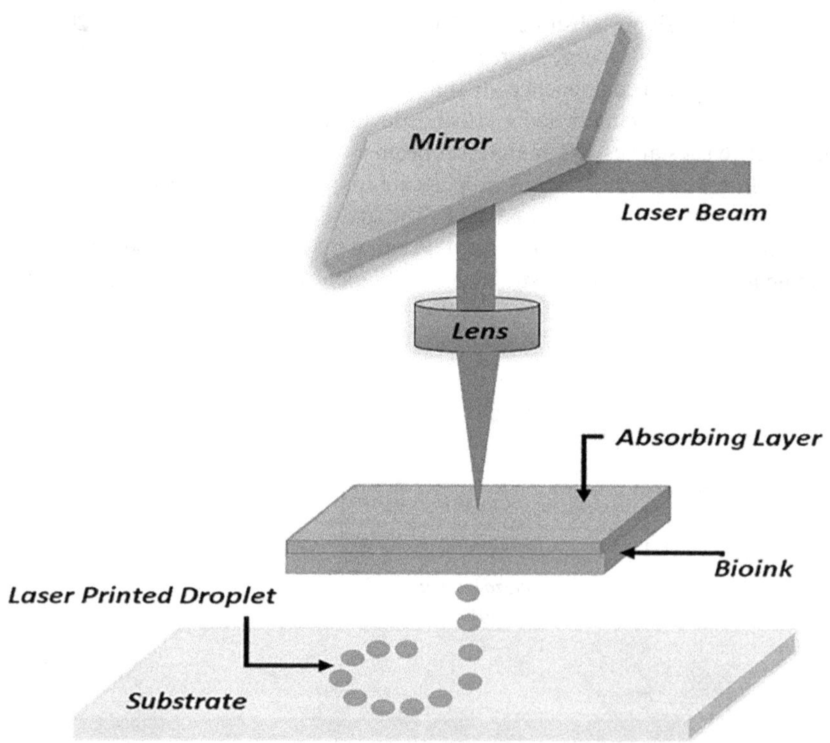

FIGURE 2.4 Schematic representation of laser-assisted bioprinting.

2.3 3D PRINTING OF HYDROGELS FOR CARTILAGE TISSUE ENGINEERING

The smooth tissue that forms the facing faces of the bones forming the joint is shiny, lacks blood vessels and nerves, and has a low chondrocyte density. It is called cartilage. Although cartilage is not a very thick structure, it prevents friction between joints and can withstand excessive loads. When cartilage is damaged in old age, trauma, joint pain, or arthritis occur. Production methods for cartilage tissue have begun to be sought in cases of damage that may occur due to its importance. Tissues with the required shape and characteristics can be printed using 3D bioprinting. Chondrocyte and MSCs for cartilage tissue are essential and important cells for cartilage regeneration (Huang, Xiong, Wang, et al., 2021).

Scaffolds should provide an environment that encourages cell attachment, migration, adhesion, proliferation, and differentiation, and the materials chosen should reflect this. Thanks to these properties, hydrogel composites and polymeric hydrogels have been preferred in recent years. Hydrogels have been proven to create the essential 3D environment for cartilage tissue regeneration in both in vitro and in vivo experiments (Sánchez-Téllez, Téllez-Jurado, & Rodríguez-Lorenzo, 2017; Nikolova & Chavali, 2019). Hydrogels are a highly suitable biomaterial that can be used to regenerate soft and hard tissues. Thanks to their mechanical hardness, elasticity, water content, bioactivity, and decomposition properties, hydrogels suitable for their purpose can be obtained by designing with appropriate material selection. In CTE, hydrogel scaffolds can be 3D printed directly from hydrogels or composite hydrogels in two ways. When compared to hybrid bioprinting, bioprinting directly from hydrogels is a comparatively simple technique. However, composite hydrogels can support 3D structures with good mechanical performance (Li, Wu, Chu, & Gelinsky, 2020). It is very critical that CTE scaffolds mechanically resemble natural cartilage properties and provide natural environmental conditions. Because they can be obtained in the desired shape and size, biomaterial-based hydrogels are frequently preferred for tissue engineering (Naghieh, Sarker, Sharma, Barhoumi, & Chen, 2020). Biomaterial-based hydrogels are hydrophilic 3D networks composed of natural or synthetic polymers such as polysaccharides and proteins that are water-soluble by chemical or physical cross-linking to form a water-insoluble hydrogel. The summary of methods, biomaterials, cell types, and bioprinting methods for 3D printing CTE is given in Table 2.1.

According to a study (Park et al., 2014), the expression levels of chondrocyte markers are higher when HA, which is very important for synovial fluid and hyaline cartilage, is used by planting chondrocytes in 3D scaffolds. In another work, chondrocytes were encapsulated in an alginate-PCL hybrid material. 3D- printed PCL stents are frequently used in cartilage engineering. PCL, on the other hand, has low cell affinity due to its hydrophobic surface. The use of biocompatible alginate hydrogels to construct exact forms in 3D-printed structures has been effective. The soft and brittle alginate can increase the weight-bearing capacity of the joints with the use of collagen hydrogel. Materials produced in this way have good mechanical stability, and cell growth can be supported and continued. As a result, chondrocytes were encapsulated using an alginate-PCL hybrid material (Schuurman et al., 2011). Yang

TABLE 2.1

Methods, Biomaterials, Cell Type and Bioprinting Methods for 3D CTE

Biomaterial	Bioprinting Method	Cell Type	References
Polycaprolactone and alginate	Extrusion-based	Chondrocyte	Cao et al. (2021)
Collagen type II hydrogel	Extrusion-based	Chondrocyte	Ren et al. (2016)
Gelatin	Extrusion-based	MSCs	Daly, Critchley, Rencsok, and Kelly et al. (2016)
Polysaccharides, gellan, alginate, and BioCartilage	Extrusion-based	Chondrocyte	Kesti et al. (2015)
Fibrinogen and fibrin	Inkjet printing	Chondrocyte	Xu et al. 2012
PCL and GelMA	Inkjet printing	MSCs and chondrocytes	Daly and Kelly (2019)
GO, chitosan, and collagen type I	Inkjet printing	Chondrocyte	Cheng et al. (2020)

et al. (2018) used 3D bio-printed CTE with collagen-alginate bioink and stated that the chondrocytes were at a good level of expansion mechanically while maintaining the phenotype. In extrusion-based bioprinting, it was observed that alginate and agarose hydrogels had a positive effect on hyaline cartilage formation when compared to other hydrogel groups. The elastic modulus of the bioink and alginate was shown to rise when PCL microfibers were added to the bioink (Mohan, Maver, Štiglic, Stana-Kleinschek, & Kargl, 2018). The fracture performance and cell viability of PEG/alginate hydrogel composites formed by 3D printing were higher than those of natural cartilage, according to the findings of another study (Huang, Xiong, Yang, et al., 2021). A composite containing agarose, alginate, GelMA, and BioINK was made, and it outperformed native cartilage (Daly et al., 2016).

2.4 3D BIOPRINTING OF CELL-LADEN HYDROGELS FOR CARTILAGE TISSUE ENGINEERING

Despite advances in medicine, it is still difficult to treat cartilage damage. Hydrogels, which can be used for both soft and hard tissue regeneration, are preferred in tissue engineering because of their mechanical hardness, elasticity, water content, bioactivity, and degradation properties. With the appropriate material selection, hydrogels with the desired properties and designs can be produced. For cell therapies, cell-loaded hydrogels have been a hope. These cell-loaded hydrogels are used in CTE (Yang, Zhang, Yue, & Khademhosseini, 2017).

Tissue engineering and cell therapy have been combined to restore cartilage damage. In this treatment, hydrogels are employed for cell transport and artificial ECM for 3D culture. Such cells as chondrocytes, preosteoblasts/osteoblasts, MSCs, and induced pluripotent stem cells (iPSCs) with chondrogenic differentiation properties are used as cell sources for cartilage repair. Autologous chondrocyte implantation is a clinically effective method for repairing cartilage damage. However, since it is difficult for orthopedic surgeons to fix the chondrocyte graft directly to the complex-shaped focal cartilage area, the delivery of chondrocytes with hydrogels has been proposed as a solution (Sharma et al., 2013).

In many studies, chondrocytes were embedded in different hydrogels, and it was observed that chondrocytes can disseminate and multiply in 3D hydrogel matrices in vitro. It has also been stated that the expression of cartilage-related proteins and genes is increased (Zeng, Yao, Wang, & Chen, 2014; Chung et al., 2014). It has been determined that hydrogels produced from various polymers respond differently during chondrocyte chondrogenesis. Studies have shown that chitosan and agarose hydrogels positively affect survival and morphology in in vitro cultures (Jin et al., 2009). Another study found that cartilage ECM, such as aggrecan and collagen type II, was generated during the maturation phase of in vitro trials, resulting in chondrogenesis (Roberts, Nicodemus, Greenwald, & Bryant, 2011).

2.5 CONCLUSION

In this review, cartilage tissue engineering, hydrogels used for cartilage tissue regeneration, 3D bioprinting techniques, and hydrogels produced by 3D techniques for cartilage tissue engineering are discussed. Hydrogels made of natural, synthetic, and both natural and synthetic materials have been produced for cartilage regeneration in the last few years. Some of these hydrogels positively affect cartilage repair and cell growth. It has been determined that hydrogels produced from natural materials are more biocompatible and have higher cell viability. The positive properties of all materials can also be used in specially designed hydrogels. Because hydrogels are not mechanically strong and have low printing performance, large cartilage tissues cannot be produced. In the future, MSC-loaded cartilage tissues can be 3D-fabricated on a large scale.

Although there are many studies on 3D bioprinting hydrogel production, some situations need to be overcome in order to implement them. The foremost of these limitations is bioink. Restrictions on its use and the absence of bioinks that meet all requirements are the reasons for this negativity. Bioinks must first be optimized. Optimization parameters are insoluble in vivo and in culture, structurally stable, supporting cell growth, non-toxic, combining with other cells, and providing vascularization. These inks can also negatively affect cell viability. Challenges for both bioinks and 3D printing remain. A future multidisciplinary collaboration will provide positive developments for many tissue and organ printing applications, including cartilage tissue engineering.

As studies on cartilage tissue engineering increase, the possibility of tissue regeneration becoming a reality also increases. Skin and scaffolds for auricular and nasal cartilage may one day be printed simultaneously using 3D printing technology. In addition, cartilage tissue engineering applications are carried out with 4D printing.

REFERENCES

Abeykoon, C., Martin, P. J., Kelly, A. L., & Brown, E. C. (2012). A review and evaluation of melt temperature sensors for polymer extrusion. *Sensors and Actuators, A: Physical*, *182*, 16–27. https://doi.org/10.1016/j.sna.2012.04.026.

Akkiraju, H., & Nohe, A. (2015). Role of chondrocytes in cartilage formation, progression of osteoarthritis and cartilage regeneration. *Journal of Developmental Biology*, *3*(4), 177–192. https://doi.org/10.3390/jdb3040177.

Akmal, M., Singh, A., Anand, A., Kesani, A., Aslam, N., Goodship, A., & Bentley, G. (2005). The effects of hyaluronic acid on articular chondrocytes. *Journal of Bone and Joint Surgery - Series B*, *87*(8), 1143–1149. https://doi.org/10.1302/0301-620X.87B8.15083.

Almeida, C. R., Serra, T., Oliveira, M. I., Planell, J. A., Barbosa, M. A., & Navarro, M. (2014). Impact of 3-D printed PLA- and chitosan-based scaffolds on human monocyte/macrophage responses: Unraveling the effect of 3-D structures on inflammation. *Acta Biomaterialia*, *10*(2), 613–622. https://doi.org/10.1016/j.actbio.2013.10.035.

Arslan, T., Ay, B., & Korkmaz, N. (2020). Deri Doku Mühendisli ğ i, (May), 0–36.

Balakrishnan, B., & Banerjee, R. (2011). Biopolymer-based hydrogels for cartilage tissue engineering. *Chemical Reviews*, *111*(8), 4453–4474. https://doi.org/10.1021/cr100123h.

Bao, W., Li, M., Yang, Y., Wan, Y., Wang, X., Bi, N., & Li, C. (2020). Advancements and frontiers in the high performance of natural hydrogels for cartilage tissue engineering. *Frontiers in Chemistry*, *8*, 53. https://doi.org/10.3389/fchem.2020.00053.

Benjamin, M., & Ralphs, J. R. (2004). Biology of fibrocartilage cells. In *International Review of Cytology* (pp. 1–46). https://doi.org/10.1016/S0074-7696(04)33001-9.

Bishop, E. S., Mostafa, S., Pakvasa, M., Luu, H. H., Lee, M. J., Wolf, J. M., … Reid, R. R. (2017). 3-D bioprinting technologies in tissue engineering and regenerative medicine: Current and future trends. *Genes and Diseases*, *4*(4), 185–195. https://doi.org/10.1016/j.gendis.2017.10.002.

Calvert, P. (2001). Inkjet printing for materials and devices. *Chemistry of Materials*, *13*(10), 3299–3305. https://doi.org/10.1021/cm0101632.

Cao, Y., Cheng, P., Sang, S., Xiang, C., An, Y., Wei, X., … Li, P. (2021). Mesenchymal stem cells loaded on 3D-printed gradient poly(ε-caprolactone)/methacrylated alginate composite scaffolds for cartilage tissue engineering. *Regenerative Biomaterials*, *8*(3), 19. https://doi.org/10.1093/rb/rbab019.

Chang, C. S., Yang, C. Y., Hsiao, H. Y., Chen, L., Chu, I. M., Cheng, M. H., & Tsao, C. K. (2018). Cultivation of auricular chondrocytes in poly(ethylene glycol)/poly(ε-caprolactone) hydrogel for tracheal cartilage tissue engineering in a rabbit model. *European Cells and Materials*, *35*, 350–364. https://doi.org/10.22203/eCM.v035a24.

Chang Yan, K., Nair, K., & Sun, W. (2010). Three dimensional multi-scale modelling and analysis of cell damage in cell-encapsulated alginate constructs. *Journal of Biomechanics*, *43*(6), 1031–1038. https://doi.org/10.1016/j.jbiomech.2009.12.018.

Cheng, Z., Xigong, L., Weiyi, D., Jingen, H., Shuo, W., Xiangjin, L., & Junsong, W. (2020). Potential use of 3D-printed graphene oxide scaffold for construction of the cartilage layer. *Journal of Nanobiotechnology*, *18*(1), 1–13. https://doi.org/10.1186/s12951-020-00655-w.

Chung, J. Y., Song, M., Ha, C. W., Kim, J. A., Lee, C. H., & Park, Y. B. (2014). Comparison of articular cartilage repair with different hydrogel-human umbilical cord blood-derived mesenchymal stem cell composites in a rat model. *Stem Cell Research and Therapy*, *5*(2), 1–13. https://doi.org/10.1186/scrt427.

Dababneh, A. B., & Ozbolat, I. T. (2014). Bioprinting technology: A current state-of-the-art review. *Journal of Manufacturing Science and Engineering, Transactions of the ASME*, *136*(6), 1–11. https://doi.org/10.1115/1.4028512.

Daly, A. C., Critchley, S. E., Rencsok, E. M., & Kelly, D. J. (2016). A comparison of different bioinks for 3D bioprinting of fibrocartilage and hyaline cartilage. *Biofabrication*, *8*(4), 1–10. https://doi.org/10.1088/1758-5090/8/4/045002.

Daly, A. C., & Kelly, D. J. (2019). Biofabrication of spatially organised tissues by directing the growth of cellular spheroids within 3D printed polymeric microchambers. *Biomaterials*, *197*(January), 194–206. https://doi.org/10.1016/j.biomaterials.2018.12.028.

Davachi, S. M., Haramshahi, S. M. A., Akhavirad, S. A., Bahrami, N., Hassanzadeh, S., Ezzatpour, S., … Bagher, Z. (2022). Development of chitosan/hyaluronic acid hydrogel scaffolds via enzymatic reaction for cartilage tissue engineering. *Materials Today Communications*, *30*(June 2021), 103230. https://doi.org/10.1016/j.mtcomm.2022.103230.

De Gans, B. J., Duineveld, P. C., & Schubert, U. S. (2004). Inkjet printing of polymers: State of the art and future developments. *Advanced Materials, 16*(3), 203–213. https://doi.org/10.1002/adma.200300385.

De Mori, A., Fernández, M. P., Blunn, G., Tozzi, G., & Roldo, M. (2018). 3D printing and electrospinning of composite hydrogels for cartilage and bone tissue engineering. *Polymers, 10*(3), 1–26. https://doi.org/10.3390/polym10030285.

Doran, P. M. (2015). *Cartilage Tissue Engineering - Methods and Protocols*. Methods in Molecular Biology, Springer, New York.

Faust, H. J., Guo, Q., & Elisseeff, J. H. (2019). *Cartilage Tissue Engineering. Principles of Regenerative Medicine*. Elsevier Inc. https://doi.org/10.1016/b978-0-12-820508-2.00004-0.

Fratzl, P. (2008). Collagen: Structure and mechanics, an introduction. In *Collagen: Structure and Mechanics* (pp. 1–13). https://doi.org/10.1007/978-0-387-73906-9_1.

Gaetani, R., Doevendans, P. A., Metz, C. H. G., Alblas, J., Messina, E., Giacomello, A., & Sluijter, J. P. G. (2012). Cardiac tissue engineering using tissue printing technology and human cardiac progenitor cells. *Biomaterials, 33*(6), 1782–1790. https://doi.org/10.1016/j.biomaterials.2011.11.003.

Gartner, L. P. (2020). *Textbook of Histology e-book* Elsevier Health Sciences.

Godoy, P., Hewitt, N. J., Albrecht, U., Andersen, M. E., Ansari, N., Bhattacharya, S., … Hengstler, J. G. (2013). Recent advances in 2D and 3D in vitro systems using primary hepatocytes, alternative hepatocyte sources and non-parenchymal liver cells and their use in investigating mechanisms of hepatotoxicity, cell signaling and ADME. *Archives of Toxicology* (Vol. 87). https://doi.org/10.1007/s00204-013-1078-5.

Guillemot, F., Souquet, A., Catros, S., & Guillotin, B. (2010). Laser-assisted cell printing: Principle, physical parameters versus cell fate and perspectives in tissue engineering. *Nanomedicine, 5*(3), 507–515. https://doi.org/10.2217/nnm.10.14.

Hacıoglu, A., Yılmazer, H., & Ustundag, C. B. (2018). 3D Printing for Tissue Engineering Applications. *Journal of Polytechnic, 0900*(1), 221–227. https://doi.org/10.2339/politeknik.389596.

Han, L., Xu, J., Lu, X., Gan, D., Wang, Z., Wang, K., … Weng, J. (2017). Biohybrid methacrylated gelatin/polyacrylamide hydrogels for cartilage repair. *Journal of Materials Chemistry B, 5*(4), 731–741. https://doi.org/10.1039/c6tb02348g.

Han, Y., Jia, B., Lian, M., Sun, B., Wu, Q., Sun, B., … Dai, K. (2021). High-precision, gelatin-based, hybrid, bilayer scaffolds using melt electro-writing to repair cartilage injury. *Bioactive Materials, 6*(7), 2173–2186. https://doi.org/10.1016/j.bioactmat.2020.12.018.

Hangody, L., Feczkó, P., Bartha, L., Bodó, G., & Kish, G. (2001). Mosaicplasty for the treatment of articular defects of the knee and ankle. In *Clinical Orthopaedics and Related Research* (pp. S328–S336). https://doi.org/10.1097/00003086-200110001-00030.

Harrison, R. H., St-Pierre, J. P., & Stevens, M. M. (2014). Tissue engineering and regenerative medicine: A year in review. *Tissue Engineering - Part B: Reviews, 20*(1), 1–16. https://doi.org/10.1089/ten.teb.2013.0668.

He, M., Zhang, B., Dou, Y., Yin, G., Cui, Y., Chen, X., … Kim, H.-Y. (2017). Fabrication and characterization of electrospun feather keratin/poly(vinyl alcohol) composite nanofibers. *RSC Advances, 7*(16), 9854–9861. https://doi.org/10.1039/C6RA25009B.

Huang, J., Xiong, J., Wang, D., Zhang, J., Yang, L., Sun, S., & Liang, Y. (2021). 3D bioprinting of hydrogels for cartilage tissue engineering. *Gels, 7*(3), 1–15. https://doi.org/10.3390/gels7030144.

Huang, J., Xiong, J., Yang, L., Zhang, J., Sun, S., & Liang, Y. (2021). Cell-free exosome-laden scaffolds for tissue repair. *Nanoscale, 13*(19), 8740–8750. https://doi.org/10.1039/d1nr01314a.

Hurst, J. M., Steadman, J. R., O'Brien, L., Rodkey, W. G., & Briggs, K. K. (2010). Rehabilitation Following Microfracture for Chondral Injury in the Knee. *Clinics in Sports Medicine, 29*(2), 257–265. https://doi.org/10.1016/j.csm.2009.12.009.

Iber, B. T., Kasan, N. A., Torsabo, D., & Omuwa, J. W. (2022). A review of various sources of chitin and chitosan in nature. *Journal of Renewable Materials*, *10*(4), 1097–1123. https://doi.org/10.32604/JRM.2022.018142.

Jin, R., Moreira Teixeira, L. S., Dijkstra, P. J., Karperien, M., van Blitterswijk, C. A., Zhong, Z. Y., & Feijen, J. (2009). Injectable chitosan-based hydrogels for cartilage tissue engineering. *Biomaterials*, *30*(13), 2544–2551. https://doi.org/10.1016/j.biomaterials.2009.01.020.

Jung, C. K. (2014). Articular cartilage: Histology and physiology. In *Techniques in Cartilage Repair Surgery* (pp. 17–21). https://doi.org/10.1007/978-3-642-41921-8_2.

Kern, S., Eichler, H., Stoeve, J., Klüter, H., & Bieback, K. (2006). Comparative analysis of mesenchymal stem cells from bone marrow, umbilical cord blood, or adipose tissue. *Stem Cells*, *24*(5), 1294–1301. https://doi.org/10.1634/stemcells.2005-0342.

Kesti, M., Eberhardt, C., Pagliccia, G., Kenkel, D., Grande, D., Boss, A., & Zenobi-Wong, M. (2015). Bioprinting complex cartilaginous structures with clinically compliant biomaterials. *Advanced Functional Materials*, *25*(48), 7406–7417. https://doi.org/10.1002/adfm.201503423.

Kyle, S., Jessop, Z. M., Al-Sabah, A., & Whitaker, I. S. (2017). 'Printability" of candidate biomaterials for extrusion based 3D printing: State-of-the-art.' *Advanced Healthcare Materials*, *6*(16), 1–16. https://doi.org/10.1002/adhm.201700264.

Li, J., Wu, C., Chu, P. K., & Gelinsky, M. (2020). 3D printing of hydrogels: Rational design strategies and emerging biomedical applications. *Materials Science and Engineering R: Reports*, *140*(November 2019), 100543. https://doi.org/10.1016/j.mser.2020.100543.

Li, X., Liu, B., Pei, B., Chen, J., Zhou, D., Peng, J., … Xu, T. (2020). Inkjet bioprinting of biomaterials. *Chemical Reviews*, *120*(19), 10793–10833. https://doi.org/10.1021/acs.chemrev.0c00008.

Lin, W., Liu, Z., Kampf, N., & Klein, J. (2020). The role of hyaluronic acid in cartilage boundary lubrication. *Cells*, *9*(7), 1606. https://doi.org/10.3390/cells9071606.

Liu, M., Zeng, X., Ma, C., Yi, H., Ali, Z., Mou, X., … He, N. (2017). Injectable hydrogels for cartilage and bone tissue engineering. *Bone Research*, *5*(November 2016). https://doi.org/10.1038/boneres.2017.14.

Makris, E. A., Gomoll, A. H., Malizos, K. N., Hu, J. C., & Athanasiou, K. A. (2015). Repair and tissue engineering techniques for articular cartilage. *Nature Reviews Rheumatology*, *11*(1), 21–34. https://doi.org/10.1038/nrrheum.2014.157.

Mobaraki, M., Ghaffari, M., Yazdanpanah, A., Luo, Y., & Mills, D. K. (2020). Bioinks and bioprinting: A focused review. *Bioprinting*, *18*(January), e00080. https://doi.org/10.1016/j.bprint.2020.e00080.

Mohan, T., Maver, T., Štiglic, A. D., Stana-Kleinschek, K., & Kargl, R. (2018). 3D bioprinting of polysaccharides and their derivatives: From characterization to application. *Fundamental Biomaterials: Polymers*. https://doi.org/10.1016/B978-0-08-102194-1.00006-2.

Murphy, S. V., & Atala, A. (2014). 3D bioprinting of tissues and organs. *Nature Biotechnology*. https://doi.org/10.1038/nbt.2958.

Naghieh, S., Sarker, M. D., Sharma, N. K., Barhoumi, Z., & Chen, X. (2020). Printability of 3D printed hydrogel scaffolds: Influence of hydrogel composition and printing parameters. *Applied Sciences (Switzerland)*, *10*(1). https://doi.org/10.3390/app10010292.

Nikolova, M. P., & Chavali, M. S. (2019). Recent advances in biomaterials for 3D scaffolds: A review. *Bioactive Materials*, *4*(October), 271–292. https://doi.org/10.1016/j.bioactmat.2019.10.005.

Ning, L., & Chen, X. (2017). A brief review of extrusion-based tissue scaffold bio-printing. *Biotechnology Journal*, *12*(8), 1–16. https://doi.org/10.1002/biot.201600671.

Norotte, C., Marga, F. S., Niklason, L. E., & Forgacs, G. (2009). Scaffold-free vascular tissue engineering using bioprinting. *Biomaterials*, *30*(30), 5910–5917. https://doi.org/10.1016/j.biomaterials.2009.06.034.

Ozbolat, I. T., & Yu, Y. (2013). Bioprinting toward organ fabrication: Challenges and future trends. *IEEE Transactions on Biomedical Engineering*, *60*(3), 691–699. https://doi.org/10.1109/TBME.2013.2243912.

Papaioannou, T. G., Manolesou, D., Dimakakos, E., Tsoucalas, G., Vavuranakis, M., & Tousoulis, D. (2019). 3D bioprinting methods and techniques: Applications on artificial blood vessel fabrication. *Acta Cardiologica Sinica*, *35*(3), 284–289. https://doi.org/10.6515/ACS.201905_35(3).20181115A.

Park, J. Y., Choi, J. C., Shim, J. H., Lee, J. S., Park, H., Kim, S. W., … Cho, D. W. (2014). A comparative study on collagen type i and hyaluronic acid dependent cell behavior for osteochondral tissue bioprinting. *Biofabrication*, *6*(3). https://doi.org/10.1088/1758-5082/6/3/035004.

Poldervaart, M. T., Wang, H., Van Der Stok, J., Weinans, H., Leeuwenburgh, S. C. G., Oner, F. C., … Alblas, J. (2013). Sustained release of BMP-2 in bioprinted alginate for osteogenicity in mice and rats. *PLoS One*, *8*(8). https://doi.org/10.1371/journal.pone.0072610.

Prajapati, V. D., & Maheriya, P. M. (2019). Hyaluronic acid as potential carrier in biomedical and drug delivery applications. *Functional Polysaccharides for Biomedical Applications*. Elsevier Ltd. https://doi.org/10.1016/B978-0-08-102555-0.00007-8.

Ren, X., Wang, F., Chen, C., Gong, X., Yin, L., & Yang, L. (2016). Engineering zonal cartilage through bioprinting collagen type II hydrogel constructs with biomimetic chondrocyte density gradient. *BMC Musculoskeletal Disorders*, *17*(1), 1–10. https://doi.org/10.1186/s12891-016-1130-8.

Rey-Rico, A., Madry, H., & Cucchiarini, M. (2016). Hydrogel-based controlled delivery systems for articular cartilage repair. *BioMed Research International*, *2016*, 1–12. https://doi.org/10.1155/2016/1215263.

Roberts, J. J., Nicodemus, G. D., Greenwald, E. C., & Bryant, S. J. (2011). Degradation improves tissue formation in (Un)loaded chondrocyte-laden hydrogels. *Clinical Orthopaedics and Related Research*, *469*(10), 2725–2734. https://doi.org/10.1007/s11999-011-1823-0.

Sánchez-Téllez, D. A., Téllez-Jurado, L., & Rodríguez-Lorenzo, L. M. (2017). Hydrogels for cartilage regeneration, from polysaccharides to hybrids. *Polymers*, *9*(12), 1–32. https://doi.org/10.3390/polym9120671.

Schuurman, W., Khristov, V., Pot, M. W., Van Weeren, P. R., Dhert, W. J. A., & Malda, J. (2011). Bioprinting of hybrid tissue constructs with tailorable mechanical properties. *Biofabrication*, *3*(2). https://doi.org/10.1088/1758-5082/3/2/021001.

Scoutaris, N., Chai, F., Maurel, B., Sobocinski, J., Zhao, M., Moffat, J. G., … Douroumis, D. (2016). Development and biological evaluation of inkjet printed drug coatings on intravascular stent. *Molecular Pharmaceutics*, *13*(1), 125–133. https://doi.org/10.1021/acs.molpharmaceut.5b00570.

Sharma, B., Fermanian, S., Gibson, M., Unterman, S., Herzka, D. A., Cascio, B., … Elisseeff, J. H. (2013). Human cartilage repair with a photoreactive adhesive-hydrogel composite. *Science Translational Medicine*, *5*(167). https://doi.org/10.1126/scitranslmed.3004838.

Silvipriya, K. S., Krishna Kumar, K., Bhat, A. R., Dinesh Kumar, B., John, A., & Lakshmanan, P. (2015). Collagen: Animal sources and biomedical application. *Journal of Applied Pharmaceutical Science*, *5*(3), 123–127. https://doi.org/10.7324/JAPS.2015.50322.

Simionescu, B. C., & Ivanov, D. (2016). Natural and synthetic polymers for designing composite materials. In *Handbook of Bioceramics and Biocomposites* (pp. 233–286). https://doi.org/10.1007/978-3-319-12460-5_11.

Tran, H. D. N., Park, K. D., Ching, Y. C., Huynh, C., & Nguyen, D. H. (2020). A comprehensive review on polymeric hydrogel and its composite: Matrices of choice for bone and cartilage tissue engineering. *Journal of Industrial and Engineering Chemistry*, *89*, 58–82. https://doi.org/10.1016/j.jiec.2020.06.017.

Tzanakakis, G., Kovalszky, I., Heldin, P., & Nikitovic, D. (2014). Proteoglycans/glycosaminoglycans: From basic research to clinical practice. *BioMed Research International*. https://doi.org/10.1155/2014/295254.

Ventura, R. D. (2021). An overview of laser-assisted bioprinting (LAB) in tissue engineering applications. *Medical Lasers, 10*(2), 76–81. https://doi.org/10.25289/ml.2021.10.2.76.

Won, Y. W., Patel, A. N., & Bull, D. A. (2014). Cell surface engineering to enhance mesenchymal stem cell migration toward an SDF-1 gradient. *Biomaterials, 35*(21), 5627–5635. https://doi.org/10.1016/j.biomaterials.2014.03.070.

Xiongfa, J., Hao, Z., Liming, Z., & Jun, X. (2018). Recent advances in 3D bioprinting for the regeneration of functional cartilage. *Regenerative Medicine, 13*(1), 73–87. https://doi.org/10.2217/rme-2017-0106.

Xu, T., Binder, K. W., Albanna, M. Z., Dice, D., Zhao, W., Yoo, J. J., & Atala, A. 2012. Hybrid printing of mechanically and biologically improved constructs for cartilage tissue engineering applications. https://doi.org/10.1088/1758–5082/5/1/015001

Xu, T., Kincaid, H., Atala, A., & Yoo, J. J. (2008). High-throughput production of single-cell microparticles using an inkjet printing technology. *Journal of Manufacturing Science and Engineering, Transactions of the ASME, 130*(2), 0210171–0210175. https://doi.org/10.1115/1.2903064.

Yang, J., Zhang, Y. S., Yue, K., & Khademhosseini, A. (2017). Cell-laden hydrogels for osteochondral and cartilage tissue engineering. *Acta Biomaterialia, 57*, 1–25. https://doi.org/10.1016/j.actbio.2017.01.036.

Yang, W., Zhu, P., Huang, H., Zheng, Y., Liu, J., Feng, L., … Guo, R. (2019). Functionalization of novel theranostic hydrogels with kartogenin-grafted USPIO nanoparticles to enhance cartilage regeneration. *ACS Applied Materials and Interfaces, 11*(38), 34744–34754. https://doi.org/10.1021/acsami.9b12288.

Yang, X., Lu, Z., Wu, H., Li, W., Zheng, L., & Zhao, J. (2018). Collagen-alginate as bioink for three-dimensional (3D) cell printing based cartilage tissue engineering. *Materials Science and Engineering C, 83*(September), 195–201. https://doi.org/10.1016/j.msec.2017.09.002.

Zeng, L., Yao, Y., Wang, D. A., & Chen, X. (2014). Effect of microcavitary alginate hydrogel with different pore sizes on chondrocyte culture for cartilage tissue engineering. *Materials Science and Engineering C, 34*(1), 168–175. https://doi.org/10.1016/j.msec.2013.09.003.

Zhang, C., Wen, X., Vyavahare, N. R., & Boland, T. (2008). Synthesis and characterization of biodegradable elastomeric polyurethane scaffolds fabricated by the inkjet technique. *Biomaterials, 29*(28), 3781–3791. https://doi.org/10.1016/j.biomaterials.2008.06.009.

Zhang, W., Lian, Q., Li, D., Wang, K., Hao, D., Bian, W., … Jin, Z. (2014). Cartilage repair and subchondral bone migration using 3d printing osteochondral composites: A one-year-period study in rabbit trochlea. *BioMed Research International, 2014*. https://doi.org/10.1155/2014/746138.

Zhang, Y., Kumar, P., Lv, S., Xiong, D., Zhao, H., Cai, Z., & Zhao, X. (2021). Recent advances in 3D bioprinting of vascularized tissues. *Materials and Design, 199*, 109398. https://doi.org/10.1016/j.matdes.2020.109398.

3 Advances in 3D Hydrogel Matrix and Their Role in Neural Tissue Engineering

Sumeyye Cesur, Tuba Bedir, Nazmi Ekren, and Oguzhan Gunduz
Marmara University

Cem Bulent Ustundag
Yildiz Technical University

CONTENTS

3.1 Introduction 38
3.2 Neural Tissue Engineering 42
3.3 Hydrogels 43
3.3.1 Polymerization 43
3.3.2 Degradation 44
3.4 Hydrogels Used for Neural Tissue Engineering 44
3.4.1 Natural Hydrogels 46
3.4.1.1 Agarose 47
3.4.1.2 Alginate 47
3.4.1.3 Collagen 47
3.4.1.4 Chitosan 48
3.4.1.5 Fibrin 48
3.4.1.6 Matrigel 48
3.4.1.7 Methylcellulose 48
3.4.1.8 Xyloglucan 49
3.4.1.9 Hyaluronic Acid 49
3.4.2 Synthetic Hydrogels 49
3.4.2.1 Poly(Lactic Acid) and Poly(Lactic-Co-Glycolic Acid) 49
3.4.2.2 Poly(Ethylene Glycol) 50
3.4.2.3 Methacrylate-Based Hydrogels 50
3.4.3 Self-assembly Peptides 50
3.4.4 Conductive Polymers 51
3.4.4.1 Polypyrrole 51
3.4.4.2 Polyaniline 51
3.4.4.3 Poly(3,4-ethylenedioxythiophene) 52

DOI: 10.1201/9781003251767-3

3.5 Criteria for Hydrogel Design 52
3.5.1 Hydrogel Mechanical Properties 52
3.5.2 Hydrogel Physical Architecture 53
3.5.3 Electrically Conductive Hydrogels 54
3.5.4 Cell Encapsulation and Transplantation with Hydrogel 54
3.5.5 Biomimetic Modification of Hydrogel 55
3.5.6 Other Factors 56
3.5.7 Neurotrophic Factor Release from Hydrogel 56
3.5.8 Drug Release from Hydrogel 58
3.6 Effect of Hydrogels on the Behavior of Neural Stem Cells 59
3.6.1 Cell Viability 59
3.6.2 Cell Adhesion 59
3.6.3 Neurite Outgrowth 60
3.6.4 Cell Proliferation 60
3.6.5 Cell Differentiation 60
3.6.6 Cell Migration 61
3.7 3D Bioprinting of Hydrogels 61
3.8 Conclusions and Future Aspects 61
References 62

3.1 INTRODUCTION

The nervous system is a network of neurons that generates and transmits information between different parts of the human body. The human nervous system is one of the most complex biological structures to emerge during development. When the system is damaged, the body's motor and sensory functions are affected (Ai et al., 2013). The nervous system is divided into two main parts: the central and peripheral nervous systems (Figure 3.1a).

The central nervous system (CNS) is the body's command center and includes the brain and spinal cord (Schmidt & Leach, 2003). The CNS, together with the peripheral system consisting of nerves and ganglia, forms the nervous system, which has an important function in body control. It receives necessary information from the senses, such as hearing, taste, smell, and touch, and sends commands to move the control glands and muscles. The CNS is affected by diseases that occur in disorders of the CNS. Disorders that occur here affect the spinal cord and brain. This can be caused by many different reasons, especially traumas and diseases (Wang et al., 2018). The PNS represents the conduit between the body and the CNS. It comprises sensory nerve cell bodies, spinal nerves, and cranial nerves (Noback et al., 2005). Peripheral nerves transmit neural messages from the sensory organs and sensory receptors in the organism to the CNS. It also transmits neural messages outward from the CNS to the glands and muscles of the body. In addition, the PNS is functionally divided into two groups: the autonomic nervous system and the somatic nervous system. The autonomic nervous system is in charge of transmitting and processing sensory inputs from internal organs, including the digestive, cardiovascular, and respiratory systems. The somatic nervous system comprises the nervous constructions of the CNS and PNS, which are in charge of the processing and transmission

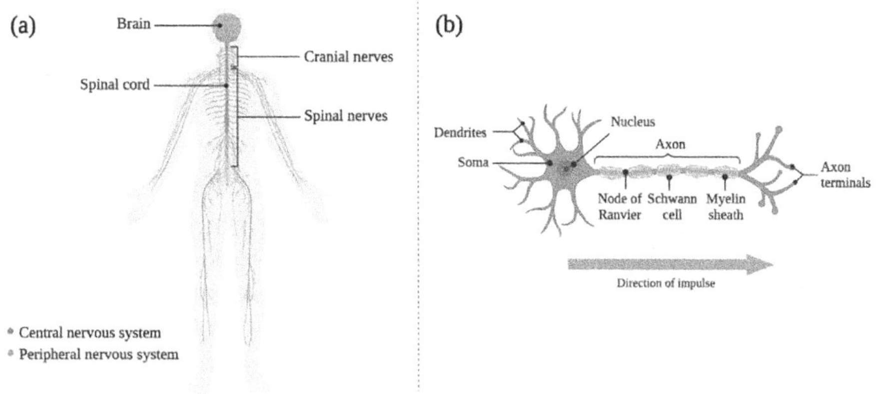

FIGURE 3.1 The important parts of the nervous system (a) and anatomy of the neuron (b).

of sensory information (conscious and unconscious), pain, vision, and unconscious muscle sensation through the body wall (Noback et al., 2005). The nervous system is composed of two cell types. These are neurons and glial cells. Millions of neurons or nerve cells and many glial cells are confined to the functional and structural tissue that is the brain, and they display a variety of forms and sizes (Figure 3.1b) (Schmidt & Leach, 2003). Neurons are the primary structural and functional units of the human nervous system. It is responsible for initiating, processing, and transmitting information (Noback et al., 2005). In addition, their function is influenced by their interaction with glial cells, which shapes the development and survival of synaptic connections and the activity of neuronal systems. Neurons consist of a cell body (soma) and its extensions, axon, and dendrites. Clusters of sensory nerve soma are found just outside the spine. Each neuron has an important process called an axon. Each axon, including its lateral branches, is usually made up of thin fibers, and each fiber is part of a synaptic connection. The other part of the neuron has dendrites. The dendrites transmit the electrical impulse from the nerve cells to the cell body, and the axon carries the impulses away. When examining nervous tissue, there are regions consisting mostly of axons and regions containing predominantly cell bodies. These two regions are often referred to as white matter (areas containing many axons) or gray matter (areas containing many dendrites and cell bodies). Glial cells, also called glia or neuroglia, are non-stimulatory, smaller cells that help neurons function. They supply structural support, nutrition, and protection for neurons. They maintain homeostatic balance and myelinated neurons (Clements et al., 2013). These functions are provided by different glial cell types. These are support cells that include microglia, oligodendrocytes, and astrocytes in the CNS and Schwann cells in the PNS. Microglia are cells called tissue macrophages of the CNS that function as representatives of the immune system in the brain. In the healthy brain, they appear in a long and elaborately branched form with multiple branches and a small cell body. Microglia degrade and clean dead cells and protect the brain from invading microorganisms (Helmut et al., 2011). Astrocytes interact with both neurons and capillaries in the CNS (Butt & Verkhratsky, 2018). Oligodendrocytes form myelin sheaths around axons in the CNS. An axon can be myelinated by a number of oligodendrocytes, and an oligodendrocyte can provide myelin for more than one neuron. This is different from PNS. Because the entire Schwann cell surrounds the axon, a single Schwann cell can provide myelin for only one axon. PNS glia consists of Schwann cells and major neuroglial cells surrounding the neuron axon. Myelin in the PNS is produced by Schwann cells. Schwann cells secrete large amounts of extracellular matrix (ECM) components. Also, Schwann cells, unlike oligodendrocytes, react violently to damage, as do astrocytes (Hof et al., 2013).

Nerve injuries can affect both the CNS and the PNS (Doblado et al., 2021). Acute traumatic injuries of the nervous system and chronic degenerative diseases lead to loss of CNS and PNS function. Injury to the CNS is one of the leading causes of permanent cognitive impairment and global death. Disturbances in the CNS resulting from neurological disorders or physical injuries often result in loss of glial support, axons, and neuronal cell bodies (Zhu et al., 2015). Physical injuries include spinal cord injuries (SCI) and traumatic brain injuries (TBI). These are not uncommon situations. Neurological disorders such as Alzheimer's disease, cerebral palsy, Parkinson's disease (PD), and multiple sclerosis are also common (Li et al., 2012). Mechanical forces related to rapid deformation of the spinal cord or brain during trauma cause axon damage (Siddique & Thakor, 2014). An SCI is a dramatic injury that is irreversible. It breaks the nerve connections between the brain and other parts of the body. In more serious cases than injury, it causes paralysis and loss of sensation. Trauma from falls can occur in a variety of ways, including car crashes, violence, and post-sport injuries (Qian et al., 2005). TBI caused by external physical exertion are injuries that cause cognitive and physical impairments. With these injuries, destruction of nerve fibers, contusions of brain tissue, brain stem injuries, and brain edema occur. TBI is mostly seen due to work accidents, traffic accidents, and falls. Headache, loss of consciousness, nausea, and cognitive effects, as well as depression and emotional and behavioral changes, are common (Hirsh et al., 2011). Neurological disorders are also common. Neurodegenerative diseases like PD, Alzheimer's disease, amyotrophic lateral sclerosis, and prion disease are serious health problems that result in cell loss in certain parts of the brain. These diseases are sneaky and progressive disorders, and their incidence is increasing day by day (Checkoway et al., 2011). PNS injury is a common worldwide clinical issue that severely affects the patient's quality of life (Gu et al., 2014). Forced traction (accidents), falls, gunshot wounds, strain injection injuries (especially the sciatic nerve is affected), ischemia (tight bandage or plaster cast), thermal injury, and metabolic diseases are among the causes of peripheral nerve injuries (Diogo et al., 2017). Due to nerve injuries, excruciating neuropathic pain develops and is so severe that it paralyzes the affected limb. It affects the patient's quality of life due to motor and sensory dysfunctions (Boni et al., 2018).

In peripheral nerves, axonal integrity is important for the propagation of the action potential across nerve cell membranes. Damage to any region along the axon's course can block nerve conduction. Myelin is also important in the transmission of the stimulus along the axon and increases the nerve conduction velocity between the myelin parts of the stimulus by jumping from one node to the other. Demyelination causes a slowdown in nerve conduction velocity by disrupting the jumping conduction. It also stops the propagation of the action potential, causing a message block.

After peripheral nerve damage due to any reason, degeneration is seen both proximally and distally to the site of the lesion.

Peripheral nerve fiber degeneration is examined in three groups:

1. Wallerian degeneration: It is the damage that occurs as a result of damage to the axon anywhere below the cell body due to various reasons and the deterioration of its integrity. There is degeneration of the distal axon and myelin sheath. The development of Wallerian degeneration can range from 4 to 21 days.
2. Axonal degeneration: It is nerve cell body and axon damage that usually develops due to metabolic and toxic causes. The first symptoms appear in the hands and feet. This condition may gradually spread proximally.
3. Segmental demyelination: Damage to Schwann cells and myelin sheath without any damage to the axon. Demyelination may occur along the entire nerve (Boni et al., 2018).

Present therapeutic attempts at CNS and PNS regeneration and repair are limited. Being able to unravel the various mechanisms for CNS and PNS injury is important for developing new therapeutic solutions (Kouyoumdjian et al., 2017). There is no clinical treatment method that will repair the CNS damage. Current treatment modalities are not sufficient to restore nerve function in the CNS. Current medical management focuses on orthopedic fixation of an unstable spine, injury prevention, rehabilitation, and the preparation of prostheses. Current treatments for spinal cord regeneration and repair are less promising. One of the treatments for SCI is the administration of the anti-inflammatory drug methylprednisolone, as acute injury occurs very quickly after the initial injury (McDonald, 1999). It is used to reduce secondary damage processes and swelling. However, this treatment causes many side effects, such as acute corticosteroid myopathy, sepsis, pneumonia, wound infection, and gastric bleeding (FitzGerald & Fawcett, 2007). Other treatments for SCI include surgery to stabilize hypothermia, rehabilitation care, and multisystem medical therapy. Many clinical treatments have improved. However, therapeutics have not made much progress in the good bridging of injured nerve spaces and the full recovery of nerve function (Liu et al., 2019). The PNS can regenerate after injury (Griffith & Naughton, 2002). PNS damage causes a significant nerve gap in which neuroraphnia (suturing of nerve stumps) is impossible. In this case, it is necessary to close the gap and support axonal regrowth by placing some kind of graft between the nerve stumps. Implantation of an autologous nerve graft, which is a functionally less important nerve segment, is considered the gold standard treatment for peripheral nerve space repair (Gu et al., 2014). However, there are inherent disadvantages to autologous nerve grafting, such as functional decline at the donor site, limited availability of nerve grafts, the need for a second surgery, and a size mismatch between donor and recipient nerves. Alternatively, allografts and xenografts are used to replace autologous nerve grafts (Vindigni et al., 2009). However, with these treatments, patients are at risk of immune- and disease-related complications (Gu et al., 2014). New neural tissue engineering strategies need to be developed as potential treatments for the clinical translation of CNS and PNS injuries due to the inadequacy of current treatments (Boni et al., 2018).

3.2 NEURAL TISSUE ENGINEERING

Neural tissue engineering aims to develop new treatment approaches for tissue damage caused by ischemia, degenerative conditions, and traumatic injuries (Joung et al., 2020). The goal of neural tissue engineering is to improve artificial biological surroundings suitable for neural tissue enlargement. Neural tissue strategies occur in a few multifaceted ways. These aim to improve three-dimensional (3D) living neural tissue that can promote neural regeneration, replace diseased or damaged neural ingredients, and repair function. Strategies in neural tissue engineering include contributions to the development of functional neural tissue from both neurons and glial cells. Also, the loss of neuronal regenerative potential during embryological development coincides with the improvement of glial cells. This emphasizes the effect of cells on the structure of the nervous system (Madhusudanan et al., 2017). Therefore, it is important to consider the neuronal and non-neuronal factors that support the extraneural matrix when planning and improving optimal tissue mimetic status for neural tissue engineering. Neural tissue engineering uses neurotrophic factors, cellular components, and biomaterials to ease neuronal regeneration and differentiation (Madhusudanan et al., 2020). Given the complex nature of the nervous system, tissue engineering strategies for successful nerve regeneration are classified as follows. These are (i) the biodegradability of the scaffold to be controlled by the body while tissue repair is taking place; (ii) biocompatibility as it promotes cell attachment, proliferation, migration, and differentiation (O'Brien, 2011); (iii) the electrical conductivity of the tissue supporting matrix; (iv) the scaffold should exhibit mechanical characteristics that resemble the neural tissue ECM (Cunha et al., 2011); and (v) contain morphological and biochemical cues for effective nerve regeneration (Bedir et al., 2020). In previous studies, these components have been used in combination or separately to support the regeneration of neurons. Among the various biomaterials, hydrogels ensure ease and flexibility in modifying the material properties to comply with neural regenerative needs (Madhusudanan et al., 2020) (Figure 3.2.).

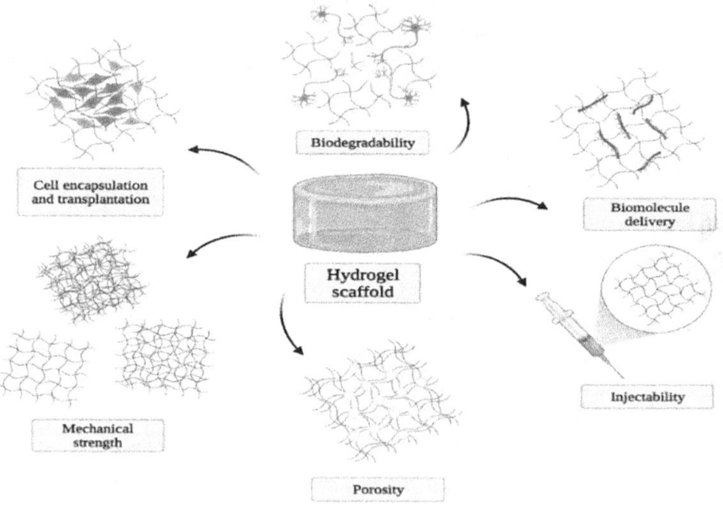

FIGURE 3.2 Schematic representation of hydrogel scaffold design criteria for neural tissue engineering.

3.3 HYDROGELS

3.3.1 POLYMERIZATION

Hydrogels are 3D hydrophilic polymer meshes with high water content in their construction (Hoffman, 2012). The chemical process by which monomers react to create a structure made of polymers is called polymerization (Aurand et al., 2012). The incorporation of water occurs throughout the gelation operation, in which a fluid polymer solution converts into a gel form by polymerizing monomers. Gelation includes the formation of covalent bonds, called crosslinks, in response to different stimuli (Carballo-Molina & Velasco, 2015). The most basic type of crosslinking happens when an amino group and an aldehyde combine to create a Schiff base, wherein dialdehyde crosslinkers like glutaraldehyde and glyoxal are utilized (Wang et al., 2004a). The binding of biofunctional molecules into hydrogels is also facilitated by crosslinking molecules. For instance, a hydrogel for neural stem cell (NSC) encapsulation has been created using a four-arm PEG tetraazide crosslinker coupled with laminin and a neurogenic factor (Li et al., 2018). Another approach is that enzymes like peroxidase and transglutaminase catalyze crosslinking reactions between polymer chains, resulting in enzymatic crosslinking. This method has been utilized to create hydrogels that are non-toxic, stable, and gel quickly (George et al., 2020). It has been indicated that transglutaminase-crosslinked HA hydrogel promotes rapid neurite development along with the creation of functional synapses and electrical connections between neurons (Broguiere et al., 2016). The critical control of the final crosslink density is achieved by covalent crosslinks. The mechanical characteristics, functionality, and rate of degradation of the hydrogel can be changed by the crosslink density (Lee & Mooney, 2001). The enhancement in the functional groups' density-like polyesters, thiols, or acrylates on the backbone of the monomer, will cause an increment in the number of crosslinks in the hydrogel and a tightening of the average network structure. Apart from chemical crosslinking, hydrogels can be created by the physical combination of constituents via hydrogen bonding at the molecular level (Lee & Mooney, 2001).

Stimuli such as pH (Chiu et al., 2009), temperature (Tate et al., 2001), ionic concentration (Nagai et al., 2006), or exposure to ultraviolet (UV) light (Chatterjee et al., 2010) affect the polymerization of hydrogels. Physical crosslinking generally takes place during pH- and temperature-dependent polymerization (Farmer et al., 2008). A variety of pH- and temperature-dependent hydrogels have been designed that can gel under the physiological conditions required for in situ polymerizations (Carballo-Molina & Velasco, 2015). In the in situ polymerization process, the unpolymerized hydrogel solution syringed into the damaged tissue polymerizes in reaction to the temperature of the body or pH difference (Nguyen & Lee, 2010). Thus, an irregularly shaped damaged area can easily be filled with hydrogel and take the shape of the recipient tissue. This process is especially effective in promoting regeneration by filling the heterogeneous defects that occur in some nervous system injuries (Macaya & Spector, 2012). Physical crosslinking has been extensively used to encourage the attachment and differentiation of neural cells, neurite extension, and the development of synaptic connections (George et al., 2020). Regarding the physical crosslinkability of hydrogels via ionic interactions, in one study, sodium alginate carboxylate groups and amino groups dispersed throughout chitosan chains were connected via ionic interactions, and the hydrogels encouraged the expansion of NSCs and olfactory coat cells (Wang et al., 2017). Photopolymerization is a quick bond-creation process that occrus when subjected to white or UV light. Polymerization of the hydrogel is achieved by adding a photoinitiator to produce reactive species, which induce the process of polymerization. However, the formation of reactive species and exposure to UV can be a problem, particularly where cells are to be added to the hydrogel, as these can cause reduced cell viability (Aurand et al., 2012). It has also been discovered that non-toxic photo-crosslinked chitosan-based hydrogels with low storage moduli that mimic soft CNS surroundings promote neurite outgrowth and the differentiation of neurons (Valmikinathan et al., 2012).

3.3.2 Degradation

Hydrogel degradation is caused by the cleavage of covalent bonds formed during polymerization. The cleavage of these bonds can be hydrolytic or enzymatic (Patterson & Hubbell, 2010). Due to the presence of high water in hydrogels subjected to *in vitro* conditions, the bond degradation is caused by hydrolysis; on the contrary, it has been shown that the main reason for the degradation of hydrogels under *in vivo* conditions is enzymatic activity (Patterson & Hubbell, 2010).

Hydrogels can be degraded through bulk or surface erosion (von Burkersroda et al., 2002). Factors such as the reach of enzymes or water into the hydrogel, the crosslink density, and the addition of degradable units determine the type of degradation. In cases where enzymes and water cannot diffuse the hydrogel due to the high crosslink density, degradation begins at the surface, and this is called surface degradation. On the other hand, the degradation that happens homogeneously in the hydrogel and is caused by the simultaneous division of the inner and outer bonds is called bulk erosion. This type of degradation is more common in hydrogels due to their rapid diffusion and high water content. It is more probable to occur, especially in hydrogels with lower crosslink density (Carballo-Molina & Velasco, 2015). The degradation rate is an important parameter in hydrogel design, both in terms of hydrogel function and host response. A slower degradation scaffold allows cells to develop their ECM and reintegrate into the host tissue. On the other hand, a rapidly degrading hydrogel helps reduce the host immune response *in vivo* (Subramanian et al., 2009).

3.4 HYDROGELS USED FOR NEURAL TISSUE ENGINEERING

Hydrogels are water-insoluble, 3D, highly hydrated polymeric materials held together by physical and/or chemical crosslinks. Physical gels are composed of molecular entanglement or secondary forces. Because physical gels are reversible, they are affected by changing conditions such as pH or temperature. Chemical gels are obtained by crosslinking polymers. There are methods for developing chemical hydrogels. The first is the direct crosslinking of water-soluble polymers without any purification procedures. The second is the polymerization of a hydrophilic monomer, called polymerization, with a crosslinking agent and then purification (Caló & Khutoryanskiy, 2015; Murphy et al., 2017). Hydrogels are porous materials with a high water content and a soft consistency. Because of these properties, they let them carry nutrients, oxygen, and soluble factors to better simulate living tissues than other biomaterials (Bordoni et al., 2020). Hydrogels have many benefits over other scaffolding materials, like low interfacial tensions, high nutrient, and oxygen permeability. Minimizes barriers to cells advancing from soft tissue to the scaffold and migrating from the scaffold to the outside of the material (Jayakumar et al., 2020). Hydrogels used in neural tissue engineering are morphologically macroporous. If the morphology of the hydrogel is degraded, it becomes macroporous to allow for neurite outgrowth. Hydrogels are mechanically similar. Flexibility can also be adjusted by controlling the hydrogels' crosslink density. Furthermore, many hydrogels offer numerous benefits, including the capacity to functionalize neural tissues for the control of proliferation, axonal extension, and neuronal cell adhesion (Nisbet et al., 2008).

The hierarchy of hydrogel structures can be classified according to different patterning levels, such as multiphase structure, single-phase alignment, and multiaxis patterning. To more accurately mimic brain tissue structure, the hydrogel construction can be altered to take the shape of a granular structure. In this multiphase construction, cells are seeded into a second phase that is rich in ECM and encircles hydrogel granules (George et al., 2020). When squeezed, granular hydrogels easily fluidize, a characteristic accepted as shear thinning (Mealy et al., 2018). This makes these systems easier to inject. Besides, fluidized hydrogel granules and cells can be blended uniformly. Having a granular construction eliminates the impact of settling after mixing. Additionally, the granules serve as a barrier that maintains cell viability throughout delivery. Also, it has been discovered that granular scaffolds stimulate the infiltration of cells and encourage vascularization *in vivo* (George et al., 2020). Anisotropic hydrogels with particles aligned along a single axis are intriguing for utilization in treatments that improve the bridging between injured parts of the CNS as well as in the creation of more accurate models of the CNS. This level of organization can be attained by aligning natural fibrous polymers, like collagen type I, where cell contact with collagen fiber bundles directs cell growth in the alignment-promoting direction (O'Rourke et al., 2017). Multiaxis patterned tissue has been produced using a variety of methods that achieve patterning at various resolutions. One approach to accomplishing this is to accumulate a pattern in the form of a basic tissue structure that is seeded layer by layer (Zhang et al., 2016). Among the techniques used, with a typical feature of 100–200 μm resolution, 3D bioprinting approaches allow quick prototyping of fully patterned hydrogel structures that can be utilized to surround and spatially arrange cells (Knowlton et al., 2018).

Hydrogels can be classified as either of natural origin or synthetic (Table 3.1.) (Perale et al., 2011). Polymers of natural origin provide properties very similar to those of living tissues, such as stimulating the cellular response. Due to its similarities with the ECM, it can also decrease the induction of immunological reactions or chronic inflammations and toxicity, which often occur thanks to synthetic polymers (Tabata, 2009). Synthetic polymers can be adjusted for degradation rate, composition, and chemical and mechanical properties (Shoichet, 2010). These different reasons make natural and synthetic biomaterials attractive for improving CNS repair and tissue regeneration: (i) porous construction allows transplantation of the cells, axon extension, and infiltration (Nisbet et al., 2008); (ii) capability to include adhesion into the hydrogel to improve tissue growth and cell attachment

TABLE 3.1
Hydrogels Used in Neural Tissue Engineering

Hydrogel Type	Origin	Characteristics	Disadvantages	References
Collagen	Natural	Biodegradable Non-cytotoxic Highly biocompatible Propes cell proliferation	Lower mechanical properties	Lee et al. (2001)
Matrigel	Natural	Biodegradable Alterable modulus properties Encourages neurite outgrowth Thermosensitive gelation	High mass changeability	Salaris et al. (2019), Zhu et al. (2019)
Poly(ethylene glycol) (PEG)	Synthetic	Biocompatible Non-cytotoxic Neuroprotective Neuro-protective Reduces cell death	Non-biodegradable Poorly adherent to protein and cells	Bjugstad et al. (2010), Laverty et al. (2004a)
Polyurethane (PU)	Synthetic	Biocompatible Biodegradable High water ingredient Elastic features Hydrogel combination probable Temperature-susceptible crosslinker	Unknown neural network compatibility	Ho and Hsu (2018), Xu and Guan (2016)
Poly(hydroxethy lmethacrylate) (pHEMA)/ Co-methylmetahcrylate (pHEMA-MMA)	Synthetic	Superior biocompatible Hydrophilic Soft and permeable High oxygen permeability	Lower biodegradable	Barui (2018), Zare et al. (2021)

(Hynd et al., 2007); (iii) the ability to include gene/drug vectors and deliver them precisely in situ (Chung & Park, 2007); and (iv) tissue-like mechanical abilities, convenient to the CNS tissue (Hejcl et al., 2008). Based on their use in SCI and repair, hydrogels are classified as natural, synthetic, and peptide hydrogels.

3.4.1 Natural Hydrogels

Natural-based hydrogels are materials with certain properties that seem to be in the ECM for neural tissue repair or are recognized by cells and are more commonly used in SCI repair (Little et al., 2008). Because these hydrogels are derived from natural sources, heterogeneity between groups can be observed and may induce immune effects in the patient to whom they are to be transplanted. Among these natural hydrogels, agarose, hyaluronic acid (HA), alginate, chitosan, collagen, matrigel, fibrin, methylcellulose, and xyloglucan will be mentioned (Assunção-Silva et al., 2015).

3.4.1.1 Agarose

Agarose obtained from red algae is in the polysaccharide group (Nisbet et al., 2008). It has mechanical properties that mimic natural tissue. Because of its porous structure, it is highly preferred in drug delivery systems (Jain et al., 2006). It is generally biocompatible with many cell types, enabling it to be used in 3D cell cultures (Stokols & Tuszynski, 2004). In addition, agarose can be used to direct neurite outgrowth and cell adhesion *in vitro* (Luo & Shoichet, 2004). In neural tissue engineering, agarose has been used with optimized gel properties such as porosity, biocompatibility, and stiffness (Stokols & Tuszynski, 2006). Bellamkonda et al. optimized a 1% w/v agarose concentration for neurite outgrowth in their study. In this prepared hydrogel, chick dorsal root ganglia (DRG) and PC12 cells were cultured for 4 days. As a result, it produced neurites on average 900 m long and 3D (Nakamoto et al., 2004). Agarose gels are preferred in gene delivery systems because they slow the release of compressed, bioactive DNA (Meilander et al., 2003). Agarose gels are particularly preferred for CNS-related diseases. This is because it can polymerize in situ to adapt to the shape of the lesion formed in the area and fill in different types of neurological defects (Jain et al., 2006).

3.4.1.2 Alginate

Alginate is a linear, anionic polysaccharide derived from the cell wall of brown algae (Rowe et al., 2009). It has been used in tissue engineering applications, for transplantation and encapsulation of the cells (Cesur, Oktar, et al., 2020). A gel is formed as a result of the interaction between divalent cations (Coviello et al., 2006). Gelation may also rely on the presence of a physical network as a result of intermolecular hydrophobic interactions between the alkyl bonds attached to the alginate (Assunção-Silva et al., 2015). In the study, Schwann cells were seeded on alginate gels. While stimulating neurite outgrowth from DRG cells within the scaffold, these cells remained alive (Mosahebi et al., 2001). As a result, alginate gels have been utilized to carry Schwann cells to a nerve-routing channel (Mosahebi et al., 2002). Besides, alginate hydrogels have also been utilized to fill gaps resulting from SCI owing to their properties like biocompatibility, low toxicity, biodegradability, and hydrophilicity (Freier et al., 2005). Diverse growth factors, like vascular endothelial growth factor (VEGF), were delivered using alginate hydrogels in *in vivo* models. Mechanical tension was applied to the hydrogel. VEGF released in excess from the hydrogels allowed for enhanced neovascularization (Lee et al., 2000).

3.4.1.3 Collagen

Collagen is the major protein in the human body, present at approximately 30% (Li et al., 2012). There are many types of collagen, and type I is the most widespread (Lee et al., 2001). Type I collagen comprises triple helices that form a fibrillar structure. The self-assembly and many important properties of type I collagen make it important for the utilization of hydrogels in the regeneration of neural tissue (O'Connor et al., 2000). A gel can be formed by changing the pH of the collagen solution (Salgado et al., 2008). Collagen-derived materials are biodegradable, non-cytotoxic, and highly biocompatible. These materials support cellular growth. Therefore, collagen is used in many applications in clinics, such as healing wound dressings, burns, tissue defects, and nerve regeneration (Lee et al., 2001). The mechanical behavior of hydrogels also affects neural function (Sundararaghavan et al., 2009). Because the mechanical behavior of collagen *in vivo* can be variable, some disadvantages, such as an antigenic response, arise if interspecies transplantation is used (Lynn et al., 2004).

3.4.1.4 Chitosan

Chitosan is an inherent polymer generated with chitin and alkalinity. Chitin is the structural polysaccharide found in many shellfish and crab shells (Chenite et al., 2000). Chitosan is biodegraded via lysozyme. With high deacetylation, there is a decrease in the rate of degradation due to the lysozyme acting on the acetylated groups (Yu et al., 2007). Chitosan does not need any additives to form a self-gel (Croisier & Jérôme, 2013). Gel formation can occur via hydrophobic interactions, hydrogen bonds, and chitosan crystallites (Chenite et al., 2000). Chitosan, which has a polycationic structure in an acidic environment, can interact with negatively charged molecules to form hydrogels (Shu & Zhu, 2002). Also, covalent bonds can be formed with metal ions to form chitosan hydrogels. These gels are not very suitable for biomedical use (Brack et al., 1997). Finally, chitosan gelation is achieved through the covalent bond between the polymer chains. Chitosan promotes growth in the culture of neurons, Schwann cells, and glia (Yuan et al., 2004). Chitosan has been used to treat spinal cord injuries and heal the sciatic nerve in dogs and rodents, according to research (Nisbet et al., 2008).

3.4.1.5 Fibrin

The fibrous protein called fibrin takes part in blood clotting. This protein is produced when it breaks down fibrinogen to form fibrin monomers during the coagulation cascade. These fibrin monomers then self-polymerize to form a 3D matrix (Mosesson, 2005). An important property of fibrin is that certain parameters such as polymerization rate and compliance can be controlled by changing the concentration of thrombin and fibrinogen. This feature allows for the formation of a solid scaffold *in vivo* while keeping the fibrin in a liquid state during injection (Sharp et al., 2012). Fibrin also has some disadvantages. Mammalian fibrin gels are easily degraded and immediately contaminated with prion proteins or blood-derived pathogens. In addition, autologous mammalian fibrinogen inhibits neurite outgrowth (Fischer et al., 2000).

3.4.1.6 Matrigel

Matrigel is a heat-sensitive, gelatinous blend excreted by mouse tumor cells. It is this protein mixture that liquefies at temperatures below 0°C and becomes solid at ambient temperatures and above. This material contains many growth factors like insulin-like growth factor-1 (IGF-1), (Fibroblast growth factor-2 FGF-2), and tissue plasminogen activator. Matrigel for CNS regeneration has multiple excellent properties (Novikova et al., 2006). Matrigel is widely utilized in both *in vitro* and *in vivo* studies. However, since it is developed from mouse tumor cells, it cannot be used in human applications (Li et al., 2012).

3.4.1.7 Methylcellulose

Cellulose is a water-insoluble, hydrophilic crystalline material. Methylcellulose is obtained by being modified with a hydrophobic side group, such as a hydrocarbon, which is water-soluble and allows heat-sensitive gelation (Desbrières et al., 2000). Methylcellulose is a cellulose-derived compound that forms a soft hydrogel at 37°C. This property enables it to be used as a biomaterial in tissue regeneration studies *in vivo* (Tate et al., 2001). When methylcellulose is injected into the damaged area of the brain, it causes a minor inflammatory response. However, it is not fully bioactive because it does not readily adsorb proteins. Adhesive molecules such as laminin need to bind to increase their bioactivity (Stabenfeldt et al., 2006).

3.4.1.8 Xyloglucan

Xyloglucan is a structural polysaccharide set in the cell wall of most herbs (Nisbet et al., 2006). To cause thermal gelation at physiological temperatures, it must have a removal rate greater than 35% and be modified with fungi-galactosidase. Removal of some of the galactose groups reduces the steric hindrance of xyloglucan (Nisbet et al., 2010). Thus, the polysaccharide chain forms hydrophobic junctions in the backbone and causes thermal gelation. The interplay of NSC cultures with the xyloglucan scaffold and the effects of xyloglucan in the controlled development of NSCs *in vitro* are also being investigated (Nisbet et al., 2008).

3.4.1.9 Hyaluronic Acid

HA is present in both the ECM and CNS of mesenchymal tissues. Like other natural biomaterials, it has a slow gelation rate and poor mechanical properties. Polyfunctional hydrazides control the chancing of the carboxylic acid groups of HA, and crosslinkable hydrogels can be produced (Prestwich et al., 1998). Subsequently, *in vivo* studies were applied. It was observed that the hydrogel inhibited the formation of the glial scar and promoted axonal extension and angiogenesis after implantation in the injured spinal cord (Hou et al., 2006).

3.4.2 Synthetic Hydrogels

Synthetic hydrogels have many prominent benefits over natural hydrogels, like designing and controlling the properties of the material and improving their biocompatibility and degradation rates. In addition, it reduces allergic risks by using an artificial biocompatible material that does not contain animal protein (Hejčl et al., 2009). Among these synthetic hydrogels, poly(lactic acid) (PLA) and poly(lactic-co-glycolic acid) (PLGA) hydrogels, poly(ethylene glycol) (PEG) hydrogels, and methacrylate-based hydrogels will be discussed.

3.4.2.1 Poly(Lactic Acid) and Poly(Lactic-Co-Glycolic Acid)

PLA/PLGA polymers are from the α-hydroxy acid class of compounds. It consists of biodegradable synthetic aliphatic polyesters (Nomura et al., 2006). To control the mechanical properties and degradation rate of these polymers, the ratio of monomer units and the molecular weight dispersion of their chains can be varied (Straley et al., 2010). PLGA and similar polymers are used in the renovation of the peripheric system of humans. The use of these polymers in CNS-related injuries is hopeful (Gautier et al., 1998). Micro- and nanoparticles of PLGA hydrogel as transport agents are utilized for applications in tissue engineering (Makadia & Siegel, 2011).

3.4.2.2 Poly(Ethylene Glycol)

Polyethylene glycol (PEG) is a hydrophilic, biocompatible, and poorly adherent polyether compound to proteins and cells (Cesur, Ulag, et al., 2020). PEG has been tested in neural tissue repair and has many properties, such as being neuroprotective. It helps reduce cell death and seal cell membranes after injury (Laverty et al., 2004). PEG hydrogels can be used as drug release vehicles due to crosslinking and can be modified to increase cell attachment (Burdick et al., 2006). Also, PEG has been found suitable for SCI studies. For treatment alone using PEG solutions, an *in vivo* model of SCI was used. The PEG solution could accelerate and improve the membrane reclosing process, enabling it to regain neuronal membrane integrity (Luo et al., 2002). In another study of SCI in dogs, PEG hydrology was used. It was observed that the use of PEG accelerated the treatment process in proportion to conventionally treated dogs (Laverty et al., 2004).

3.4.2.3 Methacrylate-Based Hydrogels

Methacrylate-based hydrogels can be adapted similarly to neural tissue. Poly(2-hydroxyethyl methacrylate and 2-hydroxyethyl methacrylate-co-methyl methacrylate) (pHEMA/pHEMA-MMA) is a synthetic polymer used generally in hydrogel form. It is frequently used because of its properties, such as being biocompatible, hydrophilic, soft, and permeable. Due to its structure, it contains water similar to living tissues (Fang et al., 2007). Like other synthetic hydrogels, their degradation rate is slow (Tsai et al., 2006). In addition, pHEMA synthesis is carried out without the use of toxic solvents and at low temperatures. Therefore, it is included in the polymer scaffold of bioactive compounds (Tsai et al., 2004). Poor cell adhesion to the hydrogel surface owing to its high hydrophilicity and low protein absorption make pHEMA-based hydrogels unsuitable for cell cultivation. But sticky protein-derived amino sugars have been modified with molecules such as collagen or oligopeptides. Thus, it greatly increased its *in vivo* and *in vitro* biocompatibility with neurons (Nisbet et al., 2008). pHEMA is highly preferred for spinal cord injuries. The pHEMA hydrogels increased axonal growth when placed in the injured spinal cord. pHEMA demonstrated good potential for neural restoration (Flynn et al., 2003).

Poly(hydroxypropyl methacrylate) (pHPMA) is a porous, non-toxic hydrogel that authorizes the transport of large and small molecules, enabling the immigration of blood vessels and cells (Woerly et al., 1999). This hydrogel is also more biocompatible than pHEMA and exhibits a resemblance to neural tissue due to its viscoelastic property (Woerly et al., 1998). The pHPMA hydrogel has been shown to aid the growth of tissue composed of axons, dendrites, blood vessels, glial cells, and ECM molecules like collagen and/or laminin (Woerly et al., 1999).

3.4.3 Self-Assembly Peptides

Self-assembly peptides (SAPs) combine to form nanostructures such as rods, sheets, and tubes. There may be amino acid sequences or monomers that allow the chemical functionality of the peptides to be presented on the surface of these structures

(Lee et al., 2019). Self-assembly of peptides is dependent on temperature, ionic strength, pH, or enzymatic triggers (Nisbet & Williams, 2012). In addition, amphiphilic molecules come together to form different nanofiber networks. SAPs also have advantages, such as being biocompatible and easy to synthesize (Silva et al., 2004). Hydrogels were formed by the self-assembly of oligopeptides, which Zhang et al. called PuraMatrix in one of the studies with SAPs. These hydrogels were found to promote both neuronal cell differentiation and attachment and neurite outgrowth (1995). In another work, Silva and colleagues improved a more complicated construction through the spontaneous assembly of peptide molecules. In addition to containing the neurite germination epitope IKVAV, the molecules also contained the Glu residue, three Gly residues, four Ala residues, and a 16-carbon alkyl tail. This encourages the self-assembly of the hydrogel through the formation of hydrogen bonds as well as unwanted contact between water molecules and hydrophobic segments (Tysseling-Mattiace et al., 2008).

3.4.4 Conductive Polymers

Conductive polymers (CPs), or backbones of polymers with slackly held electrons, are typically categorized as having both common polymeric properties and electrical characteristics resembling those of metals and semiconductors (Uz & Mallapragada, 2019). The atoms at the backbone of the material have weak bonds that allow for the delocalization and free mobility of electrons, which in turn causes the generation of electrical current through mobile charges (Le et al., 2017). Commonly used CPs are polypyrrole (PPy), polyaniline (PANI), and poly(3,4-ethylenedioxythiophene) (PEDOT) (Nezakati et al., 2018).

3.4.4.1 Polypyrrole

A conductive synthetic polymer with many uses in drug carriage and neural regeneration is polypyrrole (PPy). It has been applied to coverings for neural probes and biosensors (Sanghvi et al., 2005). The high degree of conjugation in PPy's molecular structure causes it to be extremely stiff, intractable, and difficult to process (Shi et al., 2004). According to Wang et al., PPy is an appropriate substrate for closing the peripheral nerve gap and is quite biocompatible with rat peripheral nerve tissue. They stated that there was no evidence of subacute or acute toxicity, pyretogens, hemolysis, allergies, or mutagenesis in the PPy extraction solution (2004b).

3.4.4.2 Polyaniline

PANI, also referred to as aniline black, is the oxidative polymeric byproduct of aniline under acidic circumstances. PANI can be developed in a variety of insulating forms, including the decreased leucoemeraldine base, the half-oxidized emeraldine base (PANI-emeraldine base), and the fully oxidized pernigraniline base, depending on the degree of oxidation. More proof that PANI and PANI variants can boost cell development has recently come to light (Ghasemi-Mobarakeh et al., 2011). After implanting PANI, Wang et al. looked into the *in vivo* tissue reaction and discovered no telltale signs of tissue incompatibility (Wang et al., 1999). The biocompatibility of PANI in various states was examined by Kamalesh et al. (2000), who discovered that these materials are sufficiently biocompatible to be utilized in biomedical applications.

3.4.4.3 Poly(3,4-ethylenedioxythiophene)

The most popular polythiophene derivative, poly(3,4-ethylenedioxythiophene) (PEDOT), is thought to have several unique features (Ghasemi-Mobarakeh et al., 2011). The biocompatibility of PEDOT with epithelial cells was demonstrated by Valle et al. after they examined how PEDOT films interacted with them (del Valle et al., 2007). By growing NIH3T3 fibroblasts on PEDOT films to test their biocompatibility, Luo et al. produced PEDOT films. They then implanted the films under the skin in an *in vivo* study. As a result of their findings, PEDOT films are excellent candidates for biosensing and bioengineering applications since they have good biocompatibility and an inflammatory response following implantation (Luo et al., 2008). Using the vapor phase polymerization technique, Bolin et al. created PET nanofibers that were electrospun and coated with PEDOT doped with tosylate. Their findings demonstrated outstanding neuronal cell attachment and proliferation on PEDOT-coated PET nanofibers (2009).

3.5 CRITERIA FOR HYDROGEL DESIGN

3.5.1 Hydrogel Mechanical Properties

Mechanical characteristics like elasticity and stiffness are critical design parameters to consider when forming a hydrogel. Because hydrogel's mechanical properties have a crucial role in the regulation of various cell behaviors (Discher et al., 2005). The genotype and phenotype of cells are directed by interactions between the ECM and cells and by biomechanical signals (Tibbitt & Anseth, 2009). Therefore, the design of a hydrogel with precise mechanical characteristics may influence the existence of hydrogel in the tissue or the function of the encapsulated cell (Bryant et al., 2004).

Controlling characteristics like tensile strength, compressive strength, Young's modulus (E), and failure strain determine hydrogel's elastic performance (Vedadghavami et al., 2017). Elasticity is the ability of a material to deform immediately when subjected to mechanical loading. The resistance of an elastic material to stress is defined as Young's modulus (McKee et al., 2011). Also, the intrinsic elasticity of viscoelastic materials can be determined by Young's modulus (McKee et al., 2014). The stress at the fracture point during hydrogel elongation is expressed as the tensile strength (N. et al., n.d.). Compressive strength is the capability to withstand induced loading to reduce the size (Hadryś et al., 2016). The resistance of the material to deformation when subjected to mechanical loading is described as stiffness (Pal, 2014). Various methods, such as changing the concentration of hydrogel monomers, macromers, or crosslinkers, as well as adding glycosaminoglycans involved in ECM stiffness and water absorption, are effective in modulating the elasticity of hydrogel and regulating cell behavior of the neurons (Zhou et al., 2016).

Changing the polymer content and crosslink density are factors that affect the mechanical properties of a hydrogel. The enhancement in hydrogel strength can be achieved by increasing both factors (Kong et al., 2003). Generally, softer hydrogels ideal for the brain and other soft tissues are formed with less crosslink density (Lampe et al., 2010), while stiffer hydrogels, which may be more appropriate for hard tissue applications such as bone, can produce a higher crosslink density (Moffat et al., 2008). From the point of view of neural cell types, astrocytes and oligodendrocytes desire to grow on stiffer substrates (0.5–10 kPa), while neurons prefer relatively softer surfaces (0.1–1.0 kPa) (Seidlits et al., 2010). In one study, soft substrates (0.1–0.8 kPa) resulted in an increment in neurite length in proportion to stiffer substrates (4.2–7.9 kPa) (Stukel & Willits, 2018), but neurite alignment was reported to increase with stiffness (Tuft et al., 2014).

3.5.2 Hydrogel Physical Architecture

The mesh size of the hydrogel is the distance between the crosslink points and is a physical property that contributes to hydrogel stiffness (Lin et al., 2011). It is a parameter that should be considered in the effective diffusion of nutrients and waste by cells encapsulated in the polymer matrix. Diffusion rates are also affected by the molecule's size and the hydrogel's mesh size; the larger the mesh size, the faster the diffusion or vice versa. The entry and exit of fluids and small molecules into the hydrogel are initially related to diffusion, while the degradation event is efficient following the actions of bigger molecules and cells (Bjugstad et al., 2010). Moreover, a change in the initial hydrogel composition can also result in a significant reduction in mesh size, which may prevent the ingrowth of cells in integration with the host tissue. Therefore, it may be necessary to cut many connections to supply sufficient space for cell development (Meyer et al., 2009). High uptake of water into the hydrogel can also cause an enhancement in mesh size and a consequent reduction in mechanical stability (Meyer et al., 2009). Therefore, hydrogels with appropriate mesh sizes should be designed so that larger molecules can diffuse easily and the encapsulated cells can perform their functions (Aurand et al., 2012).

The interconnected porous structure of hydrogels is crucial as it will affect nutrient and gas exchange as well as various cellular activities like cell growth, proliferation, and migration (Li et al., 2012). The porous structure can form naturally as a result of hydrogel chemistry or can be purposefully generated (Lin et al., 2011). Pores can be generated by making a complicated hydrogel with polymer areas that degrade at a quicker rate than the remainder of the hydrogel (Spiller et al., 2011). For instance, one group added an enzymatically degradable fibrin network within the PEG hydrogel, resulting in a structure of interconnected pores. They subsequently demonstrated that earlier process extension was obtained from primary neural cells encapsulated in the PEG hydrogel (Namba et al., 2009). There is a balance between macroporosity (10–400 μm) and mechanical strength. This situation could be eased by utilizing materials that have high mechanical strength by nature (Vedadghavami et al., 2017). Moreover, the characteristics and surface area of the macroporous walls can be changed by the microporous structure (2–50 μm). For example, microporosity promotes the cohesion of material when the surface interacts with the cells (Vedadghavami et al., 2017).

In addition, other features to consider are the shape and size of the hydrogel. For instance, to load an irregular-shaped lesion area, like a stroke cavity in the brain, the hydrogel can be placed in this area prior to polymerization, or a hydrogel with a very low compression modulus can be used (Emerich et al., 2010). Conversely, a thread-shaped hydrogel can be utilized as a bridge over a glial wound for the regeneration of SCI (Hejcl et al., 2008). In a hydrogel designed for brain damage, size has a significant effect. If the hydrogel has a large volume, it can adversely affect the brain by increasing the pressure on the tissue in which it is implanted. Moreover, swelling of a hydrogel causes a rise in the hydrogel's size during unconstrained hydrogel degradation. Swelling rates are defined in hydrogel studies to provide information about fluid and water uptake during the degradation of a hydrogel. Because the swelling ratio may be a necessary factor in explaining the rate of degradation (Aurand et al., 2012).

3.5.3 Electrically Conductive Hydrogels

Electrical stimulation of damaged brain tissue has been discovered to cause dramatic cellular alterations in terms of regeneration and restoration, according to research. Research has shown that a depolarizing current delivered close to damaged axons has a major impact on axonal sprouting and regeneration. This research used both *in vitro* and *in vivo* models (Goganau et al., 2018). It is amazing to note that the restoration of peripheral nerves and the spinal cord has been the primary focus of much research on the electrical stimulation of neural tissue. In the past, nerve grafts or artificial nerve conduits have been utilized to patch up gaps among injured neural tissue in SCI and peripheral nerve defect models (Arslantunali et al., 2014). Conducting hydrogels are systems that have been developed using a range of conducting materials to help the passage of ions through the supporting matrix. Understanding the character of the electrical interplay among tissues and exterior conducting materials is crucial at this point. While conventional electrical conductors like metallic electrodes only rely on mobile electrons, tissues require mobile ions as well. A current is sent to the tissue via faradic and capacitance charge transfer in response to the electrical stimulation of an electrode. While capacitance currents are produced at the electrode-tissue interface through straightforward charge separation, faradic currents are produced at the electrode-tissue contact through electrochemical processes (oxidation or reduction), which over time may be harmful to tissue. Conducting hydrogels provide a significant opportunity for material-neural interface since they have both mobile ions and electrons from conducting polymer chains, as well as increased volumetric capacitance (Peckham et al., 2013).

3.5.4 Cell Encapsulation and Transplantation with Hydrogel

Cell transplantation is a hopeful attempt at the restoration of nervous system illness, but it has limitations such as short-term cell viability, post-transplant-suited cell engraftment capability, and deficiency of cell fate control (Frisch & Francis, 1994). An effective approach to solving these problems is the use of hydrogels, which can form a private niche for cell encapsulation. In this way, hydrogels contribute to neuronal differentiation and tissue regeneration and can also decrease scarring and inflammation (Park et al., 2002). Cell transplantation with hydrogel necessitates attentive adjustment of the hydrogel microenvironment, inclusive of mechanical characteristics, cell receptor and ligand densities, and biomolecule addition (Straley et al., 2010). The natural sensitiveness of cells imposes restrictions on the choice of materials, as some chemical crosslinkers utilized to create hydrogel systems can impair the survivability of cells (Straley et al., 2010). Some natural and synthetic hydrogels have been utilized for cell encapsulation, and it has been discovered that the crosslinking degree and degradability of the hydrogel have a direct impact on the encapsulated cells (Nicodemus & Bryant, 2008). For instance, one group encapsulated fibroblast cells that secrete brain-derived neurotrophic factor (BDNF) into beads of alginate, placed them in the dorsolateral funiculus of the spinal cord, and achieved positive results. The transplanted hydrogel-cell complex induced limb motor strength improvement as well as neuritic sprouting in the damaged axons in the SCI rat model. However, there was no immunological reactivity toward the transplanted cells within the alginate beads (Tobias et al., 2005). Recently, one study has strongly indicated the use of hydrogels in the encapsulation and stimulation of progenitor cells of the nervous system to allow them to inherently differentiate into different types of cells. The researchers found that PEG hydrogel with 4-dibenzocyclooctinol (DIBO) functionalization eased the encapsulated NSCs differentiation into neurons (Li et al., 2018). This study suggested that a combination of factors such as cell encapsulation and trophic factor incorporation eased an increase in neuronal differentiation (Li et al., 2018). In addition, different origins of neural progenitor cells were also found to affect their behavior within hydrogel matrices. Evidence of this is that adult neural progenitor cells (NPCs) cultured in PEG and HA-based hydrogels demonstrated better differentiation potential as compared to neuronal progenitor cells of fetal origin (Aurand et al., 2014).

3.5.5 Biomimetic Modification of Hydrogel

Modification of many hydrogels has a significant role in promoting cell adhesion and growth in terms of neural tissue regeneration (Drotleff et al., 2004). Protein adsorption is suppressed owing to the highly hydrophilic nature of the hydrogel-forming polymers. While this is beneficial in applications where protein loss owing to adsorption is undesirable, such as controlled drug delivery, adsorbed proteins are needed for processes such as cell adhesion. If the hydrogels are not modified, the cell adhesion capacity will be very low. Therefore, hydrogels must include the corresponding receptor ligands for cell adhesion (Cui et al., 2006). In accordance with this purpose, functional peptide sequences derived from ECM proteins such as fibronectin, laminin, and collagen can be crosslinked to the hydrogel. These adhesion molecules induce the formation of focal adhesions by pioneering receptor-mediated cell adhesion (Meiners & Mercado, 2003). For example, laminin comprises three strands that present different binding sites for the receptor, and amino acid sequences that are certain, RGD, IKVAV, YIGSR, RYVVLPR, and RNIAIIIKDI, found in the binding sites of their chains are effective in cell-receptor interactions (Schense et al., 2000). Moreover, ligand selection and density are significant considerations regarding the binding of ECM domains to the hydrogel. For instance, NSC adhesion and neurite development are enhanced due to the increase in density of the RGD sequence (Gunn et al., 2005).

3.5.6 Other Factors

CNS tissue cells are sensitive to multiple signal gradients that cause cell differentiation and shape the final status of neurons and glial cells. The concentrations that make up the gradients are dynamic and spatially patterned. To maintain patterning gradients, CNS tissue needs to be compartmentalized. Culture models can be compartmentalized *in vitro* using microbioreactors, microfluidic devices, and lab-on-chip technologies (Cullen et al., 2007). With a high degree of dynamic and spatial control, microfluidic devices can be utilized to reproduce complicated *in vivo* gradient patterns. Microfluidics technology can be used to stimulate the spatial patterning of signaling elements in the neural tube (Uzel et al., 2016).

3.5.7 Neurotrophic Factor Release from Hydrogel

Apart from modulating mechanical properties and physical structure for neuronal regeneration, the incorporation of various biomolecules into the hydrogel matrix can provide a controlled release of these exogenous biomolecules (Madhusudanan et al., 2020). The delivery of biomolecules using hydrogels may offer a more favorable environment for endogenous cell regeneration. Neurotrophic factors are a class of biomolecules of interest in promoting neural tissue regeneration (Straley et al., 2010). Neuronal survival, synaptic plasticity, axonal growth, and neurotransmission can be encouraged by neurotrophic factors; therefore. they play important roles in stimulating and directing regenerative nerve growth (Jones et al., 2001). Neurotrophins such as nerve growth factor (NGF), brain-derived neurotrophic factor (BDNF), neurotrophin-3 (NT-3), neurotrophin 4/5 (NT-4/5), and glial cell line-derived growth factor (GDNF) are well-known neurotrophic factors (Deister & Schmidt, 2006; Jones et al., 2001). Some of the commonly targeted neurotrophic receptors in neural tissue engineering are p75 and tyrosine kinase receptors (Trk A, Trk B, and Trk C). Especially in the nervous system, BDNF and NGF demonstrate enhanced expression together with their receptors, while the expression of neurotrophic factors like NT-3 and Trk B is at a lower rate (Madhusudanan et al., 2020). Changes in neurotrophic factors and their receptor expression have seriously deleterious impacts on the regeneration of axons (Babensee et al., 2000). Moreover, axonal elongation is stimulated by neurotrophic factors in a chemotactic way, so these should be highly present in nervous system injuries (Murakami et al., 2002). Direct injection methods have limitations in the delivery of exogenous neurotrophic factors, such as the inability to localize these molecules to the wound region and the rapid degradation of molecules after injection (Blesch & Tuszynski, 2007). This problem can be avoided by co-administration of neurotrophic factors with hydrogels, ensuring prolonged and localized delivery. Moreover, combining the use of various neurotrophic factors has been proven to have synergistic effects (Deister & Schmidt, 2006). One group has demonstrated that PLA-PEG hydrogel formulations release NT-3 in such a way that the initial burst release is followed by a long-term release, contributing favorably to persistent neural growth (Burdick et al., 2006). Furthermore, such NT-3-containing hydrogels have been studied in the spinal cord lesion region *in vivo* studies and have demonstrated progress in axonal regeneration (Piantino et al., 2006).

Although the administration of neurotrophic factors promotes neural tissue repair through stimulation of neurite outgrowth, the intrusion environment created by the release of various inhibitory molecules into the damaged area poses a challenge (Straley et al., 2010). The glial scar is composed of connective tissue elements and astrocytes and is one of the greatest barriers to neuroregeneration. The regeneration stages are significantly influenced by molecules that act as inhibitors like chondroitin sulfate proteoglycans (CSPGs), tenascin, or ephrin-B2 (Madhusudanan et al., 2020). To inhibit or eliminate neural scar tissue's inherent resistance to the growth of axons, approaches have been devised in which therapeutics that deactivate these inhibitive agents are integrated into hydrogels to be released locally at the sites of the scar. Axonal growth in damaged nerve models has been shown to be alleviated by chondroitinase ABC (ChABC). ChABC, with poor thermal stability and high degradability, has been functionalized by applying various methods (Muir et al., 2017). For example, NT-3 and the thermally stabilized ChABC in agarose hydrogel have been found to advance the capacity of axonal regeneration and develop locomotor function in the SCI model (Lee et al., 2010a). Likewise, HA hydrogel was combined with an antibody against the Nogo receptor (NgR) and observed to increase hippocampal neuron growth *in vitro* (Wei et al., 2009) and encourage functional healing in a stroke model *in vivo* (Ma et al., 2007). Consequently, the combination of hydrogels with neurotrophic factors or other therapeutics may be a more effective approach in the treatment of nervous system injuries (Straley et al., 2010). Some hydrogels utilized to release therapeutic molecules in neural tissue engineering are mentioned in Table 3.2.

TABLE 3.2
Examples of Some Hydrogels for the Release of Therapeutic Molecules in Neural Tissue Engineering

Hydrogel	Cell Type	Neurotrophic Factor/Drug	*In vitro/ In vivo*	Results	References
Alginate	NPCs from mice embryos at day 14	BDNF or NT-3	*In vitro*	NPCs differentiated into oligodendrocytes in BDNF-containing hydrogel, whereas differentiation into neuronal fate observed in NT-3-containing hydrogel.	Shanbhag et al. (2010)
Heparin conjugated-fibrin	Dorsal root ganglia (DRGs) from chicken embryos at day 8	NT-3, NGF or BDNF	*In vitro*	Long-term release of neurotrophic factors and neurite outgrowth observed.	Sakiyama-Elbert and Hubbell (2000)

(*Continued*)

TABLE 3.2 (*Continued*)
Examples of Some Hydrogels for the Release of Therapeutic Molecules in Neural Tissue Engineering

Hydrogel	Cell Type	Neurotrophic Factor/Drug	*In vitro/ In vivo*	Results	References
Heparin conjugated-fibrin	-	NT-3	*In vivo* (Dorsal hemisection subacute SCI model)	Enhanced neural fiber density in the lesion and reduced reactive astrocyte dyeing around the lesion of subacute SCI.	Johnson et al. (2009)
Fibrin	DRGs from white leghorn chick embryos at day 10	GDNF	*In vitro*	Increased neurite extensions.	Wood et al. (2009)
Fibrin	-	NGF immobilized with heparin	*In vivo* (Sciatic nerve transection model)	A dose-dependent effect on axonal regeneration observed.	Lee et al. (2003)
Fibrin	-	NT-3	*In vivo* (SCI model)	Enhanced neuronal fiber sprouting and cell migration into the lesion but no functional motor recovery.	Taylor et al. (2006)

3.5.8 Drug Release from Hydrogel

Another strategy to enhance the efficacy of hydrogels includes their utilization as a combination of cell transporter and drug-releasing system. This is accomplished by including growth factors or special drugs in the hydrogel (Tabata, 2005). Also, these incorporated or released molecules can help binding cells grow and differentiate even further. Most delivered proteins or drug substances do not interact non-specifically with hydrogels; thus, hydrogels for such applications provide important advantages. This decreases the risk of denaturation while also allowing the easy spreading of the administered molecules to the cells or their target. Approaches such as the inclusion of soluble bioactive molecules in the polymer-solvent, the incorporation of protein-loaded microparticles for long-term delivery, or the covalent binding of growth factors to the hydrogel matrix constitute these combination systems (Holland et al., 2003, 2005).

Hydrogels in injectable form have been widely employed to release therapeutic molecules in various nervous system disorders. For example, a hydrogel composite of dopamine-loaded dextran dialdehyde and gelatin was administered to a dopamine-lacking rat model, resulting in improved motor function (Senthilkumar et al., 2007).

The therapeutic molecules' release from a hydrogel is not only affected by hydrogel properties such as mesh size and degradation but also depends on the therapeutic molecule itself. In this context, the release kinetics of the therapeutic molecule from a hydrogel are influenced by the molecule size and how the molecule is added to the hydrogel or microparticle, such as by binding or encapsulation. The easy diffusion of bigger molecules can be prohibited by a small mesh-size hydrogel, and therefore, it may be necessary to degrade the hydrogel before molecules can be released (Aurand et al., 2012). In addition, molecule polarity can be a factor influencing molecule release from a hydrogel. Hydrophilic drugs like ketoprofen, where the release rate is controlled by diffusion, have been shown to be more easily released from a hydrogel than hydrophobic drugs like spironolactone, whose release requires the degradation of hydrogel (Jeong et al., 2000). Moreover, the distribution and release of molecules from a hydrogel are highly dependent on the binding of the molecules to the polymer. When the molecule is bound, the release profile depends on the breakdown (enzymatic degradation or hydrolysis) of bonds between the hydrogel backbone and the molecule. The binding of the molecule is achieved by adding it to the hydrogel throughout the process of polymerization, the same bonds that bind the hydrogel monomers can bind drugs and other molecules (DuBose et al., 2005). Another method to administer drug release is the incorporation of drugs into microparticles and then adding them to the hydrogel matrix (Lampe et al., 2011). Various small-molecule drugs, neurotrophic factors, or peptides can be transported by microparticles. Similar to hydrogels, polymer microparticles can also be degraded at different rates and released under desired conditions when more than one therapeutic molecule is needed (Lampe et al., 2011).

3.6 EFFECT OF HYDROGELS ON THE BEHAVIOR OF NEURAL STEM CELLS

Hydrogels can provide a favorable environment for NSCs to form tissue by guiding the behavior of cells. This can be due to the easy realization of environmental sensing and response as a result of both cell-cell and cell-matrix interactions (Assunção-Silva et al., 2015).

3.6.1 Cell Viability

Cell viability is an important parameter for determining whether or not a substance is biocompatible and is also convenient for tissue engineering. In the case of hydrogels for neural tissue engineering, the concentration of hydrogels is usually the major factor affecting the viability of NSCs. Thonhoff et al. (2007) showed that lower hydrogel concentrations have a lower toxic effect on NSCs. Bioactive molecules and adhesive components can be incorporated into hydrogels to increase cell viability (Li et al., 2012).

3.6.2 Cell Adhesion

The adhesion of neural cells to the hydrogel is a crucial factor in effectively supporting neural regeneration (Straley et al., 2010). However, encouraging new tissue formation and neural cell adhesion can be hard because of the chemistry of many hydrogels. This is caused by the fact that many natural and synthetic hydrogels often inhibit protein adsorption. Chemical modifications like crosslinking ECM proteins to these non-adhesive hydrogels can promote cell growth and adhesion (Li et al., 2012). In particular, the incorporation of peptides such as RGD, IKVAV, and YIGSR into the hydrogel has been confirmed to develop the adhesion of neural cells (Li et al., 2012).

3.6.3 Neurite Outgrowth

A neurite is a projection of an axon or a dendrite from the cell body of a neuron. The primary structural elements of these neuronal extensions are neurofilament proteins, actin, and microtubules. Neurite outgrowth is a result of the actin filament's dynamic elongation and shortening (Gomez & Letourneau, 2014). Biomechanical characteristics of hydrogels as well as biochemical features like density and type of ligand have an impact on neurite outgrowth (Horn et al., 2007). The binding of cell-adhesive ligands such as RGD, IKVAV, and YIGSR to the hydrogel can enhance neurite extension. Furthermore, various combinations of these ligands were noticed to have varying degrees of effect on neurite extension (Gunn et al., 2005).

3.6.4 Cell Proliferation

Exact control of cell proliferation is essential for tissue regeneration. While most applications require increased proliferation, there are situations when less proliferation is required. The stiffness of hydrogel is one factor that influences NSC proliferation (Li et al., 2012). For instance, one group cultured adult NSCs on alginate hydrogels at different concentrations of $CaCl_2$, and the hydrogel with the lowest modulus of elasticity of 0.183 kPa found the highest cell proliferation and neuronal differentiation (Banerjee et al., 2009). It has also been reported that the conjugation of certain ligands to the hydrogel is effective in improving cell proliferation. In one study, HA hydrogels modified with RGD were demonstrated to enhance cell proliferation and extension of the neurons and obstruct glial scar development in rat brains (Cui et al., 2006).

3.6.5 Cell Differentiation

When many soluble signals are integrated into hydrogels, it has been shown to encourage the differentiation of NSCs into certain fates (Farrukh et al., 2017). In one approach, PEG hydrogel covalently functionalized with heparin, in combination with non-covalent loading and release of FGF-2, has been shown to increase neurite outgrowth, proliferation, and differentiation of encapsulated NSC (Freudenberg et al., 2009). Similarly, modification of peptide hydrogels with IKVAV has been demonstrated to support neuronal differentiation, neurite outgrowth, and cell adhesion (Mehrban et al., 2015). The stiffness of the hydrogel is also known to affect NSC differentiation. For example, adult NSCs were observed to show highly neuronal differentiation on soft gels (~0.1–0.5 kPa), while stiffer gels (~1–10 kPa) were found to increase differentiation of the glial cells (Saha et al., 2008).

3.6.6 Cell Migration

Cell migration is a crucial step for effective tissue regeneration. Factors like the pore size and pore deformability of the hydrogel and the capability of the cell to bind to the hydrogel matrix, generate contractile cytoskeleton filaments, and enhance focal adhesions play an important role in migration in hydrogels (George et al., 2020). In addition, hydrogel stiffness was also found to affect NSC migration (Hynes et al., 2009). The neural extensions are best seen when the stiffness is low, but a slightly higher stiffness is more favorable to NSC migration (Seidlits et al., 2010). The inclusion of ligands or growth factors in the hydrogel is another factor that influences the migration of neural cells. For instance, the conjugation of the RGD peptide sequence to the hydrogel resulted in improved cell viability and migration (Zhu, 2010).

3.7 3D BIOPRINTING OF HYDROGELS

Bioprinting is a method that deposits, transfers, and models biomaterials using computer-aided design. This method can be utilized to create intricate 3D constructions in which cells are layered and embedded in hydrogels, or the two are layered in tandem. The main element of 3D bioprinting is bio ink, which comprises biomaterial and live cells (Ren et al., 2021). In one study, this technique was used to model neural cells within 3D fibrin and collagen hydrogels, and high viability and improved migration were seen in the cells (Lee et al., 2010b). Recently, a photocrosslinkable bioink and a thermotherapeutic incentive bath were developed to disperse diverse neuronal populations with neurospheres and glial cell expertise while promoting the creation of self-organizing spheroids in 3D mesh topologies using integrated 3D bioprinting (Ren et al., 2021).

3.8 CONCLUSIONS AND FUTURE ASPECTS

The process of nerve regeneration after nervous system disorders is complicated and still poses a clinical challenge. In this regard, neural tissue engineering can provide effective strategies by creating a 3D biomimetic environment that can stimulate neural tissue regeneration and restore its function. In particular, hydrogel matrices have the potential to provide an appropriate substrate for axonal growth and thus overcome the difficulties associated with nerve regeneration. The versatile nature of hydrogels permits the modification of various mechanical and physical properties that can favorably affect axonal regeneration. Strategies using hydrogels alone or in combination with cells, drugs, and/or neurotrophic factors have been applied in animal models for various CNS or PNS injuries and have been proven to promote neural regeneration. However, although neural tissue regeneration is consistently achieved after hydrogel application, some factors, such as behavioral and electrophysiological tests, still yield unstable outcomes. As a result, more comprehensive studies are needed in the future for clinical applications of hydrogels.

REFERENCES

Ai, J., Kiasat-Dolatabadi, A., Ebrahimi-Barough, S., Ai, A., Lotfibakhshaiesh, N., Norouzi-Javidan, A., Saberi, H., Arjmand, B., & Aghayan, H. R. (2013). Polymeric scaffolds in neural tissue engineering: A review. *Archives of Neuroscience*, *1*(1), 15–20. https://doi.org/10.5812/archneurosci.9144.

Arslantunali, D., Dursun, T., Yucel, D., Hasirci, N., & Hasirci, V. (2014). Peripheral nerve conduits: Technology update. In *Medical Devices: Evidence and Research*. https://doi.org/10.2147/MDER.S59124.

Assunção-Silva, R. C., Gomes, E. D., Sousa, N., Silva, N. A., & Salgado, A. J. (2015). Hydrogels and cell based therapies in spinal cord injury regeneration. *Stem Cells International*, *2015*. https://doi.org/10.1155/2015/948040.

Aurand, E. R., Lampe, K. J., & Bjugstad, K. B. (2012). Defining and designing polymers and hydrogels for neural tissue engineering. *Neuroscience Research*, *72*(3), 199–213. https://doi.org/10.1016/j.neures.2011.12.005.

Aurand, E. R., Wagner, J. L., Shandas, R., & Bjugstad, K. B. (2014). Hydrogel formulation determines cell fate of fetal and adult neural progenitor cells. *Stem Cell Research*, *12*(1), 11–23. https://doi.org/https://doi.org/10.1016/j.scr.2013.09.013.

Babensee, J. E., McIntire, L. V., & Mikos, A. G. (2000). Growth factor delivery for tissue engineering. *Pharmaceutical Research*, *17*(5), 497–504. https://doi.org/10.1023/A:1007502828372.

Banerjee, A., Arha, M., Choudhary, S., Ashton, R. S., Bhatia, S. R., Schaffer, D. V., & Kane, R. S. (2009). The influence of hydrogel modulus on the proliferation and differentiation of encapsulated neural stem cells. *Biomaterials*, *30*(27), 4695–4699. https://doi.org/https://doi.org/10.1016/j.biomaterials.2009.05.050.

Barui, A. (2018). Synthetic polymeric gel. In *Polymeric Gels*. https://doi.org/10.1016/b978-0-08-102179-8.00003-x.

Bedir, T., Ulag, S., Ustundag, C. B., & Gunduz, O. (2020). 3D bioprinting applications in neural tissue engineering for spinal cord injury repair. *Materials Science and Engineering C*, *110*, 110741. https://doi.org/10.1016/j.msec.2020.110741.

Bjugstad, K. B., Lampe, K., Kern, D. S., & Mahoney, M. (2010). Biocompatibility of poly(ethylene glycol)-based hydrogels in the brain: An analysis of the glial response across space and time. *Journal of Biomedical Materials Research: Part A*, *95*(1), 79–91. https://doi.org/10.1002/jbm.a.32809.

Blesch, A., & Tuszynski, M. H. (2007). Transient growth factor delivery sustains regenerated axons after spinal cord injury. *The Journal of Neuroscience: The Official Journal of the Society for Neuroscience*, *27*(39), 10535–10545. https://doi.org/10.1523/JNEUROSCI.1903–07.2007.

Bolin, M. H., Svennersten, K., Wang, X., Chronakis, I. S., Richter-Dahlfors, A., Jager, E. W. H., & Berggren, M. (2009). Nano-fiber scaffold electrodes based on PEDOT for cell stimulation. *Sensors and Actuators, B: Chemical*. https://doi.org/10.1016/j.snb.2009.04.062.

Boni, R., Ali, A., Shavandi, A., & Clarkson, A. N. (2018). Current and novel polymeric biomaterials for neural tissue engineering. *Journal of Biomedical Science*, *25*(1), 1–21. https://doi.org/10.1186/s12929-018-0491-8.

Bordoni, M., Scarian, E., Rey, F., Gagliardi, S., Carelli, S., Pansarasa, O., & Cereda, C. (2020). Biomaterials in neurodegenerative disorders: A promising therapeutic approach. *International Journal of Molecular Sciences*. https://doi.org/10.3390/ijms21093243.

Brack, H. P., Tirmizi, S. A., & Risen, W. M. (1997). A spectroscopic and viscometric study of the metal ion-induced gelation of the biopolymer chitosan. *Polymer*. https://doi.org/10.1016/S0032-3861(96)00780-X.

Broguiere, N., Isenmann, L., & Zenobi-Wong, M. (2016). Novel enzymatically cross-linked hyaluronan hydrogels support the formation of 3D neuronal networks. *Biomaterials*, *99*, 47–55. https://doi.org/https://doi.org/10.1016/j.biomaterials.2016.04.036.

Bryant, S. J, Bender, R. J., Durand, K. L., & Anseth, K. S. (2004). Encapsulating chondrocytes in degrading PEG hydrogels with high modulus: Engineering gel structural changes to facilitate cartilaginous tissue production. *Biotechnology and Bioengineering*, *86*(7), 747–755. https://doi.org/10.1002/bit.20160.

Burdick, J. A., Ward, M., Liang, E., Young, M. J., & Langer, R. (2006). Stimulation of neurite outgrowth by neurotrophins delivered from degradable hydrogels. *Biomaterials*, *27*(3), 452–459. https://doi.org/https://doi.org/10.1016/j.biomaterials.2005.06.034.

Butt, A., & Verkhratsky, A. (2018). Neuroglia: Realising their true potential. *Brain and Neuroscience Advances*. https://doi.org/10.1177/2398212818817495.

Caló, E., & Khutoryanskiy, V. V. (2015). Biomedical applications of hydrogels: A review of patents and commercial products. *European Polymer Journal*, *65*, 252–267. https://doi.org/10.1016/j.eurpolymj.2014.11.024.

Carballo-Molina, O. A., & Velasco, I. (2015). Hydrogels as scaffolds and delivery systems to enhance axonal regeneration after injuries. *Frontiers in Cellular Neuroscience*, *9*, 1–12. https://doi.org/10.3389/fncel.2015.00013.

Cesur, S., Oktar, F. N., Ekren, N., Kilic, O., Alkaya, D. B., Seyhan, S. A., Ege, Z. R., Lin, C.-C., Kuruca, S. E., Erdemir, G., & Gunduz, O. (2020). Preparation and characterization of electrospun polylactic acid/sodium alginate/orange oyster shell composite nanofiber for biomedical application. *Journal of the Australian Ceramic Society*, *56*(2), 533–543. https://doi.org/10.1007/s41779-019-00363-1.

Cesur, S., Ulag, S., Ozak, L., Gumussoy, A., Arslan, S., Yilmaz, B. K., Ekren, N., Agirbasli, M., Kalaskar, D. M., & Gunduz, O. (2020). Production and characterization of elastomeric cardiac tissue-like patches for Myocardial Tissue Engineering. *Polymer Testing*, *90*, 106613. https://doi.org/https://doi.org/10.1016/j.polymertesting.2020.106613.

Chatterjee, K., Lin-Gibson, S., Wallace, W. E., Parekh, S. H., Lee, Y. J., Cicerone, M. T., Young, M. F., & Simon, C. G. (2010). The effect of 3D hydrogel scaffold modulus on osteoblast differentiation and mineralization revealed by combinatorial screening. *Biomaterials*, *31*(19), 5051–5062. https://doi.org/10.1016/j.biomaterials.2010.03.024.

Checkoway, H., Lundin, J. I., & Kelada, S. N. (2011). Neurodegenerative diseases. In *IARC Scientific Publications*. https://doi.org/10.1071/rdv24n1ab251.

Cheng, T.-Y., Chen, M.-H., Chang, W.-H., Huang, M.-Y., & Wang, T.-W. (2013). Neural stem cells encapsulated in a functionalized self-assembling peptide hydrogel for brain tissue engineering. *Biomaterials*, *34*(8), 2005–2016. https://doi.org/https://doi.org/10.1016/j.biomaterials.2012.11.043.

Chenite, A., Chaput, C., Wang, D., Combes, C., Buschmann, M. D., Hoemann, C. D., Leroux, J. C., Atkinson, B. L., Binette, F., & Selmani, A. (2000). Novel injectable neutral solutions of chitosan form biodegradable gels in situ. *Biomaterials*. https://doi.org/10.1016/S0142-9612(00)00116-2.

Chiu, Y. L., Chen, S. C., Su, C. J., Hsiao, C. W., Chen, Y. M., Chen, H. L., & Sung, H. W. (2009). pH-triggered injectable hydrogels prepared from aqueous N-palmitoyl chitosan: In vitro characteristics and in vivo biocompatibility. *Biomaterials*, *30*(28), 4877–4888. https://doi.org/10.1016/j.biomaterials.2009.05.052.

Chung, H. J., & Park, T. G. (2007). Surface engineered and drug releasing pre-fabricated scaffolds for tissue engineering. In *Advanced Drug Delivery Reviews*. https://doi.org/10.1016/j.addr.2007.03.015.

Clements, I. P., Munson, J. M., & Bellamkonda, R. V. (2013). Neuronal tissue engineering. In Biomaterials science (pp. 1291–1306). Academic Press.

Coviello, T., Matticardi, P., & Alhaique, F. (2006). Drug delivery strategies using polysaccharidic gels. *Expert Opinion on Drug Delivery*. https://doi.org/10.1517/17425247.3.3.395.

Croisier, F., & Jérôme, C. (2013). Chitosan-based biomaterials for tissue engineering. *European Polymer Journal*. https://doi.org/10.1016/j.eurpolymj.2012.12.009.

Cui, F. Z., Tian, W. M., Hou, S. P., Xu, Q. Y., & Lee, I.-S. (2006). Hyaluronic acid hydrogel immobilized with RGD peptides for brain tissue engineering. *Journal of Materials Science. Materials in Medicine*, *17*(12), 1393–1401. https://doi.org/10.1007/s10856-006-0615-7.

Cullen, D. K., Vukasinovic, J., Glezer, A., & LaPlaca, M. C. (2007). Microfluidic engineered high cell density three-dimensional neural cultures. *Journal of Neural Engineering*, *4*(2), 159–172. https://doi.org/10.1088/1741–2560/4/2/015. clemen

Cunha, C., Panseri, S., & Antonini, S. (2011). Emerging nanotechnology approaches in tissue engineering for peripheral nerve regeneration. *Nanomedicine: Nanotechnology, Biology, and Medicine*, *7*(1), 50–59. https://doi.org/10.1016/j.nano.2010.07.004.

Deister, C., & Schmidt, C. E. (2006). Optimizing neurotrophic factor combinations for neurite outgrowth. *J. Neural Eng.*, *3*, 172–179. https://doi.org/10.1088/1741-2560/3/2/011.

del Valle, L. J., Aradilla, D., Oliver, R., Sepulcre, F., Gamez, A., Armelin, E., Alemán, C., & Estrany, F. (2007). Cellular adhesion and proliferation on poly(3,4-ethylenedioxythiophene): Benefits in the electroactivity of the conducting polymer. *European Polymer Journal*. https://doi.org/10.1016/j.eurpolymj.2007.03.050.

Desbrières, J., Hirrien, M., & Ross-Murphy, S. B. (2000). Thermogelation of methylcellulose: Rheological considerations. *Polymer*. https://doi.org/10.1016/S0032-3861(99)00413-9.

Diogo, C. C., Camassa, J. A., Pereira, J. E., da Costa, L. M., Filipe, V., Couto, P. A., Geuna, S., Maurício, A. C., & Varejão, A. S. (2017). The use of sheep as a model for studying peripheral nerve regeneration following nerve injury: Review of the literature. *Neurological Research*. https://doi.org/10.1080/01616412.2017.1331873.

Discher, D. E., Janmey, P., & Wang, Y.-L. (2005). Tissue cells feel and respond to the stiffness of their substrate. *Science (New York, N.Y.)*, *310*(5751), 1139–1143. https://doi.org/10.1126/science.1116995.

Doblado, L. R., Martínez-Ramos, C., & Pradas, M. M. (2021). Biomaterials for neural tissue engineering. *Frontiers in Nanotechnology*, *3*(April). https://doi.org/10.3389/fnano.2021.643507.

Drotleff, S., Lungwitz, U., Breunig, M., Dennis, A., Blunk, T., Tessmar, J., & Göpferich, A. (2004). Biomimetic polymers in pharmaceutical and biomedical sciences. *European Journal of Pharmaceutics and Biopharmaceutics: Official Journal of Arbeitsgemeinschaft Fur Pharmazeutische Verfahrenstechnik e.V*, *58*(2), 385–407. https://doi.org/10.1016/j.ejpb.2004.03.018.

DuBose, J. W., Cutshall, C., & Metters, A. T. (2005). Controlled release of tethered molecules via engineered hydrogel degradation: Model development and validation. *Journal of Biomedical Materials Research. Part A*, *74*(1), 104–116. https://doi.org/10.1002/jbm.a.30307.

Emerich, D. F., Silva, E., Ali, O., Mooney, D., Bell, W., Yu, S. J., Kaneko, Y., & Borlongan, C. (2010). Injectable VEGF hydrogels produce near complete neurological and anatomical protection following cerebral ischemia in rats. *Cell Transplantation*, *19*(9), 1063–1071. https://doi.org/10.3727/096368910X498278.

Fang, D., Pan, Q., & Rempel, G. L. (2007). Preparation and morphology study of microporous poly(HEMA-MMA) particles. *Journal of Applied Polymer Science*. https://doi.org/10.1002/app.24941.

Farmer, T. G., Edgar, T. F., & Peppas, N. A. (2008). In vivo simulations of the intravenous dynamics of submicrometer particles of pH-responsive cationic hydrogels in diabetic patients. *Industrial and Engineering Chemistry Research*, *47*(24), 10053–10063. https://doi.org/10.1021/ie070957b.

Farrukh, A., Ortega, F., Fan, W., Marichal, N., Paez, J. I., Berninger, B., del Campo, A., & Salierno, M. J. (2017). Bifunctional hydrogels containing the laminin motif IKVAV promote neurogenesis. *Stem Cell Reports*, *9*(5), 1432–1440. https://doi.org/https://doi.org/10.1016/j.stemcr.2017.09.002.

Fischer, M. B., Roeckl, C., Parizek, P., Schwarz, H. P., & Aguzzi, A. (2000). Binding of disease-associated prion protein to plasminogen. *Nature*. https://doi.org/10.1038/35044100.

FitzGerald, J., & Fawcett, J. (2007). Repair in the central nervous system. *Journal of Bone and Joint Surgery - Series B*. https://doi.org/10.1302/0301-620X.89B11.19651.

Flynn, L., Dalton, P. D., & Shoichet, M. S. (2003). Fiber templating of poly(2-hydroxyethyl methacrylate) for neural tissue engineering. *Biomaterials*, *24*(23), 4265–4272. https://doi.org/10.1016/S0142-9612(03)00334-X.

Freier, T., Montenegro, R., Koh, H. S., & Shoichet, M. S. (2005). Chitin-based tubes for tissue engineering in the nervous system. *Biomaterials*. https://doi.org/10.1016/j.biomaterials.2004.11.040.

Freudenberg, U., Hermann, A., Welzel, P. B., Stirl, K., Schwarz, S. C., Grimmer, M., Zieris, A., Panyanuwat, W., Zschoche, S., Meinhold, D., Storch, A., & Werner, C. (2009). A starPEG–heparin hydrogel platform to aid cell replacement therapies for neurodegenerative diseases. *Biomaterials*, *30*(28), 5049–5060. https://doi.org/https://doi.org/10.1016/j.biomaterials.2009.06.002.

Frisch, S. M., & Francis, H. (1994). Disruption of epithelial cell-matrix interactions induces apoptosis. *The Journal of Cell Biology*, *124*(4), 619–626. https://doi.org/10.1083/jcb.124.4.619.

Gautier, S. E., Oudega, M., Fragoso, M., Chapon, P., Plant, G. W., Bunge, M. B., & Parel, J. M. (1998). Poly(α-hydroxyacids) for application in the spinal cord: Resorbability and biocompatibility with adult rat schwann cells and spinal cord. *Journal of Biomedical Materials Research*. https://doi.org/10.1002/(SICI)1097-4636(19981215)42:4<642::AID-JBM22>3.0.CO;2-K.

George, J., Hsu, C. C., Nguyen, L. T. B., Ye, H., & Cui, Z. (2020). Neural tissue engineering with structured hydrogels in CNS models and therapies. *Biotechnology Advances*, *42*(March 2019). https://doi.org/10.1016/j.biotechadv.2019.03.009.

Ghasemi-Mobarakeh, L., Prabhakaran, M. P., Morshed, M., Nasr-Esfahani, M. H., Baharvand, H., Kiani, S., Al-Deyab, S. S., & Ramakrishna, S. (2011). Application of conductive polymers, scaffolds and electrical stimulation for nerve tissue engineering. *Journal of Tissue Engineering and Regenerative Medicine*, *5*(4). https://doi.org/10.1002/term.383.

Goganau, I., Sandner, B., Weidner, N., Fouad, K., & Blesch, A. (2018). Depolarization and electrical stimulation enhance in vitro and in vivo sensory axon growth after spinal cord injury. *Experimental Neurology*. https://doi.org/10.1016/j.expneurol.2017.11.011.

Gomez, T. M., & Letourneau, P. C. (2014). Actin dynamics in growth cone motility and navigation. *Journal of Neurochemistry*, *129*(2), 221–234. https://doi.org/10.1111/jnc.12506.

Griffith, L. G., & Naughton, G. (2002). Tissue engineering - Current challenges and expanding opportunities. *Science*. https://doi.org/10.1126/science.1069210.

Gu, X., Ding, F., & Williams, D. F. (2014). Neural tissue engineering options for peripheral nerve regeneration. *Biomaterials*. https://doi.org/10.1016/j.biomaterials.2014.04.064.

Gunn, J. W., Turner, S. D., & Mann, B. K. (2005). Adhesive and mechanical properties of hydrogels influence neurite extension. *Journal of Biomedical Materials Research: Part A*, *72*(1), 91–97. https://doi.org/10.1002/jbm.a.30203.

Hadryś D., Węgrzyn, T., Piwnik, J., Wszołek, L., & Węgrzyn, D. (2016). Compressive strength of steel frames after welding with micro-jet cooling. *Archives of Metallurgy and Materials*, *61*(1), 123–126. https://doi.org/10.1515/amm-2016-0023.

Hejcl, A., Lesný, P., Prádný, M., Michálek, J., Jendelová, P., Stulík, J., & Syková, E. (2008). Biocompatible hydrogels in spinal cord injury repair. *Physiological Research*, *57*(Suppl 3), S121–S132. https://doi.org/10.33549/physiolres.931606.

Hejčl, A., Lesný, P., Přádný, M., Šedý, J., Zámečník, J., Jendelová, P., Michálek, J., & Syková, E. (2009). Macroporous hydrogels based on 2-hydroxyethyl methacrylate. Part 6: 3D hydrogels with positive and negative surface charges and polyelectrolyte complexes in spinal cord injury repair. *Journal of Materials Science: Materials in Medicine*. https://doi.org/10.1007/s10856-009-3714-4.

Helmut, K., Hanisch, U. K., Noda, M., & Verkhratsky, A. (2011). Physiology of microglia. *Physiological Reviews*. https://doi.org/10.1152/physrev.00011.2010.

Hirsh, A. T., Braden, A. L., Craggs, J. G., & Jensen, M. P. (2011). Psychometric properties of the Community Integration Questionnaire in a heterogeneous sample of adults with physical disability. *Archives of Physical Medicine and Rehabilitation*. https://doi.org/10.1016/j.apmr.2011.05.004.

Ho, L., & Hsu, S.-H. (2018). Cell reprogramming by 3D bioprinting of human fibroblasts in polyurethane hydrogel for fabrication of neural-like constructs. *Acta Biomaterialia*. https://doi.org/10.1016/j.actbio.2018.01.044.

Hof, P. R., Kidd, G., DeFelipe, J., de Vellis, J., Gama Sosa, M. A., Elder, G. A., & Trapp, B. D. (2013). Cellular Components of Nervous Tissue. In *Fundamental Neuroscience: Fourth Edition*. https://doi.org/10.1016/B978–0–12–385870–2.00003–2

Hoffman, A. S. (2012). Hydrogels for biomedical applications. *Advanced Drug Delivery Reviews*, *64*, 18–23. https://doi.org/10.1016/j.addr.2012.09.010.

Holland, T. A., Tabata, Y., & Mikos, A. G. (2003). In vitro release of transforming growth factor-beta 1 from gelatin microparticles encapsulated in biodegradable, injectable oligo(poly(ethylene glycol) fumarate) hydrogels. *Journal of Controlled Release : Official Journal of the Controlled Release Society*, *91*(3), 299–313. https://doi.org/10.1016/s0168-3659(03)00258-x.

Holland, T. A., Tabata, Y., & Mikos, A. G. (2005). Dual growth factor delivery from degradable oligo(poly(ethylene glycol) fumarate) hydrogel scaffolds for cartilage tissue engineering. *Journal of Controlled Release : Official Journal of the Controlled Release Society*, *101*(1–3), 111–125. https://doi.org/10.1016/j.jconrel.2004.07.004.

Horn, E. M., Beaumont, M., Shu, X. Z., Harvey, A., Prestwich, G. D., Horn, K. M., Gibson, A. R., Preul, M. C., & Panitch, A. (2007). Influence of cross-linked hyaluronic acid hydrogels on neurite outgrowth and recovery from spinal cord injury. *Journal of Neurosurgery. Spine*, *6*(2), 133–140. https://doi.org/10.3171/spi.2007.6.2.133.

Hou, S., Tian, W., Xu, Q., Cui, F., Zhang, J., Lu, Q., & Zhao, C. (2006). The enhancement of cell adherence and inducement of neurite outgrowth of dorsal root ganglia co-cultured with hyaluronic acid hydrogels modified with Nogo-66 receptor antagonist in vitro. *Neuroscience*. https://doi.org/10.1016/j.neuroscience.2005.09.029.

Hynd, M. R., Turner, J. N., & Shain, W. (2007). Applications of hydrogels for neural cell engineering. *Journal of Biomaterials Science, Polymer Edition*. https://doi.org/10.1163/156856207782177909.

Hynes, S. R., Rauch, M. F., Bertram, J. P., & Lavik, E. B. (2009). A library of tunable poly(ethylene glycol)/poly(L-lysine) hydrogels to investigate the material cues that influence neural stem cell differentiation. *Journal of Biomedical Materials Research. Part A*, *89*(2), 499–509. https://doi.org/10.1002/jbm.a.31987.

Jain, A., Kim, Y.-T., McKeon, R. J., & Bellamkonda, R. V. (2006). In situ gelling hydrogels for conformal repair of spinal cord defects, and local delivery of BDNF after spinal cord injury. *Biomaterials*, *27*(3), 497–504. https://doi.org/10.1016/j.biomaterials.2005.07.008.

Jayakumar, A., Jose, V. K., & Lee, J. M. (2020). Hydrogels for medical and environmental applications. *Small Methods*, *4*(3). https://doi.org/10.1002/smtd.201900735.

Jeong, B., Bae, Y. H., & Kim, S. W. (2000). Drug release from biodegradable injectable thermosensitive hydrogel of PEG-PLGA-PEG triblock copolymers. *Journal of Controlled Release : Official Journal of the Controlled Release Society*, *63*(1–2), 155–163. https://doi.org/10.1016/s0168-3659(99)00194-7.

Johnson, P. J., Parker, S. R., & Sakiyama-Elbert, S. E. (2009). Controlled release of neurotrophin-3 from fibrin-based tissue engineering scaffolds enhances neural fiber sprouting following subacute spinal cord injury. *Biotechnology and Bioengineering*, *104*(6), 1207–1214. https://doi.org/https://doi.org/10.1002/bit.22476.

Jones, L. L., Oudega, M., Bunge, M. B., & Tuszynski, M. H. (2001). Neurotrophic factors, cellular bridges and gene therapy for spinal cord injury. *The Journal of Physiology*, *533* (Pt 1), 83–89. https://doi.org/10.1111/j.1469-7793.2001.0083b.x.

Joung, D., Lavoie, N. S., Guo, S. Z., Park, S. H., Parr, A. M., & McAlpine, M. C. (2020). 3D printed neural regeneration devices. *Advanced Functional Materials*. https://doi.org/10.1002/adfm.201906237.

Kamalesh, S., Tan, P., Wang, J., Lee, T., Kang, E. T., & Wang, C. H. (2000). Biocompatibility of electroactive polymers in tissues. *Journal of Biomedical Materials Research*. https://doi.org/10.1002/1097-4636(20001205)52:3<467::AID-JBM4>3.0.CO;2-6.

Knowlton, S., Anand, S., Shah, T., & Tasoglu, S. (2018). Bioprinting for neural tissue engineering. *Trends in Neurosciences*, *41*(1), 31–46. https://doi.org/10.1016/j.tins.2017.11.001.

Kong, H., Lee, K., & Mooney, D. (2003). Nondestructively probing the cross-linking density of polymeric hydrogels. *Macromolecules*, *36*. https://doi.org/10.1021/ma034865j.

Kouyoumdjian, J. A., Graça, C. R., & Ferreira, V. F. M. (2017). Peripheral nerve injuries: A retrospective survey of 1124 cases. *Neurology India*. https://doi.org/10.4103/neuroindia.NI_987_16.

Lampe, K. J., Kern, D. S., Mahoney, M. J., & Bjugstad, K. B. (2011). The administration of BDNF and GDNF to the brain via PLGA microparticles patterned within a degradable PEG-based hydrogel: Protein distribution and the glial response. *Journal of Biomedical Materials Research. Part A*, *96*(3), 595–607. https://doi.org/10.1002/jbm.a.33011.

Lampe, K. J., Mooney, R. G., Bjugstad, K. B., & Mahoney, M. J. (2010). Effect of macromer weight percent on neural cell growth in 2D and 3D nondegradable PEG hydrogel culture. *Journal of Biomedical Materials Research. Part A*, *94*(4), 1162–1171. https://doi.org/10.1002/jbm.a.32787.

Laverty, P. H., Leskovar, A., Breur, G. J., Coates, J. R., Bergman, R. L., Widmer, W. R., Toombs, J. P., Shapiro, S., & Borgens, R. B. (2004). A preliminary study of intravenous surfactants in paraplegic dogs: Polymer therapy in canine clinical SCI. *Journal of Neurotrauma*. https://doi.org/10.1089/neu.2004.21.1767.

Le, T. H., Kim, Y., & Yoon, H. (2017). Electrical and electrochemical properties of conducting polymers. *Polymers*. https://doi.org/10.3390/polym9040150.

Lee, A. C., Yu, V. M., Lowe, J. B., Brenner, M. J., Hunter, D. A., Mackinnon, S. E., & Sakiyama-Elbert, S. E. (2003). Controlled release of nerve growth factor enhances sciatic nerve regeneration. *Experimental Neurology*, *184*(1), 295–303. https://doi.org/https://doi.org/10.1016/S0014-4886(03)00258-9.

Lee, C. H., Singla, A., & Lee, Y. (2001). Biomedical applications of collagen. *International Journal of Pharmaceutics*. https://doi.org/10.1016/S0378-5173(01)00691-3.

Lee, H., McKeon, R. J., & Bellamkonda, R. V. (2010a). Sustained delivery of thermostabilized chABC enhances axonal sprouting and functional recovery after spinal cord injury. *Proceedings of the National Academy of Sciences*, *107*(8), 3340 LP–3345. https://doi.org/10.1073/pnas.0905437106.

Lee, K. Y., & Mooney, D. J. (2001). Hydrogels for tissue engineering. *Chemical Reviews*, *101*(7), 1869–1879. https://doi.org/10.1021/cr000108x.

Lee, K. Y., Peters, M. C., Anderson, K. W., & Mooney, D. J. (2000). Controlled growth factor release from synthetic extracellular matrices. *Nature*. https://doi.org/10.1038/35050141.

Lee, S., Trinh, T. H. T., Yoo, M., Shin, J., Lee, H., Kim, J., Hwang, E., Lim, Y. B., & Ryou, C. (2019). Self-assembling peptides and their application in the treatment of diseases. *International Journal of Molecular Sciences*. https://doi.org/10.3390/ijms20235850.

Lee, Y.-B., Polio, S., Lee, W., Dai, G., Menon, L., Carroll, R. S., & Yoo, S.-S. (2010b). Bio-printing of collagen and VEGF-releasing fibrin gel scaffolds for neural stem cell culture. *Experimental Neurology*, *223*(2), 645–652. https://doi.org/10.1016/j.expneurol.2010.02.014.

Li, H., Zheng, J., Wang, H., Becker, M. L., & Leipzig, N. D. (2018). Neural stem cell encapsulation and differentiation in strain promoted crosslinked polyethylene glycol-based hydrogels. *Journal of Biomaterials Applications*, *32*(9), 1222–1230. https://doi.org/10.1177/0885328218755711.

Li, X., Katsanevakis, E., Liu, X., Zhang, N., & Wen, X. (2012). Engineering neural stem cell fates with hydrogel design for central nervous system regeneration. *Progress in Polymer Science*, *37*(8), 1105–1129. https://doi.org/10.1016/j.progpolymsci.2012.02.004.

Lin, S., Sangaj, N., Razafiarison, T., Zhang, C., & Varghese, S. (2011). Influence of physical properties of biomaterials on cellular behavior. *Pharmaceutical Research*, *28*(6), 1422–1430. https://doi.org/10.1007/s11095-011-0378-9.

Little, L., Healy, K. E., & Schaffer, D. (2008). Engineering biomaterials for synthetic neural stem cell microenvironments. *Chemical Reviews*. https://doi.org/10.1021/cr078228t.

Liu, Z., Yang, Y., He, L., Pang, M., Luo, C., Liu, B., & Rong, L. (2019). High-dose methylprednisolone for acute traumatic spinal cord injury: A meta-analysis. *Neurology*. https://doi.org/10.1212/WNL.0000000000007998.

Luo, J., Borgens, R., & Shi, R. (2002). Polyethylene glycol immediately repairs neuronal membranes and inhibits free radical production after acute spinal cord injury. *Journal of Neurochemistry*. https://doi.org/10.1046/j.1471-4159.2002.01160.x.

Luo, S. C., Ali, E. M., Tansil, N. C., Yu, H. H., Gao, S., Kantchev, E. A. B., & Ying, J. Y. (2008). Poly(3,4-ethylenedioxythiophene) (PEDOT) nanobiointerfaces: Thin, ultrasmooth, and functionalized PEDOT films with in vitro and in vivo biocompatibility. *Langmuir*. https://doi.org/10.1021/la800333g.

Luo, Y., & Shoichet, M. S. (2004). A photolabile hydrogel for guided three-dimensional cell growth and migration. *Nature Materials*, *3*(4), 249–254. https://doi.org/10.1038/nmat1092.

Lutolf, M. P., Lauer-Fields, J. L., Schmoekel, H. G., Metters, A. T., Weber, F. E., Fields, G. B., & Hubbell, J. A. (2003). Synthetic matrix metalloproteinase-sensitive hydrogels for the conduction of tissue regeneration: Engineering cell-invasion characteristics. *Proceedings of the National Academy of Sciences of the United States of America*, *100*(9), 5413–5418. https://doi.org/10.1073/pnas.0737381100.

Lynn, A. K., Yannas, I. V., & Bonfield, W. (2004). Antigenicity and immunogenicity of collagen. *Journal of Biomedical Materials Research - Part B Applied Biomaterials*. https://doi.org/10.1002/jbm.b.30096.

Ma, J., Tian, W. M., Hou, S. P., Xu, Q. Y., Spector, M., & Cui, F. Z. (2007). An experimental test of stroke recovery by implanting a hyaluronic acid hydrogel carrying a Nogo receptor antibody in a rat model. *Biomedical Materials*, *2*(4), 233–240. https://doi.org/10.1088/1748-6041/2/4/005.

Macaya, D., & Spector, M. (2012). Injectable hydrogel materials for spinal cord regeneration: A review. *Biomedical Materials*, *7*(1). https://doi.org/10.1088/1748-6041/7/1/012001.

Madhusudanan, P., Raju, G., & Shankarappa, S. (2020). Hydrogel systems and their role in neural tissue engineering. *Journal of the Royal Society, Interface*, *17*(162), 20190505. https://doi.org/10.1098/rsif.2019.0505.

Madhusudanan, P., Reade, S., & Shankarappa, S. A. (2017). Neuroglia as targets for drug delivery systems: A review. *Nanomedicine: Nanotechnology, Biology, and Medicine*. https://doi.org/10.1016/j.nano.2016.08.013.

Makadia, H. K., & Siegel, S. J. (2011). Poly Lactic-co-Glycolic Acid (PLGA) as biodegradable controlled drug delivery carrier. *Polymers*. https://doi.org/10.3390/polym3031377.

McDonald, J. W. (1999). Repairing the damaged spinal cord. *Scientific American*. https://doi.org/10.1038/scientificamerican0999-64.

McKee, C. T., Last, J. A., Russell, P., & Murphy, C. J. (2011). Indentation versus tensile measurements of young's modulus for soft biological tissues. *Tissue Engineering Part B: Reviews*, *17*(3), 155–164. https://doi.org/10.1089/ten.teb.2010.0520.

McKee, J. R., Hietala, S., Seitsonen, J., Laine, J., Kontturi, E., & Ikkala, O. (2014). Thermoresponsive nanocellulose hydrogels with tunable mechanical properties. *ACS Macro Letters*, *3*(3), 266–270. https://doi.org/10.1021/mz400596g.

Mealy, J. E., Chung, J. J., Jeong, H.-H., Issadore, D., Lee, D., Atluri, P., & Burdick, J. A. (2018). Injectable granular hydrogels with multifunctional properties for biomedical applications. *Advanced Materials*, *30*(20), 1705912. https://doi.org/https://doi.org/10.1002/adma.201705912.

Mehrban, N., Zhu, B., Tamagnini, F., Young, F. I., Wasmuth, A., Hudson, K. L., Thomson, A. R., Birchall, M. A., Randall, A. D., Song, B., & Woolfson, D. N. (2015). Functionalized α-helical peptide hydrogels for neural tissue engineering. *ACS Biomaterials Science & Engineering*, *1*(6), 431–439. https://doi.org/10.1021/acsbiomaterials.5b00051.

Meilander, N. J., Pasumarthy, M. K., Kowalczyk, T. H., Cooper, M. J., & Bellamkonda, R. V. (2003). Sustained release of plasmid DNA using lipid microtubules and agarose hydrogel. *Journal of Controlled Release*. https://doi.org/10.1016/S0168-3659(03)00007-5.

Meiners, S., & Mercado, M. L. T. (2003). Functional peptide sequences derived from extracellular matrix glycoproteins and their receptors: Strategies to improve neuronal regeneration. *Molecular Neurobiology*, *27*(2), 177–196. https://doi.org/10.1385/MN:27: 2: 177.

Meyer, U., Handschel, J., Meyer, T., & Wiesmann, H. P. (2009). *Fundamentals of Tissue Engineering and Regenerative Medicine*. Springer, Berlin. https://doi.org/10.1155/2014/431540.

Moffat, K. L., Sun, W.-H. S., Pena, P. E., Chahine, N. O., Doty, S. B., Ateshian, G. A., Hung, C. T., & Lu, H. H. (2008). Characterization of the structure-function relationship at the ligament-to-bone interface. *Proceedings of the National Academy of Sciences of the United States of America*, *105*(23), 7947–7952. https://doi.org/10.1073/pnas.0712150105.

Mosahebi, A., Simon, M., Wiberg, M., & Terenghi, G. (2001). A novel use of alginate hydrogel as Schwann cell matrix. *Tissue Engineering*. https://doi.org/10.1089/107632701753213156.

Mosahebi, A., Fuller, P., Wiberg, M., & Terenghi, G. (2002). Effect of allogeneic schwann cell transplantation on peripheral nerve regeneration. *Experimental Neurology*. https://doi.org/10.1006/exnr.2001.7846.

Mosesson, M. W. (2005). Fibrinogen and fibrin structure and functions. *Journal of Thrombosis and Haemostasis*. https://doi.org/10.1111/j.1538-7836.2005.01365.x.

Muir, E., Raza, M., Ellis, C., Burnside, E., Love, F., Heller, S., Elliot, M., Daniell, E., Dasgupta, D., Alves, N., Day, P., Fawcett, J., & Keynes, R. (2017). Trafficking and processing of bacterial proteins by mammalian cells: Insights from chondroitinase ABC. *PLoS ONE*, *12*(11). https://doi.org/10.1371/journal.pone.0186759.

Murakami, Y., Furukawa, S., Nitta, A., & Furukawa, Y. (2002). Accumulation of nerve growth factor protein at both rostral and caudal stumps in the transected rat spinal cord. *Journal of the Neurological Sciences*, *198*(1–2), 63–69. https://doi.org/10.1016/s0022-510x(02)00080-1.

Murphy, A. R., Laslett, A., O'Brien, C. M., & Cameron, N. R. (2017). Scaffolds for 3D in vitro culture of neural lineage cells. *Acta Biomaterialia*. https://doi.org/10.1016/j.actbio.2017.02.046.

Nagai, Y., Unsworth, L. D., Koutsopoulos, S., & Zhang, S. (2006). Slow release of molecules in self-assembling peptide nanofiber scaffold. *Journal of Controlled Release*, *115*(1), 18–25. https://doi.org/10.1016/j.jconrel.2006.06.031.

Nakamoto, T., Kain, K. H., & Ginsberg, M. H. (2004). Neurobiology: New connections between integrins and axon guidance. *Current Biology*. https://doi.org/10.1016/S0960-9822(04)00035-1.

Namba, R. M., Cole, A. A., Bjugstad, K. B., & Mahoney, M. J. (2009). Development of porous PEG hydrogels that enable efficient, uniform cell-seeding and permit early neural process extension. *Acta Biomaterialia*, *5*(6), 1884–1897. https://doi.org/10.1016/j.actbio.2009.01.036.

Nezakati, T., Seifalian, A., Tan, A., & Seifalian, A. M. (2018). Conductive polymers: Opportunities and challenges in biomedical applications. *Chemical Reviews*. https://doi.org/10.1021/acs.chemrev.6b00275.

Nguyen, M. K., & Lee, D. S. (2010). Injectable biodegradable hydrogels. *Macromolecular Bioscience*, *10*(6), 563–579. https://doi.org/10.1002/mabi.200900402.

Nicodemus, G. D., & Bryant, S. J. (2008). Cell encapsulation in biodegradable hydrogels for tissue engineering applications. *Tissue Engineering Part B: Reviews*, *14*(2), 149–165. https://doi.org/10.1089/ten.teb.2007.0332.

Nisbet, D. R., Crompton, K. E., Hamilton, S. D., Shirakawa, S., Prankerd, R. J., Finkelstein, D. I., Horne, M. K., & Forsythe, J. S. (2006). Morphology and gelation of thermosensitive xyloglucan hydrogels. *Biophysical Chemistry*. https://doi.org/10.1016/j.bpc.2005.12.005.

Nisbet, D. R., Crompton, K. E., Horne, M. K., Finkelstein, D. I., & Forsythe, J. S. (2008). Neural tissue engineering of the CNS using hydrogels. *Journal of Biomedical Materials Research - Part B Applied Biomaterials*. https://doi.org/10.1002/jbm.b.31000.

Nisbet, D. R., Rodda, A. E., Horne, M. K., Forsythe, J. S., & Finkelstein, D. I. (2010). Implantation of functionalized thermally gelling xyloglucan hydrogel within the brain: Associated neurite infiltration and inflammatory response. *Tissue Engineering - Part A*. https://doi.org/10.1089/ten.tea.2009.0677.

Nisbet, D. R., & Williams, R. J. (2012). Self-assembled peptides: Characterisation and in vivo response. *Biointerphases*. https://doi.org/10.1007/s13758-011-0002-x.

Noback, C. R., Strominger, N. L., Demarest, R. J., & Ruggiero, D. A. (2005). *The Human Nervous System: Structure and Function: Sixth Edition*. https://doi.org/10.1007/978-1-59259-730-7.

Nomura, H., Tator, C. H., & Shoichet, M. S. (2006). Bioengineered strategies for spinal cord repair. *Journal of Neurotrauma*. https://doi.org/10.1089/neu.2006.23.496.

Novikova, L. N., Mosahebi, A., Wiberg, M., Terenghi, G., Kellerth, J. O., & Novikov, L. N. (2006). Alginate hydrogel and matrigel as potential cell carriers for neurotransplantation. *Journal of Biomedical Materials Research - Part A*. https://doi.org/10.1002/jbm.a.30603.

O'Brien, F. J. (2011). Biomaterials & scaffolds for tissue engineering. *Materials Today*, *14*(3), 88–95. https://doi.org/https://doi.org/10.1016/S1369-7021(11)70058-X.

O'Connor, S. M., Stenger, D. A., Shaffer, K. M., Maric, D., Barker, J. L., & Ma, W. (2000). Primary neural precursor cell expansion, differentiation and cytosolic Ca^{2+} response in three-dimensional collagen gel. *Journal of Neuroscience Methods*. https://doi.org/10.1016/S0165-0270(00)00303-4.

O'Rourke, C., Lee-Reeves, C., Drake, R. A. L., Cameron, G. W. W., Loughlin, A. J., & Phillips, J. B. (2017). Adapting tissue-engineered in vitro CNS models for high-throughput study of neurodegeneration. *Journal of Tissue Engineering*. https://doi.org/10.1177/2041731417697920.

Pal, S. (2014). *Mechanical Properties of Biological Materials BT - Design of Artificial Human Joints & Organs* (S. Pal (ed.); pp. 23–40). Springer US. https://doi.org/10.1007/978-1-4614-6255-2_2.

Park, K. I., Teng, Y. D., & Snyder, E. Y. (2002). The injured brain interacts reciprocally with neural stem cells supported by scaffolds to reconstitute lost tissue. *Nature Biotechnology*, *20*(11), 1111–1117. https://doi.org/10.1038/nbt751.

Patterson, J., & Hubbell, J. A. (2010). Enhanced proteolytic degradation of molecularly engineered PEG hydrogels in response to MMP-1 and MMP-2. *Biomaterials*, *31*(30), 7836–7845. https://doi.org/10.1016/j.biomaterials.2010.06.061.

Peckham, P. H., Ackermann, D. M., & Moss, C. W. (2013). The role of biomaterials in stimulating bioelectrodes. In *Biomaterials Science: An Introduction to Materials: Third Edition*. https://doi.org/10.1016/B978-0-08-087780-8.00084-X.

Perale, G., Rossi, F., Sundstrom, E., Bacchiega, S., Masi, M., Forloni, G., & Veglianese, P. (2011). Hydrogels in spinal cord injury repair strategies. *ACS Chemical Neuroscience*. https://doi.org/10.1021/cn200030w.

Piantino, J., Burdick, J. A., Goldberg, D., Langer, R., & Benowitz, L. I. (2006). An injectable, biodegradable hydrogel for trophic factor delivery enhances axonal rewiring and improves performance after spinal cord injury. *Experimental Neurology*, *201*(2), 359–367. https://doi.org/https://doi.org/10.1016/j.expneurol.2006.04.020.

Prestwich, G. D., Marecak, D. M., Marecek, J. F., Vercruysse, K. P., & Ziebell, M. R. (1998). Controlled chemical modification of hyaluronic acid: Synthesis, applications, and biodegradation of hydrazide derivatives. *Journal of Controlled Release*. https://doi.org/10.1016/S0168-3659(97)00242-3.

Qian, T., Guo, X., Levi, A. D., Vanni, S., Shebert, R. T., & Sipski, M. L. (2005). High-dose methylprednisolone may cause myopathy in acute spinal cord injury patients. 199–203. https://doi.org/10.1038/sj.sc.3101681.

Ren, Y., Yang, X., Ma, Z., Sun, X., Zhang, Y., Li, W., Yang, H., Qiang, L., Yang, Z., Liu, Y., Deng, C., Zhou, L., Wang, T., Lin, J., Li, T., Wu, T., & Wang, J. (2021). Developments and opportunities for 3D bioprinted organoids. *International Journal of Bioprinting*, *7*(3), 364. https://doi.org/10.18063/ijb.v7i3.364.

Rowe, R.C., Sheskey, P.J. and Quinn, M.E. (2009) Handbook of Pharmaceutical Excipients. 6th Edition, Pharmaceutical Press, 506–509.

Saha, K., Keung, A. J., Irwin, E. F., Li, Y., Little, L., Schaffer, D. V., & Healy, K. E. (2008). Substrate modulus directs neural stem cell behavior. *Biophysical Journal*, *95*(9), 4426–4438. https://doi.org/https://doi.org/10.1529/biophysj.108.132217.

Sakiyama-Elbert, S. E., & Hubbell, J. A. (2000). Controlled release of nerve growth factor from a heparin-containing fibrin-based cell ingrowth matrix. *Journal of Controlled Release*, *69*(1), 149–158. https://doi.org/https://doi.org/10.1016/S0168-3659(00)00296-0.

Salaris, F., Colosi, C., Brighi, C., Soloperto, A., de Turris, V., Benedetti, M. C., Ghirga, S., Rosito, M., Di Angelantonio, S., & Rosa, A. (2019). 3D bioprinted human cortical neural constructs derived from induced pluripotent stem cells. *Journal of Clinical Medicine*. https://doi.org/10.3390/jcm8101595.

Salgado, A. J., Sousa, N., Silva, N. A., Neves, N. M., & Reis, R. L. (2008). Hydrogels for spinal cord injury regeneration. *Natural-Based Polymers for Biomedical Applications*. https://doi.org/10.1533/9781845694814.4.570.

Sanghvi, A. B., Miller, K. P. H., Belcher, A. M., & Schmidt, C. E. (2005). Biomaterials functionalization using a novel peptide that selectively binds to a conducting polymer. *Nature Materials*. https://doi.org/10.1038/nmat1397.

Schense, J. C., Bloch, J., Aebischer, P., & Hubbell, J. A. (2000). Enzymatic incorporation of bioactive peptides into fibrin matrices enhances neurite extension. *Nature Biotechnology*, *18*(4), 415–419. https://doi.org/10.1038/74473.

Schmidt, C. E., & Leach, J. B. (2003). Neural tissue engineering: Strategies for repair and regeneration. *Annual Review of Biomedical Engineering*, *5*(1), 293–347. https://doi.org/10.1146/annurev.bioeng.5.011303.120731.

Seidlits, S. K., Khaing, Z. Z., Petersen, R. R., Nickels, J. D., Vanscoy, J. E., Shear, J. B., & Schmidt, C. E. (2010). The effects of hyaluronic acid hydrogels with tunable mechanical properties on neural progenitor cell differentiation. *Biomaterials*, *31*(14), 3930–3940. https://doi.org/10.1016/j.biomaterials.2010.01.125.

Senthilkumar, K. S., Saravanan, K. S., Chandra, G., Sindhu, K. M., Jayakrishnan, A., & Mohanakumar, K. P. (2007). Unilateral implantation of dopamine-loaded biodegradable hydrogel in the striatum attenuates motor abnormalities in the 6-hydroxydopamine model of hemi-parkinsonism. *Behavioural Brain Research*, *184*(1), 11–18. https://doi.org/https://doi.org/10.1016/j.bbr.2007.06.025.

Shanbhag, M. S., Lathia, J. D., Mughal, M. R., Francis, N. L., Pashos, N., Mattson, M. P., & Wheatley, M. A. (2010). Neural progenitor cells grown on hydrogel surfaces respond to the product of the transgene of encapsulated genetically engineered fibroblasts. *Biomacromolecules*, *11*(11), 2936–2943. https://doi.org/10.1021/bm100699q.

Sharp, K. G., Dickson, A. R., Marchenko, S. A., Yee, K. M., Emery, P. N., Laidmåe, I., Uibo, R., Sawyer, E. S., Steward, O., & Flanagan, L. A. (2012). Salmon fibrin treatment of spinal cord injury promotes functional recovery and density of serotonergic innervation. *Experimental Neurology*. https://doi.org/10.1016/j.expneurol.2012.02.016.

Shi, G., Rouabhia, M., Wang, Z., Dao, L. H., & Zhang, Z. (2004). A novel electrically conductive and biodegradable composite made of polypyrrole nanoparticles and polylactide. *Biomaterials*. https://doi.org/10.1016/j.biomaterials.2003.09.032.

Shoichet, M. S. (2010). Polymer scaffolds for biomaterials applications. *Macromolecules*. https://doi.org/10.1021/ma901530r.

Shu, X. Z., & Zhu, K. J. (2002). Controlled drug release properties of ionically cross-linked chitosan beads: The influence of anion structure. *International Journal of Pharmaceutics*. https://doi.org/10.1016/S0378-5173(01)00943-7.

Siddique, R., & Thakor, N. (2014). Investigation of nerve injury through microfluidic devices. *Journal of the Royal Society Interface*. https://doi.org/10.1098/rsif.2013.0676.

Silva, G. A., Czeisler, C., Niece, K. L., Beniash, E., Harrington, D. A., Kessler, J. A., & Stupp, S. I. (2004). Selective differentiation of neural progenitor cells by high-epitope density nanofibers. *Science*. https://doi.org/10.1126/science.1093783.

Spiller, K. L., Holloway, J. L., Gribb, M. E., & Lowman, A. M. (2011). Design of semi-degradable hydrogels based on poly(vinyl alcohol) and poly(lactic-co-glycolic acid) for cartilage tissue engineering. *Journal of Tissue Engineering and Regenerative Medicine*, *5*(8), 636–647. https://doi.org/https://doi.org/10.1002/term.356.

Stabenfeldt, S. E., Garcia, A. J., & LaPlaca, M. C. (2006). Thermoreversible laminin-functionalized hydrogel for neural tissue engineering. *Journal of Biomedical Materials Research - Part A*. https://doi.org/10.1002/jbm.a.30638.

Stokols, S., & Tuszynski, M. H. (2004). The fabrication and characterization of linearly oriented nerve guidance scaffolds for spinal cord injury. *Biomaterials*. https://doi.org/10.1016/j.biomaterials.2004.01.041.

Stokols, S., & Tuszynski, M. H. (2006). Freeze-dried agarose scaffolds with uniaxial channels stimulate and guide linear axonal growth following spinal cord injury. *Biomaterials*. https://doi.org/10.1016/j.biomaterials.2005.06.039.

Straley, K. S., Foo, C. W. P., & Heilshorn, S. C. (2010). Biomaterial design strategies for the treatment of spinal cord injuries. *Journal of Neurotrauma*, *27*(1), 1–19. https://doi.org/10.1089/neu.2009.0948.

Stukel, J. M., & Willits, R. K. (2018). The interplay of peptide affinity and scaffold stiffness on neuronal differentiation of neural stem cells. *Biomedical Materials (Bristol, England)*, *13*(2), 24102. https://doi.org/10.1088/1748-605X/aa9a4b.

Subramanian, A., Krishnan, U. M., & Sethuraman, S. (2009). Development of biomaterial scaffold for nerve tissue engineering: Biomaterial mediated neural regeneration. *Journal of Biomedical Science*, *16*, 108. https://doi.org/10.1186/1423-0127-16-108.

Sundararaghavan, H. G., Monteiro, G. A., Firestein, B. L., & Shreiber, D. I. (2009). Neurite growth in 3D collagen gels with gradients of mechanical properties. *Biotechnology and Bioengineering*. https://doi.org/10.1002/bit.22074.

Tabata, Y. (2005). Significance of release technology in tissue engineering. *Drug Discovery Today*, *10*(23–24), 1639–1646. https://doi.org/10.1016/S1359-6446(05)03639-1.

Tabata, Y. (2009). Biomaterial technology for tissue engineering applications. *Journal of the Royal Society Interface*. https://doi.org/10.1098/rsif.2008.0448.focus.

Tate, M. C., Shear, D. A., Hoffman, S. W., Stein, D. G., & LaPlaca, M. C. (2001). Biocompatibility of methylcellulose-based constructs designed for intracerebral gelation following experimental traumatic brain injury. *Biomaterials*, *22*(10), 1113–1123. https://doi.org/10.1016/S0142-9612(00)00348-3.

Taylor, S. J., Rosenzweig, E. S., McDonald, J. W., & Sakiyama-Elbert, S. E. (2006). Delivery of neurotrophin-3 from fibrin enhances neuronal fiber sprouting after spinal cord injury. *Journal of Controlled Release*, *113*(3), 226–235. https://doi.org/https://doi.org/10.1016/j.jconrel.2006.05.005.

Thonhoff, J. R., Lou, D. I., Jordan, P. M., Zhao, X., & Wu, P. (2007). Compatibility of human fetal neural stem cells with hydrogel biomaterials in vitro. *Brain Research, 1187*, 42–51. https://doi.org/10.1016/j.brainres.2007.10.046.

Tibbitt, M. W., & Anseth, K. S. (2009). Hydrogels as extracellular matrix mimics for 3D cell culture. *Biotechnology and Bioengineering, 103*(4), 655–663. https://doi.org/https://doi.org/10.1002/bit.22361.

Tobias, C. A., Han, S. S. W., Shumsky, J. S., Kim, D., Tumolo, M., Dhoot, N. O., Wheatley, M. A., Fischer, I., Tessler, A., & Murray, M. (2005). Alginate encapsulated BDNF-producing fibroblast grafts permit recovery of function after spinal cord injury in the absence of immune suppression. *Journal of Neurotrauma, 22*(1), 138–156. https://doi.org/10.1089/neu.2005.22.138.

Tsai, E. C., Dalton, P. D., Shoichet, M. S., & Tator, C. H. (2004). Synthetic hydrogel guidance channels facilitate regeneration of adult rat brainstem motor axons after complete spinal cord transection. *Journal of Neurotrauma*. https://doi.org/10.1089/0897715041269687.

Tsai, E. C., Dalton, P. D., Shoichet, M. S., & Tator, C. H. (2006). Matrix inclusion within synthetic hydrogel guidance channels improves specific supraspinal and local axonal regeneration after complete spinal cord transection. *Biomaterials*. https://doi.org/10.1016/j.biomaterials.2005.07.025.

Tuft, B. W., Zhang, L., Xu, L., Hangartner, A., Leigh, B., Hansen, M. R., & Guymon, C. A. (2014). Material stiffness effects on neurite alignment to photopolymerized micropatterns. *Biomacromolecules, 15*(10), 3717–3727. https://doi.org/10.1021/bm501019s.

Tysseling-Mattiace, V. M., Sahni, V., Niece, K. L., Birch, D., Czeisler, C., Fehlings, M. G., Stupp, S. I., & Kessler, J. A. (2008). Self-assembling nanofibers inhibit glial scar formation and promote axon elongation after spinal cord injury. *Journal of Neuroscience*. https://doi.org/10.1523/JNEUROSCI.0143-08.2008.

Uz, M., & Mallapragada, S. K. (2019). Conductive polymers and hydrogels for neural tissue engineering. *Journal of the Indian Institute of Science*. https://doi.org/10.1007/s41745-019-00126-8.

Uzel, S. G. M., Amadi, O. C., Pearl, T. M., Lee, R. T., So, P. T. C., & Kamm, R. D. (2016). Simultaneous or sequential orthogonal gradient formation in a 3D cell culture microfluidic platform. *Small, 12*(5), 612–622. https://doi.org/https://doi.org/10.1002/smll.201501905.

Valmikinathan, C. M., Mukhatyar, V. J., Jain, A., Karumbaiah, L., Dasari, M., & Bellamkonda, R. V. (2012). Photocrosslinkable chitosan based hydrogels for neural tissue engineering. *Soft Matter, 8*(6), 1964–1976. https://doi.org/10.1039/c1sm06629c.

Vedadghavami, A., Minooei, F., Mohammadi, M. H., Khetani, S., Rezaei Kolahchi, A., Mashayekhan, S., & Sanati-Nezhad, A. (2017). Manufacturing of hydrogel biomaterials with controlled mechanical properties for tissue engineering applications. *Acta Biomaterialia, 62*(July 2018), 42–63. https://doi.org/10.1016/j.actbio.2017.07.028.

Vindigni, V., Cortivo, R., Iacobellis, L., Abatangelo, G., & Zavan, B. (2009). Hyaluronan benzyl ester as a scaffold for tissue engineering. *International Journal of Molecular Sciences, 10*(7), 2972–2985. https://doi.org/10.3390/ijms10072972.

von Burkersroda, F., Schedl, L., & Göpferich, A. (2002). Why degradable polymers undergo surface erosion or bulk erosion. *Biomaterials, 23*(21), 4221–4231. https://doi.org/https://doi.org/10.1016/S0142-9612(02)00170-9.

Wang, C. H., Dong, Y. Q., Sengothi, K., Tan, K. L., & Kang, E. T. (1999). In-vivo tissue response to polyaniline. *Synthetic Metals*. https://doi.org/10.1016/S0379-6779(98)01006-6.

Wang, G., Wang, X., & Huang, L. (2017). Feasibility of chitosan-alginate (Chi-Alg) hydrogel used as scaffold for neural tissue engineering: A pilot study in vitro. *Biotechnology and Biotechnological Equipment, 31*(4), 766–773. https://doi.org/10.1080/13102818.2017.1332493.

Wang, T., Turhan, M., & Gunasekaran, S. (2004a). Selected properties of pH-sensitive, biodegradable chitosan–poly(vinyl alcohol) hydrogel. *Polymer International, 53*(7), 911–918. https://doi.org/https://doi.org/10.1002/pi.1461.

Wang, X., Gu, X., Yuan, C., Chen, S., Zhang, P., Zhang, T., Yao, J., Chen, F., & Chen, G. (2004b). Evaluation of biocompatibility of polypyrrole in vitro and in vivo. *Journal of Biomedical Materials Research - Part A*. https://doi.org/10.1002/jbm.a.20065.

Wang, Y., Tan, H., & Hui, X. (2018). Biomaterial scaffolds in regenerative therapy of the central nervous system. *BioMed Research International*. https://doi.org/10.1155/2018/7848901.

Wei, Y.-T., Sun, X.-D., Xia, X., Cui, F.-Z., He, Y., Liu, B.-F., & Xu, Q.-Y. (2009). Hyaluronic acid hydrogel modified with nogo-66 receptor antibody and poly(L-Lysine) enhancement of adherence and survival of primary hippocampal neurons. *Journal of Bioactive and Compatible Polymers*, *24*(3), 205–219. https://doi.org/10.1177/0883911509102266.

Woerly, S., Petrov, P., Syková, E., Roitbak, T., Simonová, Z., & Harvey, A. R. (1999). Neural tissue formation within porous hydrogels implanted in brain and spinal cord lesions: Ultrastructural, immunohistochemical, and diffusion studies. *Tissue Engineering*. https://doi.org/10.1089/ten.1999.5.467.

Woerly, S., Pinet, E., De Robertis, L., Bousmina, M., Laroche, G., Roitback, T., Vargová, L., & Syková, E. (1998). Heterogeneous PHPMA hydrogels for tissue repair and axonal regeneration in the injured spinal cord. *Journal of Biomaterials Science. Polymer Edition*, *9*(7), 681–711. https://doi.org/10.1163/156856298x00091.

Wood, M. D., Borschel, G. H., & Sakiyama-Elbert, S. E. (2009). Controlled release of glial-derived neurotrophic factor from fibrin matrices containing an affinity-based delivery system. *Journal of Biomedical Materials Research Part A*, *89A*(4), 909–918. https://doi.org/https://doi.org/10.1002/jbm.a.32043.

Xu, Y., & Guan, J. (2016). Interaction of cells with polyurethane scaffolds. In *Advances in Polyurethane Biomaterials*. https://doi.org/10.1016/B978-0-08-100614-6.00018-4

Yang, C. Y., Song, B., Ao, Y., Nowak, A. P., Abelowitz, R. B., Korsak, R. A., Havton, L. A., Deming, T. J., & Sofroniew, M. V. (2009). Biocompatibility of amphiphilic diblock copolypeptide hydrogels in the central nervous system. *Biomaterials*, *30*(15), 2881–2898. https://doi.org/10.1016/j.biomaterials.2009.01.056.

Yu, L. M. Y., Kazazian, K., & Shoichet, M. S. (2007). Peptide surface modification of methacrylamide chitosan for neural tissue engineering applications. *Journal of Biomedical Materials Research - Part A*. https://doi.org/10.1002/jbm.a.31069.

Yuan, Y., Zhang, P., Yang, Y., Wang, X., & Gu, X. (2004). The interaction of Schwann cells with chitosan membranes and fibers in vitro. *Biomaterials*. https://doi.org/10.1016/j.biomaterials.2003.11.029.

Zare, M., Bigham, A., Zare, M., Luo, H., Rezvani Ghomi, E., & Ramakrishna, S. (2021). Phema: An overview for biomedical applications. *International Journal of Molecular Sciences*. https://doi.org/10.3390/ijms22126376.

Zhang, S., Holmes, T. C., DiPersio, C. M., Hynes, R. O., Su, X., & Rich, A. (1995). Self-complementary oligopeptide matrices support mammalian cell attachment. *Biomaterials*. https://doi.org/10.1016/0142-9612(95)96874-Y.

Zhang, Z. N., Freitas, B. C., Qian, H., Lux, J., Acab, A., Trujillo, C. A., Herai, R. H., Huu, V. A. N., Wen, J. H., Joshi-Barr, S., Karpiak, J. V., Engler, A. J., Fu, X. D., Muotri, A. R., & Almutairi, A. (2016). Layered hydrogels accelerate iPSC-derived neuronal maturation and reveal migration defects caused by MeCP2 dysfunction. *Proceedings of the National Academy of Sciences of the United States of America*. https://doi.org/10.1073/pnas.1521255113.

Zhong, J., Chan, A., Morad, L., Kornblum, H. I., Fan, G., & Carmichael, S. T. (2010). Hydrogel matrix to support stem cell survival after brain transplantation in stroke. *Neurorehabilitation and Neural Repair*, *24*(7), 636–644. https://doi.org/10.1177/1545968310361958.

Zhou, W., Stukel, J. M., Cebull, H. L., & Willits, R. K. (2016). Tuning the mechanical properties of poly(Ethylene Glycol) microgel-based scaffolds to increase 3D schwann cell proliferation. *Macromolecular Bioscience*, *16*(4), 535–544. https://doi.org/https://doi.org/10.1002/mabi.201500336.

Zhu, J. (2010). Bioactive modification of poly(ethylene glycol) hydrogels for tissue engineering. *Biomaterials*, *31*(17), 4639–4656. https://doi.org/10.1016/j.biomaterials.2010.02.044.

Zhu, M., Wang, Y., Ferracci, G., Zheng, J., Cho, N. J., & Lee, B. H. (2019). Gelatin methacryloyl and its hydrogels with an exceptional degree of controllability and batch-to-batch consistency. *Scientific Reports*. https://doi.org/10.1038/s41598-019-42186-x.

Zhu, W., Castro, N. J., & Zhang, L. G. (2015). *Nanotechnology and 3D Bioprinting for Neural Tissue Regeneration* (1st Ed.). Elsevier Inc. https://doi.org/10.1016/B978-0-12-800547-7/00014-X.

4 Evolution of Biogenic Synthesized Scaffolds for Tissue Engineering Applications

Deepa Suhag and Yogita Basnal
Amity University, Haryana, India

CONTENTS

4.1 Introduction 78
4.1.1 Tissue Engineering 78
4.2 History of Biogenic Materials in Tissue Engineering/Reconstruction 79
4.2.1 Details of Biogenic Materials 80
4.2.1.1 Nacre Teeth from Sea Shell 80
4.2.1.2 Silicone Ball 81
4.2.1.3 Calcium Carbonate 81
4.2.1.4 Calcium Phosphate 82
4.2.1.5 Silk 82
4.2.1.6 Alginate 82
4.2.1.7 Chitosan 83
4.2.1.8 Collagen 83
4.2.1.9 Fibrin 84
4.2.1.10 Polyesters 84
4.2.2 Scaffold-Based Tissue Engineering 84
4.2.2.1 Scaffolds 84
4.2.2.2 Key Factors to Keep in Mind While Designing Optimal Scaffolds for Tissue Engineering Are 85
4.2.2.3 The Scaffolds Meant for Tissue Engineering Can Be Broadly Categorized under the Following Three Types 86
4.2.2.4 On the Basis of Origin and Chemical Composition, the Scaffolding Biomaterials Can Further Be Classified under Three Categories Which Are 87
4.2.3 Scaffold-Free Approach 87
4.2.4 Cells, Scaffolds, Biochemical Cues and Tissue Engineering 88
4.2.4.1 Characteristic Features of Cells Used in Tissue Engineering 88

DOI: 10.1201/9781003251767-4

4.2.4.2 Various Cell Types Used in Tissue Engineering and Their Classification Based on Different Criterion 90
4.3 Wound Healing Process: Acute and Chronic Wounds 91
4.4 Conclusion and Future Perspectives 92
References...93

4.1 INTRODUCTION

Tissue engineering is a multidisciplinary science that is now considered as a distinct branch in the field of science and technology and primarily relies on scaffolds, which can be of natural, semi-synthetic or synthetic origin.[1] In tissue engineering, the main focus is on scaffold development techniques to create physical templates to grow lost and damaged portions of the body.[2] Scaffolds are made up of materials that are analogous to the natural extracellular matrix (ECM) of our body.[1] Naturally occurring materials form scaffolds that have biocompatibility, biodegradability and non-toxicity and are therefore able to mimic natural ECM efficiently.[3]

Knowledge of the historical aspect of scaffolds, especially biogenic synthesized scaffolds for tissue engineering, is imminent because having sufficient knowledge of the evolution of biogenic platforms will aid in spearheading research in this area of science and provide future directions in the field of tissue engineering. Therefore, in this chapter, we understand how biogenic synthesized biomaterials have evolved over time. In the past, people belonging to the Mayan civilization used nacre teeth, which are made up of aragonite (calcium carbonate), for dental implants because they helped in the synthesis of vertebrate bones by producing calcium phosphate.[4,5] Subsequently, in 1891, a cemented ivory ball, which is another biogenic material, was employed by a German professor named Themistocles Glück for creating the ball-and-socket joint of the hip.[6] After some years, in 1939, cellophane was used for blood vessel replacement.[7] Here it is pertinent to mention that natural polymers such as silk, chitosan, etc. are some common polymers that are the main constituents of biogenic synthesized 3D scaffolds.[8,9] Also, the role of polyesters, which contain ester groups and are derived from plants and bacteria, cannot be overlooked when it comes to tissue engineering applications. Polyhydroxyalkanoates (PHAs) and polyhydroxybutyrate (PHB) are two such materials that are widely used in the fabrication of matrices required for tissue repair as well as organ transplant and ossification, respectively.[10]

4.1.1 Tissue Engineering

Trauma, diseases and congenital defects are the three main causes that lead to the damage and degeneration of human body tissues.[11,12] After the damage, it becomes necessary to initiate the repair, regeneration and even replacement of the injured/lost tissue with the help of some sophisticated biological substitutes so as to restore the function of the lost tissue. It can be accomplished with the help of tissue engineering, which is also known as regenerative medicine.[12] Living organisms have the innate ability to regenerate some of their body parts with the help of the molecular processes taking place inside their bodies, which are in turn directed by the body's genetic programming. In situ tissue regeneration is an approach in which the body's innate regenerative capability is integrated with engineered substitutes for tissue regeneration.[13] Tissue engineering is a multifaceted branch of science that integrates the principles of engineering and life sciences, i.e., the body's innate regenerative ability, to develop sophisticated scaffolds that can mimic natural body machinery to regenerate, restore and replace damaged tissue.[14] In addition to this, tissue engineering applies principles of some other branches of science including material sciences and medicine. After applying the knowledge of all the required branches of science, a tissue engineer must be able to either replace portions of lost tissues of organs such as the pancreas, cartilage, liver, heart, kidney, etc. or regenerate the complete organ.[3] A tissue engineer must integrate the knowledge of an engineer, a cell and molecular biologist, an immunologist, a material scientist and a surgeon to develop suitable scaffolds for tissue regeneration.[15] The knowledge of cell and molecular biology helps him understand the important molecular, biological, chemical and cellular events that are required for tissue and organ development. Material sciences are an integral part of tissue engineering because studying the material properties of tissues to be replaced helps in designing tissue substitutes with matching properties. The knowledge of engineering is useful in designing cost-effective bioreactors as well as biomaterials for growth and development of the lost tissue in vitro. As soon as the engineered tissue/organ is implanted into the injured body of the patient, the tissue engineer is required to closely monitor the activities of bioactive molecules, various cell types, and engineered tissues in speeding up the healing processes in vivo, just as a surgeon does.[3] Lastly, the tissue engineer needs to play the role of an immunologist because immune cells play a major role in wound healing and tissue damage. A close monitoring of the interaction of designed biomaterials and immune cells is therefore a very important aspect of tissue engineering.[12] Currently, tissue engineering is being used to engineer almost every tissue and organ of the body, including vital organs such as the kidney, intestine, heart muscles and valves, skin, pancreas and liver. Attempts are being made to engineer parts of connective tissues, including ligaments, tendon, bones and cartilage. Till now, organs such as the bladder, skin, airways (i.e. trachea and larynx), and bone implants have been successfully engineered.[3]

4.2 HISTORY OF BIOGENIC MATERIALS IN TISSUE ENGINEERING/RECONSTRUCTION

Tissue engineering has been in practice even before the term "tissue engineering" was officially coined in 1988 at a National Science Foundation workshop.[11] The idea of tissue engineering has fascinated humans since ancient times. One such example is that of the fabled Prometheus. According to Greek mythology, Prometheus (the god of fire) stole the secret of fire to introduce it to humans, and was tortured for this by Zeus by being chained to a mountain peak. Every day, an eagle was sent by Zeus to feast on chained Prometheus's liver as a part of the punishment. However, overnight, Prometheus's liver regenerated, and his ordeal would resume the next morning.[16] Ancient literature is full of the regenerative potential of claws, limbs, liver and antlers. Aristotle (384–322 BC) observed regenerative

TABLE 4.1
Tabulated Representation of History of Biogenic Materials

S. No.	Year	Material/Biomaterial	Application
1.	600 AD	Nacre teeth from seashell	Bone graft substitution[26]
2.	1891	Natural ivory	Femoral heads[6]
3.	1960	Silicone ball	Heart valve[28]
4.	1961	Silicone gel	Breast implants[30]
5.	1990s	Calcium carbonate	Bone graft application[31]
6.	1920	Calcium phosphate	Ossification[33]
7.	18th century	Silk	Tendon tissue engineering[9]
8.	1983	Alginate	Wound dressing material[37]
9.	1926	Chitosan	In the form of membrane[8]
10.	20th century	Collagen	As a biomaterial[56]
11.	1909	Fibrin	As a hemostat[64]
12.	1996	Polyesters (Polyhydroxyalkanoates)	Orthopedic and regeneration purposes[10]

capability in lizards and snakes, which could re-grow amputated parts. Abraham Trembley, in 1740, successfully developed a nine-headed hydra.[17] A pathologist, Rudolf Virchow (1821–1902), studied cells and subsequently established that tissue regeneration has something to do with cell proliferation.[18] It was only after the invention of the microscope in the 1600s, that Robert Hooke was able to discover cells; prior to this, until the mid-seventeenth century, scientists were unaware of the existence of cells.[19] Later on, in 1838, Matthias Jakob Schleiden, a German botanist, in collaboration with Theodor Schwann, a German zoologist, formulated the cell theory, and it was only after that modern biology could progress.[20] By the early nineteenth century, we were able to grow mammalian animal cells in test tubes.[21] In the early 1930s, Charles Lindbergh, a famous aviator, and Alexis Carrel, the 1912 Nobel Prize winner in Physiology and Medicine, were able to culture whole organs successfully. Lindbergh contributed as a bioengineer because he invented a sophisticated system known as the "bombeador of perfusión" that could maintain adult tissues such as cardiac tissue alive for so many weeks.[22] In the 1960s, the discovery of growth factors was a major breakthrough in the field of tissue engineering.[23] In Table 4.1, some important biogenic synthesized biomaterials are enlisted in the chronological order of their uses.

4.2.1 Details of Biogenic Materials

4.2.1.1 Nacre Teeth from Sea Shell

Nacre, or mother of pearl, is naturally found in the shell material of mollusks.[24] Mostly, it comprises two layers with typical microstructures. One of the layers is the calcite layer, whereas another layer, which is the inner layer, is aragonite.[25] Calcite and aragonite are two polymorphs of calcium carbonate.[5] Nacre is filled with calcium carbonate crystallized in a matrix made up of protein and polysaccharide.[24] It is a well-known fact that the shells of invertebrates can trigger bone formation, but nacre can do osteoinduction as well as osteointegration. The use of nacre from seashells for dental implants was first done by people belonging to the Mayan civilization in 600 AD. Nowadays, the same kind of procedure is termed as osseointegration.[26] Nacre induces osteogenesis by the production of calcium phosphate, which is the main constituent of bones. Mayan people exploited this property of nacre for dental implants, which is confirmed by the discovery of Mayan skulls with shell dental implants.[5] The capability of nacre to get incorporated into bone tissue and induce differentiation of stem cells into osteoblasts can be utilized in biomedical fields such as orthopedic or dental areas.[25]

4.2.1.2 Silicone Ball

Naturally, silicon is extracted from the endo- and exoskeletons of marine organisms.[27] A silicone ball was used in tissue engineering for the first time in 1960 by Starr and M. Lowell Edwards when it was successfully implanted into the mitral and aortic valve.[28] The silicone elastomer rubber ball showed promising results because of its small size, which made it very easy to place it inside the heart itself.[29] The function of the heart valves is to allow the flow of blood unidirectionally throughout the day without any backflow. During this course, the heart valves passively open and close over 100 000 times per day. But a diseased heart valve is unable to perform its function, which leads to backflow of blood, which can result in abnormal pressure gradients in the heart.[28] The main advantage of using silicone-based heart valves is that they are quite flexible and biocompatible. But their low durability, thickening, tearing and thrombosis formation are limitations in their usage in heart tissue engineering applications.[29] In addition to this, silicon is known to play an important role during the initial stage of bone mineralization because it promotes calcium phosphate precipitation during the process. It also plays an important role in improving the quality of the ECM by facilitating the interaction of collagen and proteoglycans. Other functions of silicone include the differentiation of stem cells in osteoblasts as well as osteocytes. It also serves an inhibitory function by restricting the formation of osteoclasts and bone resorption.[27] Silicone has great mechanical properties and chemical stability. Being inert in nature and hydrophobic, it is highly biocompatible. Silicone has therefore found application in various tissue engineering applications, such as medical inserts, urinary catheters, reconstructive gel fillers and metatarsophalangeal joint implants in bone tissue engineering. But silicone implants are susceptible to microbial infection, which limits their application as a biomaterial.[30]

4.2.1.3 Calcium Carbonate

Biogenic calcium carbonate is harnessed from mussels, sea coral, egg shells and nacre venus verrucosa. The commercial use of calcium carbonate initially started in the 1990s. The stony skeleton of corals is highly porous. Surprisingly, the pore structure of corals resembles trabecular bone, due to which it has found application in bone grafts, i.e. in bone tissue engineering. This porous three-dimensional (3D) structure triggers hard tissue growth as soon as it is resorbed, and subsequently, new bone replaces it. But its low mechanical strength makes it unsuitable for those applications that require load bearing.[31]

4.2.1.4 Calcium Phosphate

Clams, corals, cuttlefish, red algae, sea urchins, sponges, etc. are some of the natural sources of biogenic calcium phosphates.[32] Biomaterials consisting of calcium phosphate were used in tissue engineering for the first time in 1920 by Albee for human bone recovery. It has been widely used in tissue engineering for the last 50 years.[33] Their potential to chemically bind with hard tissue and provide stability to the damaged bone makes them a promising biomaterial for bone implantation. They have the potential to upregulate osteogenesis, and they can also get incorporated into defects in the form of granules. As scaffolding biomaterials, they allow rapid passage of large amounts of cells onto their surface and also promote cell proliferation.[34,35] Their great biocompatibility, osteoconductive and osteoinductive potential make them one of the best candidates as a scaffolding material for bone tissue engineering. However, their weak resorption and brittleness limit their use in bone tissue engineering applications.[32,34]

4.2.1.5 Silk

Silk was first used in biomedical applications in the 18th century as a suturing material.[9] However, nowadays it has found an application as a scaffolding biomaterial too. Naturally, silkworms, spiders, scorpions, mites and flies are the major sources of silk.[36] Silk has excellent mechanical properties, biocompatibility, low toxicity and porosity, due to which it is extensively used in various tissue engineering applications. In bone tissue engineering applications, they are known to induce cell attachment, cell differentiation and calcium phosphate deposition, which ultimately lead to calcification. Apart from this, scaffolding materials made up of silk fibroin have also been used in heart muscle regeneration, i.e. cardiac tissue regeneration, hepatic tissue regeneration, bladder tissue regeneration, ocular tissue regeneration, vascular tissue regeneration, neural tissue regeneration, skin tissue regeneration, cartilage tissue regeneration, ligament and tendon tissue regeneration, tracheal tissue regeneration and eardrum tissue regeneration. But their brittleness is a restraint in their usage as a scaffolding material in tissue engineering applications.[9,36]

4.2.1.6 Alginate

Alginate as a wound dressing material was first introduced in 1983. Alginate is a natural, linear and hydrophilic polysaccharide that is extracted from the cell walls of marine algae and some bacteria.[37–42] Sodium alginate is another linear copolymer.[43] Both sodium alginate and alginate are copolymers of β-(1 → 4) linked d-mannuronic acid (M) and α-(1 → 4) linked l-guluronic acid (G) units.[44] Upon hydration, alginate gets converted into a gel state.[38] It is quite economic, has high water absorbing potential, is biocompatible, easy to process and is ubiquitous.[40] It is widely used in wound healing in the form of hydrogels. Apart from this, it is also being used in bone tissue engineering.[41] But it has low mechanical strength because of the reversibility of the interlinking bonds, a higher degradation rate and its hydrophilic nature, which makes it non-adhesive.[45] Slow hemostasis and the inability to restrict pathogen infections are some other flaws associated with alginate-based scaffolds.[40] Sodium alginate-based hydrogels are also appropriate as wound healing scaffolds because they exhibit good biocompatibility.[42]

4.2.1.7 Chitosan

The first incidence of chitosan being used commercially was reported in 1926, when it was used in the form of membranes.[8] Chitosan is a biopolymer derived from the natural polymer chitin, which is extracted from the shells of crustaceans, insect exoskeletons and fungal cell walls, where it is known to provide strength and stability.[46–49] In contrast to this, chitosan is naturally found only in the cell walls of certain fungus.[49] After cellulose, chitosan is the second most ubiquitous polysaccharide that is found naturally.[50] Chitin is a derivative of glucose and is a hydrophobic linear homopolymer with a high molecular weight.[49,51] Chitosan is a suitable candidate for designing scaffolds that are used in tissue engineering applications because of its porous structure, gel-forming characteristics, biocompatibility, biodegradability, antimicrobial activity, non-toxicity, mucoadhesive properties, analgesic characteristics and adjustable viscosity. [48,49,52,53] Also, upon degradation, it generates harmless amino sugars in the human body.[48] It is easily metabolized in the human body with the help of lysozyme and certain other enzymes.[46] Chitosan-based scaffolds play a vital role in each stage of wound healing. The reason why it is suitable for scaffolding material in tissue engineering applications is because it has good mechanical properties, porosity, biocompatibility, wound healing potential and tissue replacement ability.[8] In view of the aforementioned properties, it has been exploited in the fields of bone tissue engineering, cartilage tissue engineering and neural tissue engineering.[54] The reason why neat chitosan is not used for developing hydrogels is because of its brittleness and low mechanical properties, but these disadvantages can be easily overcome by blending chitosan with certain synthetic polymers.[55]

4.2.1.8 Collagen

The first ever use of a collagen-based biomaterial dates back to the early twentieth century.[56] In the body, fibroblasts are known to synthesize collagen, which mainly serves the function of supporting and maintaining structural integrity.[57,58] Apart from this, it also regulates tissue development and provides shape, texture and resilience.[58] During wound healing, it helps in the initiation of cellular and molecular cascades, which are essential for tissue regeneration and wound debridement and ultimately results into wound healing.[57]

Collagen is a type of fibrous protein that has a helical structure.[58,59] It is the most abundant protein found in the bodies of mammals and accounts for approximately one-third of all the body proteins in all vertebrates.[58,60] So far, 29 different types of collagen proteins have been identified. Bovine, porcine, equine and avian are the terrestrial vertebrates from which collagen is mainly extracted. Besides this, some aquatic animals, such as fish, as well as tiny invertebrates like jellyfish, squid and sponges, are also sources of collagen protein.[61] Among all types of collagen, collagen type I is the most abundant constituent of the ECM of skin, bone and tendon.[59] Collagen protein, whether extracted from terrestrial or aquatic animals, has a common structure in which three alpha chains are coiled in a right-handed manner to form triple helices.[61] Collagen, being highly biocompatible, biodegradable and least immunogenic as compared to other natural polymers, is of immense use for developing biomaterials that are meant for tissue substitution, tissue regeneration, matrix remodeling and tissue repair.[58,60] Additionally, collagen also has fibril-synthesizing self-assembling characteristics, which make it a suitable biomaterial for making wound healing scaffolds.[60] Apart from this, it is also used for dermal, cardiovascular and connective tissue engineering applications.[56] Collagen is able to perform all the aforementioned functions because of its ability to promote cross-linking; however, due to its poor thermal stability, mechanical strength, antibacterial properties and enzymatic resistance, its use in biomedical applications such as wound healing dressing material is not recommended.[57,60,62] Marine collagen is often preferred over mammalian collagen by researchers because of two main reasons: one is that marine collagen restricts the transmission of infection. Another reason is associated with religious beliefs.[63] It is a common observation that at the time of extraction, the natural cross-linking and self-assembling properties of collagen are compromised, which leads to a reduction in mechanical strength and less stability in the extracted collagen as compared to the collagen that is found naturally in the body of the organism from which it is extracted.[60]

4.2.1.9 Fibrin

The first use of fibrin was made by Bergel in 1909 as a hemostat. Subsequently, Medawar and Matras used it as an adhesive in 1940 and for nerve attachment in 1972, respectively. Later on, in 1998, it was declared as the first sealant material for hemostatic application by the Food and Drug Administration (FDA) in the USA.[64]

4.2.1.10 Polyesters

Polyhydoxyalkanoates (PHAs), which are a type of polyesters, were first used in tissue engineering in 1996 for orthopedic and regeneration purposes. Poly(3-hydroxybutyrate-co-3-hydroxyvalerate) (PHBV), which is a PHA copolyester, was made to transform into 3D foams so as to regenerate chondrocytes and osteoblasts.[10] Beijerinck was the first person to notice PHAs as inclusion bodies inside the bacteria.[65]

4.2.2 Scaffold-Based Tissue Engineering

4.2.2.1 Scaffolds

The central purpose of a scaffold is to provide a platform for supportive and conductive matrices for ideal tissue reconstruction. Such biogenic scaffolds are ideally 3D matrices that can imitate natural ECM to temporarily facilitate cell migration and proliferation and their differentiation by providing a desired environment leading to the formation of desired tissue and organ types.[66] In a scaffold-based approach, a template is required to facilitate cell adherence, proliferation and migration for the ultimate regeneration of 3D tissues.[2] An ideal template/scaffolding material must have a biocompatible, mechanically stable and porous structure that can facilitate gaseous exchange and transport of nutrients and metabolites effectively. They should also be porous or permeable structures for establishing interpenetrating networks for optimal tissue development by providing structural support as well as a biochemical environment for promoting angiogenesis, nerve formation, muscle regeneration and bone regeneration. Table 4.2 represents how engineered tissues mimic the function of the natural ECM of the body.

4.2.2.2 Key Factors to Keep in Mind While Designing Optimal Scaffolds for Tissue Engineering Are

i. Mechanical properties, which include stiffness and elastic modulus;
ii. Physicochemical requirements such as porosity, rate of degradation and surface chemistry;

TABLE 4.2
ECM Function Inside Natural Body and the Analogous Function of the Engineered Scaffolding Material in Various Tissues

S. No.	Function of ECM in Native Tissues	Analogous Functions of Scaffolding Material in Engineered Tissues	Biological, Architectural and Mechanical Features of Scaffolding Biomaterial
1.	Provide structural support to residing cells	Give structural support to the exogenous cells so that they can attach and then grow, migrate and also differentiate, in vivo as well as in vitro	Must have binding sites for various cells, porosity and interconnecting junctions meant for cell migration and diffusion of nutrients. Must be resistant to immediate biodegradation
2.	Imparts mechanical property	Contributes to the shape and mechanical stability at the defective site within the tissue. Confers rigidity and stiffness to the engineered tissue	Must have good mechanical strength to fill up the void created due to injury/disease and must be capable of stimulating the native tissue
3.	Provides biological signals/cue so that cell can respond to the microenvironment	Proactively interacts with the cells so as to promote cell proliferation and differentiation	Must provide biological signals such as binding sites for cell adhesion and physical cues like surface topography
4.	Reservoir of biological cue such as growth factors	Acts as a delivery vehicle for growth-stimulating factors that are provided exogenously	Must be able to retain microstructures and other factors pertaining to the matrix via bioactive agents of scaffolding material
5.	Generate a flexible environment to promote processes such as remodeling during wound healing	Generation of a void 3D space so as to facilitate vascularization and generation of new tissue during the remodeling process	Must have porosity in the form of microstructures that allow diffusion of nutrients and metabolites, a controlled rate of degradation in the designed matrix and the degraded product must be biocompatible[1]

iii. Biological requirements such as cell adhesion, vascularization and biocompatibility[67];
iv. Surface to volume ratio, physical properties such as shape, structure and molecular weight and chemical behavior, i.e. chemical composition of the polymer used[68];
v. Other considerations include sterility and cost-effectiveness.[67]

4.2.2.3 The Scaffolds Meant for Tissue Engineering Can Be Broadly Categorized under the Following Three Types

i. Fibrous scaffolds

Fibrous biomaterials are of immense use in tissue engineering applications. The structure and diameter of the fiber play a very important role in scaffolding because they directly impact the behavior of the surrounding cells. The pore size of scaffolding biomaterials plays a very important role because it regulates the organization and activities of cells. The fibrous scaffolding material is quite efficient at mimicking the native ECM, which comprises proteinaceous fibers like collagen, elastin, fibronectin and laminin.

ii. Porous scaffolds

Porous scaffolding biomaterials are very efficient in transforming cells into biofunctional tissues because their large surface area is perfect for efficient attachment of cells such as fibroblasts, chondrocytes, etc. In porous scaffolds, the pores within are interconnected in a proper manner, which is of immense use because the interconnected networks allow infiltration of host cells, neo-vascularization and also promote the cell proliferation and ultimately their differentiation. All these features of porous scaffolds promote development of cells into functional tissues. The fabrication of the porous scaffolds can be done with the help of various techniques such as particulate leaching, freeze drying, phase separation, etc. Various natural and synthetic materials are used for developing porous scaffolding templates.

iii. Hydrogels

Hydrogels comprise polymer chains that form jelly-like structures and tend to swell manifold when they are placed in aqueous solutions. Owing to their swelling properties and hydrophilic nature, they are very efficient at retaining large amounts of water. At the same time, they are highly biocompatible. Their structure resembles natural tissues, which allows them to trap cells and give those cells the required structure and growth signal to develop into biofunctional structures. They are highly permeable to oxygen and nutrients and display low interfacial tension, which helps in migration of cells. It is very easy to modulate their elasticity because it depends on the type of cross-linking networks that are used to synthesize the hydrogels. The polymer networks in hydrogels can be covalently linked. Some common natural biomaterials that are used for synthesizing hydrogels are polysaccharides such as agarose, hyaluronan, alginate, methylcellulose, xyloglucan, etc. Synthetic materials commonly used for developing hydrogels are methacrylate, polyethylene glycol, etc.[3]

4.2.2.4 On the Basis of Origin and Chemical Composition, the Scaffolding Biomaterials Can Further Be Classified under Three Categories Which Are

i. Natural scaffolding material

These biomaterials are derived from living organisms. The main advantage of using such biomaterials is that they are highly biocompatible, least immunogenic, non-toxic, easily available and easy to harness from natural resources.. Their disposal is also easy because they are easily decomposed into carbon dioxide and water with the help of microbes.

ii. Synthetic scaffolding material

Synthetic biomaterials, on the other hand, have a consistent composition, large-scale production is easy and they are very cost-effective. They can be given any desired shape, and their mechanical properties can also be easily modulated.[68] They have precise control over pore size and degradation rate, display hydrophobicity and have good mechanical properties.[3] But they may produce inflammatory responses, which is not desirable.[68] Also, they require biomolecules to exhibit their biological function without their incorporation into biomolecules, they cannot perform their biological function, and their degradation products are very toxic.[3]

iii. Biosynthetic/Semi-synthetic/Hybrid scaffolding material

Both natural and synthetic biomaterials have their limitations. So, in order to overcome their limitations, biosynthetic polymers are developed. They possess features of both synthetic and natural biomaterials. In these materials, synthetic materials are functionalized via their modification with biopolymers.[69] Natural polymers have poor thermal stability, mechanical strength and enzymatic resistance.[60] Natural polymers also lack antibacterial properties.[54] But by blending/cross-linking natural materials with certain synthetic polymers with the help of chemical, physical or biological methods, it can be made a suitable candidate for biomedical applications because this type of cross-linking enhances mechanical as well as thermal stability, mechanical and tensile strength, and stiffness of natural biomaterials and reduces their enzymatic degradation.[60] Figure 4.1 represents the classification of various types of scaffolding materials and their common examples.

4.2.3 Scaffold-Free Approach

The scaffold-free approach, on the other hand, is a bottom-up approach that, instead of employing scaffolds, relies upon the innate ability of cells to grow and transform into 3D tissue and organ-like aggregates by self-assembly.[71] Cell sheets, spheroids and, contemporarily, tissue strands are being used as powerful tools to develop into tissue- and organ-like structures that facilitate ECM production.[2] But certain limitations of this type of tissue engineering approach, which include disorderly rates of degradation, immune reactions and the production of toxic degradation products, limit its use as a tissue engineering application.[72]

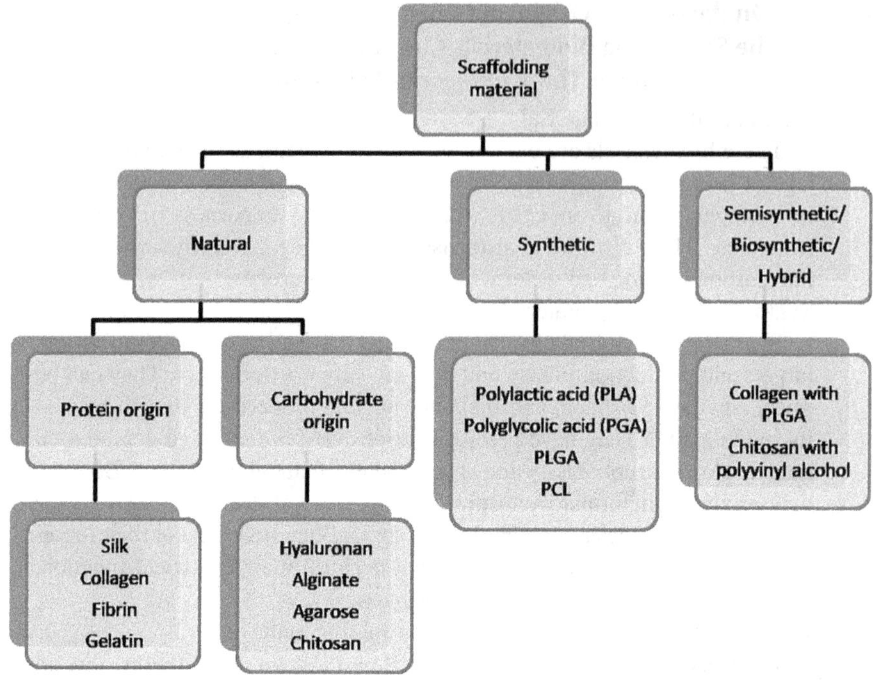

FIGURE 4.1 Flow chart for the classification of various types of scaffolding materials.[68,70]

4.2.4 Cells, Scaffolds, Biochemical Cues and Tissue Engineering

Cells, scaffolds and biochemical cues are generally considered as tissue engineering triad because they play a major role in regenerative medicine and tissue engineering.[1] Tissue engineering essentially has these three components. Living cells are required to promote the development of new tissue: an engineered template or porous scaffold is required to create a 3D environment to facilitate cell attachment and migration, their proliferation and their restructuring into 3D tissue-like structures. Multiple biological cues such as growth factors, cytokines, hormones such as corticosteroids, cell surface receptors to which the hormones bind to generate a response by initiating a signal transduction cascade, etc. are also essential to trigger the regeneration of new tissue constructs (Figure 4.2).

In addition to this, some other considerations of tissue engineering that cannot be overlooked are assembly methods and patient safety.

To sum up, the overall considerations of tissue engineering can be listed as represented in Figure 4.3[73, 74]:

4.2.4.1 Characteristic Features of Cells Used in Tissue Engineering

The building blocks of all the tissues are cells, and after an injury, when a tissue heals and regenerates, cells play a very important role.[73] In general, based on the type of system, the cells serve a variety of functions, including protein synthesis and the secretion of ECM. The cells used in tissue engineering must have the following characteristics:

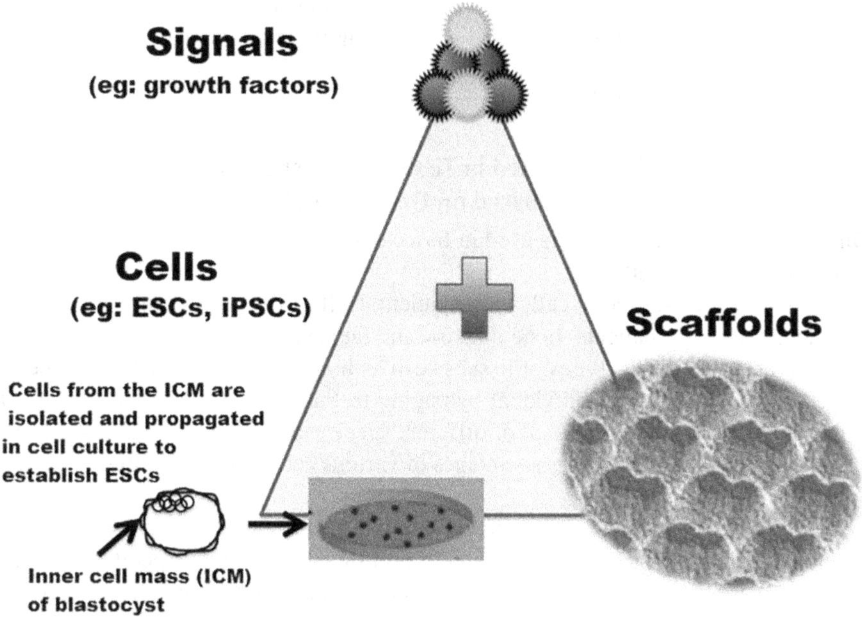

FIGURE 4.2 Important aspects of tissue engineering: Cells termed as embryonic stem cells (ESCs) and induced pluripotent stem cells (iPSCs), scaffolds and biochemical cues.[72]

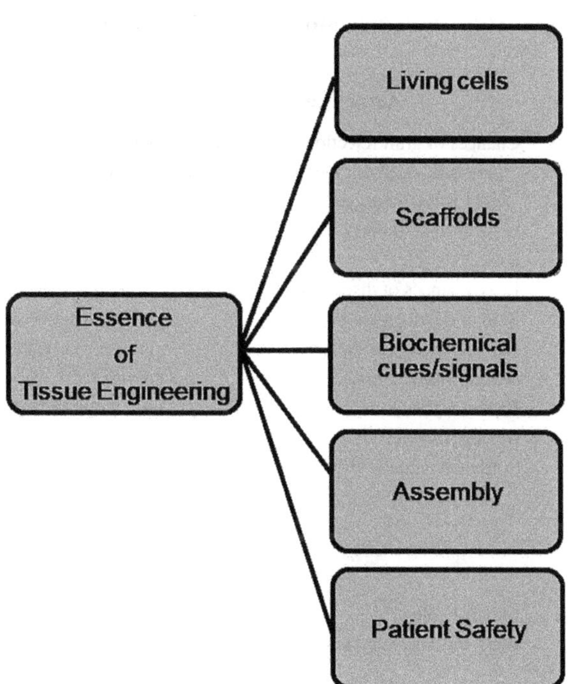

FIGURE 4.3 Various aspects of tissue engineering.

i. Expandability, which implies they must be available in sufficient amounts;
ii. Must be capable of surviving and maintaining function for an overall period of time;
iii. Must be compatible, i.e. non-immunogenic.[3]

4.2.4.2 Various Cell Types Used in Tissue Engineering and Their Classification Based on Different Criterion

On the basis of source, the cells used in tissue engineering can be **autologous, allogenic or xenogenic cells**.

The autologous source of cells is the patient itself.[72] Most commonly, mesenchymal stem cells from patients' bone marrow and fat serve the purpose, as they easily differentiate into various types of tissues such as bone, cartilage, etc. The source of allogenic cells is a donor individual belonging to the same species. The source of xenogenic cells is a donor animal of different species such as pig.[3,72] Table 4.3 summarizes the advantages and disadvantages of various cell sources required for tissue engineering.

On the basis of the extent of differentiation, the cells can be classified as tissue-specific differentiated cells, progenitor cells and stem cells. Tissue-specific differentiated cells are harvested from adult or neonatal tissue. Using them is advantageous because they are fully differentiated, so their separate differentiation into specific

TABLE 4.3
Tabulated Comparisons between Autologous, Allogenic, and Xenogenic Cell Sources

S. No.	Source	Advantages	Disadvantages
1.	Autologous	Chances of graft rejection are remote so there is no need of employing immune suppressive therapy; No ethical restraints; Biocompatible; Least chances of disease transmission; Rate of degradation is low; Less or no legal complications	Donor site morbidity, i.e. the donor site will have injury; Extraction of sufficient amount of cells is a difficult task; Two different operative sites get generated – the donor site and the recipient site which leads to greater risk and additional cost
2.	Allogenic	No morbidity at donor site; Highly viable donor cells; Healthy tissues; Sufficient amount of tissue is available	Provisional; Immunosuppressive therapy may be required; Risky because disease transmission may occur; More legal implication; Challenges such as ethical and psychological[74]
3.	Xenogenic	Reliable cells; Cells will be available in abundance	Higher risk of pathogen, i.e. zoonotic infection; Highest chances of immune rejection[3]

tissues is not required, due to which they already know how to perform their functions. For example, cardiomyocytes beat spontaneously. Another advantage of using tissue-specific differentiated cells is that they mostly have surface markers, due to which their purified population can be extracted easily. But they are fewer in quantity, and their ability to display proliferation is less as compared to stem cells and progenitor cells, which limits their use in tissue engineering. Progenitor cells are extracted from a fully grown adult individual, after which they can differentiate into a specific cell type, but they are more specific as compared to stem cells.[3] They have limited potency, and their self-renewal potential is also lower. Their function within the body is to replace dead or damaged cells at the site of injury. They perform this function by migrating to the injury site and differentiating into the target cells. Their potency totally depends upon the parent stem cell from which they have regenerated as well as their niche. But their expansion potential is less as compared to that of stem cells. Maintaining blood, intestinal and skin tissue is their most important role.[3,74] Stem cells are undifferentiated/unspecialized cells that after cell division, can reproduce themselves, i.e. they are capable of self-renewal, and their daughter cells have the potential to differentiate into multiple cell types.[3,75] The main advantage of using stem cells is their ability to proliferate indefinitely.[3] Stem cells can be further classified on the basis of their differentiation potential. Stem cells can be embryonic stem cells (ESCs), adult stems or induced pluripotent stem cells (iPS cells or iPSCs).[3] ESCs are extracted from an embryonic stage, and this is the reason why they can be differentiated into any cell type of the three germ layers. It can develop into the interior stomach lining, gastrointestinal tract and lungs, which are derived from endoderm; mesodermal cell types, which can be muscle, bone, and blood; and urogenital and ectodermal cell types, which include epidermal tissues and cells of the nervous system. But ethically, their use is prohibited.[73] iPS cells or iPSCs and mature somatic cells are differentiated, but they can be reprogrammed into a pluripotent state by means of transcription factors such as oct4, sox2, klf4 and c-myc. Once they are reprogrammed, they exhibit unusual self-renewal and the capability to differentiate into multiple cell lineages.[76] Adult stem cells are multipotent cells, which implies that they can regenerate various cell types, including bone, cartilage, and muscle tissue.[3,73] They are isolated from various adult tissues such as the brain, skin, muscle, bone marrow and many other specific organs.[72] The advantage of these cells is that using them is a straight-forward approach and does not lead to teratoma formation. Another advantage of using them is that they do not raise ethical issues.[3]

4.3 WOUND HEALING PROCESS: ACUTE AND CHRONIC WOUNDS

The type of wound dressing or scaffolding that is selected for a particular wound totally depends upon the type, depth, location and extent of the wound. The amount of exudates/pus, infection and wound adhesion are some additional factors that need to be taken into consideration while selecting a wound dressing. Based on the healing process and duration of healing, wounds can be categorized into two categories: (i) acute wounds and (ii) chronic wounds.

Acute wounds often occur due to unexpected accidents or surgical injuries.[77] They are comparatively easy to heal and often take a normal healing path during recovery. The duration of their healing process is around 8–12 weeks after infliction.[78] The chronic wounds on, the other hand, are acquired due to burns, ulcers, and pressure sores.[77,79] These chronic wounds are not only more complex but also more severe. They often lead to trauma and inflammation at the wound site.[78] In the case of chronic wounds, the normal healing path is disrupted, which makes the healing of such wounds a really difficult task.[80] The healing of such wounds doesn't occur in a timely manner and therefore requires long-term medical treatments, which ultimately result in financial burdens on the inflicted individual.[79,78] The wounds can be treated more effectively as well as economically by incorporating tissue engineering as a point of intervention, wherein appropriate scaffolds that have the potential to mimic the ECM of the damaged tissue are incorporated for tissue reconstruction and regeneration.[81]

4.4 CONCLUSION AND FUTURE PERSPECTIVES

The primary purpose of this chapter was to shed light on the current state of tissue engineering and discuss the biogenic evolution of scaffolds, which have assisted in successfully transforming tissue regeneration as a procedure, while highlighting the different types of cells and scaffolds/scaffold-free platforms available for performing tissue engineering. Appropriate selection of biomaterials as scaffolds for re-engineering of damaged tissue is key, as the scaffold would decide the fate of tissue regeneration and eventual wound healing and reconstruction. Moreover, another pivotal aspect of tissue engineering is the cell source and its point of origin.

Additionally, historical development of scaffolds has been discussed in detail, with special emphasis being laid on biogenic scaffolds. All scaffolds, be they natural, synthetic and/or biosynthetic, each have their own set of advantages and disadvantages. Synthetic biomaterials have high reproducibility and are usually mechanically more stable. However, their non-biofunctionality is their major drawback and limits their use as a preferred scaffolding material. In view of their high biocompatibility, low immunogenicity, and minimal to negligible toxicity, biogenically synthesized scaffolds are considered as one of the most promising biomaterials for tissue engineering applications. In the current day and age, however, biosynthetic scaffolds are garnering a lot of attention as preferable scaffolding materials. This rise in popularity of biosynthetic biomaterials may be attributed to their dual nature, wherein they have the plausible potential of overcoming drawbacks suffered by synthetic as well as natural scaffolding materials individually. Therefore, in view of these observations, numerous attempts are being made to exploit the novel attributes of synthetic as well as biogenic scaffolds so as to develop ideal biosynthetic scaffolds with varied morphologies for a host of tissue engineering and reconstruction applications. However, there still remain several loopholes that need to be addressed before they can be employed at the clinical level, such as biodegradability, mechanical competence, immune-compatibility and induction of vascularization.

In view of the above, efforts need to be made to enhance the thermal stability, mechanical strength, antimicrobial activity and downregulate the enzymatic digestion of biogenic synthesized scaffolding biomaterials so that they can fit into the current commercial production needs. Another major challenge in tissue engineering is the lack of expertise and know-how required to grow thick tissues, where the intrinsic capillary network is lacking. Due to the lack of such a capillary network, the supply of nutrients, oxygen and waste removal is hindered in these tissues. In addition to this, governmental regulation, ethical issues and acceptance by the general public are some other restraints on bioengineered tissues and organs. In short, it would be safe to say that the biggest challenge is to mimic what happens naturally, i.e. ECM mimicking, without overstepping ethical boundaries.

REFERENCES

1. Leong BPCÆKW. Scaffolding in tissue engineering: General approaches and tissue-specific considerations. 2008;17. doi:10.1007/s00586-008-0745-3.
2. Ovsianikov A., Khademhosseini A., Mironov V. The synergy of scaffold-based and scaffold-free tissue engineering strategies. *Trends Biotechnol.* 2018;36(4):348–357. doi:10.1016/j.tibtech.2018.01.005.
3. Chiu L.L.Y., Chu Z., Radisic M. *2.07 Tissue Engineering*. Published online 2011.
4. Ratner B.D., Bryant S.J. Biomaterials: Where we have been and where we are going. *Annu Rev Biomed Eng.* 2004;6(1):41–75. doi:10.1146/annurev.bioeng.6.040803.140027.
5. Alakpa E.V., Burgess K.E.V., Chung P., et al. Nacre topography produces higher crystallinity in bone than chemically induced osteogenesis. *ACS Nano.* 2017;11(7):6717–6727. doi:10.1021/acsnano.7b01044.
6. Gluck T., Brand R.A. The classic: Report on the positive results obtained by the modern surgical experiment regarding the suture and replacement of defects of superior tissue, as well as the utilization of re-absorbable and living tamponade in surgery. *Clin Orthop Relat Res.* 2011;469(6):1528–1535. doi:10.1007/s11999-011-1837-7.
7. Todros S., Todesco M., Bagno A. Biomaterials and Their Biomedical Applications: From Replacement to Regeneration. Published online 2021.
8. Croisier F., Jérôme C. Chitosan-based biomaterials for tissue engineering. *Eur Polym J.* 2013;49(4):780–792. doi:10.1016/j.eurpolymj.2012.12.009.
9. Salehi S., Koeck K., Scheibel T. Spider silk for tissue engineering applications. *Molecules.* 2020;25(3). doi:10.3390/molecules25030737.
10. Chen G.-Q., Wu Q. The application of polyhydroxyalkanoates as tissue engineering materials. *Biomaterials.* 2005;26:6565–6578. doi:10.1016/j.biomaterials.2005.04.036.
11. Brien F.J.O. Biomaterials & scaffolds Every day thousands of surgical procedures are performed to replace. *Mater Today.* 2011;14(3):88–95. doi:10.1016/S1369-7021(11)70058-X.
12. Sadtler K., Singh A., Wolf M.T., Wang X., Pardoll D.M., Elisseeff J.H. Design, clinical translation and immunological response of biomaterials in regenerative medicine. 2016. doi:10.1038/natrevmats.2016.40.
13. Gaharwar A.K., Singh I., Khademhosseini A. Engineered biomaterials for in situ tissue regeneration. *Nat Rev Mater.* doi:10.1038/s41578-020-0209-x.
14. Vacan J.P., Langer R. Tissue engineering: The design and fabrication of living replacement devices for surgical reconstruction and transplantation. 1999:1–3.
15. Wolfe P.S., Sell S.A., Bowlin G.L. Natural and Synthetic Scaffolds. Published online 2011. doi:10.1007/978-3-642-02824-3.
16. Ankoma-Sey V. Hepatic regeneration - Revisiting the myth of prometheus. *News Physiol Sci.* 1999;14(4):149–155. doi:10.1152/physiologyonline.1999.14.4.149.
17. Odelberg S.J. Unraveling the molecular basis for regenerative cellular plasticity. *PLoS Biol.* 2004;2(8):2–5. doi:10.1371/journal.pbio.0020232.

18. Schultz M. Photo quiz. *Emerg Infect Dis.* 2008;14(9):1479–1481. doi:10.3201/eid1409.080667.
19. Gest H. Homage to Robert Hooke (1635-1703): New insights from the recently discovered Hooke Folio. *Perspect Biol Med.* 2009; 52(3):392–399. doi: 10.1353/pbm.0.0096. PMID: 19684374.
20. Mazzarello P. A unifying concept: The history of cell theory. *Nat Cell Biol.* 1999;1(1):E13–E15. doi:10.1038/8964.
21. Biggers J.D. IVF and embryo transfer: Historical origin and development. *Reprod Biomed Online.* 2012;25(2):118–127. doi:10.1016/j.rbmo.2012.04.011.
22. Dennis R.G., Smith B., Philp A., Donnelly K., Baar K., Donnelly K. Bioreactors for Guiding Muscle Tissue Growth and Development:1–41. doi:10.1007/10
23. Loo S., Kam A., Li B.B., Feng N., Wang X., Tam J.P. Discovery of hyperstable noncanonical plant-derived epidermal growth factor receptor agonist and analogs. Published online 2021. doi: 10.1021/acs.jmedchem.1c00551.
24. Jackson A.P., Vincent J.F.V., Turner R.M. The mechanical design of nacre. *Proc R Soc London Ser B Biol Sci.* 1988;234(1277):415–440. doi:10.1098/rspb.1988.0056.
25. Luz G.M., Mano J.F. Biomimetic design of materials and biomaterials inspired by the structure of nacre. *Philos Trans R Soc A Math Phys Eng Sci.* 2009;367(1893):1587–1605. doi:10.1098/rsta.2009.0007.
26. Turksen, K. (Ed.). (2019). *Cell Biology and Translational Medicine, Volume 4: Stem Cells and Cell Based Strategies in Regeneration (Advances in Experimental Medicine and Biology,* Vol. 1119). Springer.
27. Le T.D.H., Bonani W., Speranza G., et al. Processing and characterization of diatom nanoparticles and microparticles as potential source of silicon for bone tissue engineering. *Mater Sci Eng C.* 2016;59:471–479. doi:10.1016/j.msec.2015.10.040.
28. Nachlas A.L.Y., Li S., Davis M.E. Developing a clinically relevant tissue engineered heart valve—A review of current approaches. *Adv Healthc Mater.* 2017;6(24):1–30. doi:10.1002/adhm.201700918.
29. Taghizadeh B., Ghavami L., Derakhshankhah H., et al. Biomaterials in valvular heart diseases. *Front Bioeng Biotechnol.* 2020;8:1–20. doi:10.3389/fbioe.2020.529244.
30. Zare M., Ghomi E.R., Venkatraman P.D., Ramakrishna S. Silicone-based biomaterials for biomedical applications: Antimicrobial strategies and 3D printing technologies. *J Appl Polym Sci.* 2021;1–18. doi:10.1002/app.50969.
31. Macha I.J., Ben-Nissan B. Marine skeletons: Towards hard tissue repair and regeneration. *Mar Drugs.* 2018;16(7):1–11. doi:10.3390/md16070225.
32. Clarke S.A., Walsh P., Maggs C.A., Buchanan F. Designs from the deep: Marine organisms for bone tissue engineering. *Biotechnol Adv.* 2011;29(6):610–617. doi:10.1016/j.biotechadv.2011.04.003.
33. Bakheet M.A., Saeed M.A., Isa A.R.B.M., Sahnoun R. *First Principles Study of the Physical Properties of Pure and Doped Calcium Phosphate Biomaterial for Tissue Engineering.* Elsevier Inc.; 2016. doi:10.1016/B978-0-323-42862-0.00007-9.
34. Fahmy M.D., Jazayeri H.E., Razavi M., Masri R., Tayebi L. Three-dimensional bioprinting materials with potential application in preprosthetic surgery. *J Prosthodont.* 2016;25(4):310–318. doi:10.1111/jopr.12431.
35. Wu J., Yin N., Chen S., Weibel D.B., Wang H. Simultaneous 3D cell distribution and bioactivity enhancement of bacterial cellulose (BC) scaffold for articular cartilage tissue engineering. *Cellulose.* 2019;26(4):2513–2528. doi:10.1007/s10570-018-02240-9.
36. Kundu B., Rajkhowa R., Kundu S.C., Wang X. Silk fibroin biomaterials for tissue regenerations. *Adv Drug Deliv Rev.* 2013;65(4):457–470. doi:10.1016/j.addr.2012.09.043.
37. Sahoo D.R., Biswal T. Alginate and its application to tissue engineering. *SN Appl Sci.* 2021;3(1):1–19. doi:10.1007/s42452-020-04096-w.

38. Grijalvo S., Nieto-Díaz M., Maza R.M., Eritja R., Díaz D.D. Alginate hydrogels as scaffolds and delivery systems to repair the damaged spinal cord. *Biotechnol J.* 2019;14(12):1–8. doi:10.1002/biot.201900275.
39. Bakhiet E.K., Hassan M.A., Hassan H.R., Ali S.G. Statistical optimization studies for polyhydroxybutyrate (PHB) production by novel Bacillus subtilis using agricultural and industrial wastes. *Int J Environ Sci Technol.* 2018. doi:10.1007/s13762-018-1900-y.
40. He Y., Zhao W., Dong Z., et al. A biodegradable antibacterial alginate/carboxymethyl chitosan/Kangfuxin sponges for promoting blood coagulation and full-thickness wound healing. *Int J Biol Macromol.* 2021;167:182–192. doi:10.1016/j.ijbiomac.2020.11.168.
41. Chen G.Q., Zhang J. Microbial polyhydroxyalkanoates as medical implant biomaterials. *Artif Cells Nanomed Biotechnol.* 2018;46(1):1–18. doi:10.1080/21691401.2017.1371185.
42. Zhang X., Li Y., Ma Z., He D., Li H. Modulating degradation of sodium alginate/bioglass hydrogel for improving tissue infiltration and promoting wound healing. *Bioact Mater.* 2021;6(11):3692–3704. doi:10.1016/j.bioactmat.2021.03.038.
43. Yadav C., Chhajed M., Choudhury P., et al. Bio-extract amalgamated sodium alginate-cellulose nanofibres based 3D-sponges with interpenetrating BioPU coating as potential wound care scaffolds. *Mater Sci Eng C.* 2021;118(August 2020):111348. doi:10.1016/j.msec.2020.111348.
44. Andriamanantoanina H., Rinaudo M. Relationship between the molecular structure of alginates and their gelation in acidic conditions. *Polym Int.* 2010;59(11):1531–1541. doi:10.1002/pi.2943.
45. Yang B., Yao F., Ye L., et al. A conductive PEDOT/alginate porous scaffold as a platform to modulate the biological behaviors of brown adipose-derived stem cells. *Biomater Sci.* 2020;8(11):3173–3185. doi:10.1039/c9bm02012h.
46. Ahmed S., Ikram S. Chitosan based scaffolds and their applications in wound healing. *Achiev Life Sci.* 2016;10(1):27–37. doi:10.1016/j.als.2016.04.001.
47. Antipova C.G., Lukanina K.I., Krasheninnikov S.V., et al. Study of highly porous poly-l-lactide-based composites with chitosan and collagen. *Polym Adv Technol.* 2021;32(2):853–860. doi:10.1002/pat.5136.
48. Islam M.M., Shahruzzaman M., Biswas S., Nurus Sakib M., Rashid T.U. Chitosan based bioactive materials in tissue engineering applications-A review. *Bioact Mater.* 2020;5(1):164–183. doi:10.1016/j.bioactmat.2020.01.012.
49. Singh R., Shitiz K., Singh A. Chitin and chitosan: Biopolymers for wound management. *Int Wound J.* 2017;14(6):1276–1289. doi:10.1111/iwj.12797.
50. Eivazzadeh-Keihan R., Radinekiyan F., Aliabadi H.A.M., et al. Chitosan hydrogel/silk fibroin/Mg(OH)2 nanobiocomposite as a novel scaffold with antimicrobial activity and improved mechanical properties. *Sci Rep.* 2021;11(1):1–13. doi:10.1038/s41598-020-80133-3.
51. Liu H., Wang C., Li C., et al. A functional chitosan-based hydrogel as a wound dressing and drug delivery system in the treatment of wound healing. *RSC Adv.* 2018;8(14):7533–7549. doi:10.1039/c7ra13510f.
52. Du X., Wu L., Yan H., et al. Microchannelled alkylated chitosan sponge to treat non-compressible hemorrhages and facilitate wound healing. *Nat Commun.* 2021;12(1):1–16. doi:10.1038/s41467-021-24972-2.
53. Liu F., Li W., Liu H., et al. Preparation of 3D printed chitosan/polyvinyl alcohol double network hydrogel scaffolds. *Macromol Biosci.* 2021;21(4):1–10. doi:10.1002/mabi.202000398.
54. de Sousa Victor R., da Cunha Santos A.M., de Sousa B.V., de Araújo Neves G., de Lima Santana L.N., Menezes R.R. A review on Chitosan's uses as biomaterial: Tissue engineering, drug delivery systems and cancer treatment. *Materials (Basel).* 2020;13(21):1–71. doi:10.3390/ma13214995.

55. Jafari A., Hassanajili S., Azarpira N., Bagher Karimi M., Geramizadeh B. Development of thermal-crosslinkable chitosan/maleic terminated polyethylene glycol hydrogels for full thickness wound healing: In vitro and in vivo evaluation. *Eur Polym J.* 2019;118: 113–127. doi:10.1016/j.eurpolymj.2019.05.046.
56. Copes F., Pien N., Van Vlierberghe S., Boccafoschi F., Mantovani D. Collagen-based tissue engineering strategies for vascular medicine. *Front Bioeng Biotechnol.* 2019;7: 1–15. doi:10.3389/fbioe.2019.00166.
57. Homaeigohar S., Boccaccini A.R. Antibacterial biohybrid nanofibers for wound dressings. *Acta Biomater.* 2020;107:25–49. doi:10.1016/j.actbio.2020.02.022.
58. Coelho R.C.G., Marques A.L.P., Oliveira S.M., et al. Extraction and characterization of collagen from Antarctic and Sub-Antarctic squid and its potential application in hybrid scaffolds for tissue engineering. *Mater Sci Eng C.* 2017;78:787–795. doi:10.1016/j.msec.2017.04.122.
59. Chaudhari A.A., Vig K., Baganizi D.R., et al. Future prospects for scaffolding methods and biomaterials in skin tissue engineering: A review. *Int J Mol Sci.* 2016;17(12). doi:10.3390/ijms17121974.
60. Gu L, Shan T, Ma Y., Tay F.R., Niu L. Novel biomedical applications of crosslinked collagen. *Trends Biotechnol.* 2019;37(5):464–491. doi:10.1016/j.tibtech.2018.10.007.
61. Gaspar-Pintiliescu A., Anton E.D., Iosageanu A., et al. Enhanced wound healing activity of undenatured type I collagen isolated from discarded skin of black sea gilthead bream (Sparus aurata) conditioned as 3D porous dressing. *Chem Biodivers.* 2021;18(8). doi:10.1002/cbdv.202100293.
62. David G., Bargan A.I., Drobota M., Bele A., Rosca I. Comparative investigation of collagen-based hybrid 3d structures for potential biomedical applications. *Materials (Basel).* 2021;14(12). doi:10.3390/ma14123313.
63. Ramanathan G., Seleenmary Sobhanadhas L.S., Sekar Jeyakumar G.F., Devi V., Sivagnanam U.T., Fardim P. Fabrication of biohybrid cellulose acetate-collagen bilayer matrices as nanofibrous spongy dressing material for wound-healing application. *Biomacromolecules.* 2020;21(6):2512–2524. doi:10.1021/acs.biomac.0c00516.
64. Spotnitz W.D. Fibrin sealant: The only approved hemostat, sealant, and adhesive—a laboratory and clinical perspective. *ISRN Surg.* 2014;2014:1–28. doi:10.1155/2014/203943.
65. Thorat Gadgil B.S., Killi N., Rathna G.V.N. Polyhydroxyalkanoates as biomaterials. *Medchemcomm.* 2017;8(9):1774–1787. doi:10.1039/c7md00252a.
66. Li B, Moriarty TF, Webster T, Xing M, editors. Racing for the surface: Antimicrobial and interface tissue engineering. Morgantown, WV, USA: Springer; 2020 Feb 28; https://doi.org/10.1007/978-3-030-34471-9.
67. Nikolova M.P., Chavali M.S. Bioactive materials recent advances in biomaterials for 3D scaffolds: A review. *Bioact Mater.* 2019;4:271–292. doi:10.1016/j.bioactmat.2019.10.005.
68. Park J.Y., Park S.H., Kim M.G., Park S.-H., Yoo T.H., Kim M.S. Biomimetic scaffolds for bone tissue engineering. Published online 2018:109–121. doi:10.1007/978-981-13-0445-3.
69. Carlini A.S., Adamiak L., Gianneschi N.C. Biosynthetic Polymers as Functional Materials. Published online 2016. doi:10.1021/acs.macromol.6b00439.
70. Alaribe F.N., Manoto S.L., Motaung S.C.K.M. Scaffolds from biomaterials: Advantages and limitations in bone and tissue engineering. Published online 2016. doi:10.1515/biolog-2016-0056.
71. De Pieri A. Scaffold-free cell-based tissue engineering therapies: Advances, shortfalls and forecast. *NPJ Regen Med.* Published online 2021. doi:10.1038/s41536-021-00133-3.
72. Akter F. *Principles of Tissue Engineering.* Elsevier; 2016. doi:10.1016/B978-0-12-805361-4.00002-3.
73. Belleghem SMVAN, Mahadik B. *Overview of Tissue Engineering.* Fourth Edition. Elsevier; 2006. doi:10.1016/B978-0-12-816137-1.00081-7.

74. Whitaker I.S. Tissue-engineered solutions in plastic and reconstructive surgery: Principles and practice. 2017;4. doi:10.3389/fsurg.2017.00004.
75. Zech N. Adult stem cell Manipulation and possible clinical perspectives. *Journal für Reproduktionsmedizin und Endokrinologie-Journal of Reproductive Medicine and Endocrinology*. 2004;1(2):91-9.
76. Chandra P.K., Soker S., Atala A. *Tissue Engineering: Current Status and Future Perspectives*. INC doi:10.1016/B978-0-12-818422-6.00004-6.
77. Rezvani Ghomi E., Khalili S., Nouri Khorasani S., Esmaeely Neisiany R., Ramakrishna S. Wound dressings: Current advances and future directions. *J Appl Polym Sci*. 2019;136(27):1–12. doi:10.1002/app.47738.
78. Kang Il J., Park K.M. Advances in gelatin-based hydrogels for wound management. *J Mater Chem B*. 2021;9(6):1503–1520. doi:10.1039/d0tb02582h.
79. Okur M.E., Karantas I.D., Şenyiğit Z., Üstündağ Okur N., Siafaka P.I. Recent trends on wound management: New therapeutic choices based on polymeric carriers. *Asian J Pharm Sci*. 2020;15(6):661–684. doi:10.1016/j.ajps.2019.11.008.
80. Subramaniam T., Fauzi M.B., Lokanathan Y., Law J.X. The role of calcium in wound healing. *Int J Mol Sci*. 2021;22(12). doi:10.3390/ijms22126486.
81. Cui N., Dai C.Y., Mao X., et al. Poloxamer-based scaffolds for tissue engineering applications: A review. *Gels*. 2022;8(6):1–24. doi:10.3390/gels8060360.

5 3D Bioprinting of Hydrogels for Bones and Skin Tissue Regeneration

Sümeyra Ayan
Yildiz Technical University and Marmara Research Center TUBITAK

Rıdvan Yıldırım
Yildiz Technical University and Marmara University

Nazmi Ekren and Oguzhan Gunduz
Marmara University

Cem Bulent Ustundag
Yildiz Technical University

CONTENTS

5.1 Introduction 100
5.2 Hydrogels Used in 3D Bioprinting 101
  5.2.1 Natural Hydrogels 102
    5.2.1.1 Decellularized Hydrogel 102
    5.2.1.2 Protein-Based Hydrogels 102
    5.2.1.3 Polysaccharide-Based Hydrogels 103
  5.2.2 Synthetic Hydrogels 104
    5.2.2.1 Poly(Ethylene Glycol) 104
    5.2.2.2 Poly(Vinyl Alcohol) 105
    5.2.2.3 Poly(2-Hydroxyethyl Methacrylate) 105
    5.2.2.4 Polyacrylamides 105
    5.2.2.5 Copolymeric Hydrogels 106
  5.2.3 Composite Hydrogels 106
5.3 Hydrogels for Bone Regeneration 107
  5.3.1 3D Bioprinting of Cell-Laden Hydrogels 108
    5.3.1.1 Polymer-Based Cell-Laden Hydrogels 108
    5.3.1.2 Composite Cell-Laden Hydrogels 110
  5.3.2 3D Bioprinting of Acellular Hydrogels 112
    5.3.2.1 Polymer-Based Acellular Hydrogels 112

DOI: 10.1201/9781003251767-5

5.3.2.2 Composite Acellular Hydrogels 113
5.4 Hydrogels for Skin Tissue Regeneration 114
5.5 Conclusion and Future Perspectives 119
References 120

5.1 INTRODUCTION

The 3D bioprinting is highly used in order to develop neither tissue nor organ structures to mimic native tissues in regenerative medicine tissue engineering (TE) (Cui et al., 2017; Gopinathan and Noh, 2018). The first commercialization of the 3D printing process was published by Charles Hull in 1980 (Shahrubudin et al., 2019). Compared to traditional scaffold fabrication techniques (such as phase separation, molding, etc.), the 3D printing technique is more advantageous to use since microscale structures can be programmed easily and flexibly, providing freedom to design in 3D space. Various materials, such as metals and polymers, are suitable for the 3D printing technique. Nevertheless, the use of conductive polymers in 3D printing is limited due to the extensive effort and insufficient 3D printability of existing conductive polymer inks (Fang et al., 2022; Yuk et al., 2020). With the emergence of various 3D bioprinting technological methods, bioinks designed according to the requirements of specific injury sites are being developed to mimic natural tissue properties and support biofunctionality to support bioprinting requirements (Decante et al., 2021).

3D printers, which produce solid objects of almost any shape starting with a digital model, are used in many fields today, although they were once an ambitious empty dream (Aimar et al., 2019; Mao et al., 2020). Research on the 3D printing technology for medical applications can be divided into four areas as: (i) direct suppression of tissues and organs with full life functions, (ii) personalized production of permanent non-bioactive implants, (iii) the production of locally biodegradable and bioactive scaffolds, and (iv) the production of models of pathological organs to aid in preoperative planning and surgical treatment analysis (Derby, 2012; Saunders et al., 2008; Xu et al., 2013; Yan et al., 2018).

3D printers can be basically classified as inkjet-, light-assisted-, or extrusion-based printers. In inkjet-based bioprinters, bioprinting is performed by creating droplets with thermal or piezoelectric stimulation as a driving force. High cell viability can be achieved with this type of bioprinter. While temperature-sensitive materials can be degraded in thermal-based bioprinters, the applied frequencies (15–25 kHz) in piezoelectric-based bioprinters can damage cells. In this type of printer, the bioink to be used should have a low viscosity. In light-assisted bioprinters, bioprinting can be done by reflecting the light in a layer-by-layer manner on a screen, while in cases where a laser is used as a light source, printing is performed with the movement of the laser point on a surface. In the layer-by-layer method, the pattern is either created on micromirrors (based on dynamic light processing (DLP)) or on a monochrome LCD display. Laser-based printers have a very high resolution, while DLP and LCD-based ones have a relatively lower resolution. While the resolution of the printer can be increased by using the digital micromirror device (DMD), which allows high-resolution printing with the developing technology, the resolution can also be increased by reducing the layer area with the help of lenses. On the other hand, using high-resolution monochrome LCD displays, more sensitive and precise printing can be obtained. The light source used in these methods should not be in the UV region which can damage the cells. The viscosity of the material used should be low or medium (1–300 mPa·s). In addition, the material must be capable of curing with light. With this technique, bioprinting can be performed at high cell viability (min 95%). In extrusion-based methods, a cartridge loaded with bioink is compressed by pneumatic or mechanical (piston- or screw-based) driving forces. Shear stress may affect the survival of cells at the needle tip when a narrow needle tip is used, depending on the type of polymer employed in the bioink. However, higher cell viability can be achieved when needles with larger tips are used. In this case, the resolution of the printed sample decreases. Since bioinks with a wide viscosity range can be bioprinted, this bioprinting technique is widely used in BTE research (Yazdanpanah et al., 2022).

Clinically, the autologous split-thickness skin graft remains the gold standard for comprehensive wound treatments (Masri et al., 2022). There are some situations that limit the clinical applications of 3D printing technologies. These include the inability to make 3D structures with interconnected microchannels for the transport of suitable materials and the difficulty of producing organs (i.e. skin, bone, etc.) suitable for their mechanical properties, anatomical structures, and biological functions (Zhou et al., 2020).

5.2 HYDROGELS USED IN 3D BIOPRINTING

The rheological properties of the material are very important for the effective attachment of cells to the surface of the scaffold obtained by the use of 3D printers. Increasing research in recent years has focused on the use of different forms of hydrogels for bioprinting with cells (Vrana et al., 2022). Hydrogels are able to be made by the radiation method in different ways, containing irradiation of pure polymers, neither monomers nor solutions of polymers (Rosiak and Yoshii, 1999). Hydrogels have a soft texture due to their high-water content, have little friction with the surrounding tissues, and show low adhesion to the mucosal surface and tissues. Due to their water-holding properties in hydrogels' structures, they are able to be used for the removal of body fluids. They are inert in biological reactions. Similarities with living tissues create many opportunities for applications in medicine (Ulusoy and Dikmen, 2020). While hydrogels are widely used in biomedical engineering because of their structural resemblance to the hydrated structures of the human body, the properties of hydrogels must be improved because of their disadvantages: uncontrolled release and mechanical stiffness of hydrophilic molecules. Intelligent hydrogel systems that respond to a variety of stimuli (i.e. ions, pH, light, and temperature) are being developed and explored extensively in tissue regeneration. Nowadays, smart hydrogels that can be applied to 3D printing have received a lot of attention (Choi et al., 2021). Hydrogels used in 3D bioprinting are classified into three main categories: natural hydrogels, synthetic hydrogels, and composite hydrogels.

5.2.1 Natural Hydrogels

Natural hydrogels, whose unique features include biocompatibility, low cytotoxicity, biodegradability, and similarity to the physiological environment, have some limitations, such as not having strong mechanical properties and not being easily controlled. To overcome these usage limitations, composite polymers of natural hydrogels are created (Catoira et al., 2019; Karoyo and Wilson, 2021; Li et al., 2019). Natural hydrogels are classified into three main categories: decellularized hydrogels, protein-based hydrogels, and polysaccharides, as shown in Figure 5.1.

5.2.1.1 Decellularized Hydrogel

Decellularized extracellular matrix (dECM) has attracted great interest in dECM hydrogels as an innovative technique for TE because of their biocompatibility and unique biological activity (Hussein et al., 2020; Tsui et al., 2021; Zhang et al., 2021b). The dECM hydrogel, a mixture of different proteins in the ECM of a natural tissue/organ, has a regenerative potential up to ten times higher than conventional commercial hydrogels made from other biocompatible materials, with a variety of damaged tissue types including the heart, nerve, cartilage, muscle, kidney, skin, and vessels (Ha et al., 2021; Hernandez et al., 2020; Li et al., 2020b; Peng et al., 2021; Rao et al., 2021).

5.2.1.2 Protein-Based Hydrogels

Protein-based materials are able to be used to change various biochemical and rheological properties of bioinks. These materials can be renewable, environmentally friendly, and highly sensitive (often heat labile) comparison with synthetic polymers. This makes it difficult to extract and purify proteins (Veiga et al., 2021). Collagen (Col), elastin, gelatin, and silk fibrin are examples of proteins that are used in TE.

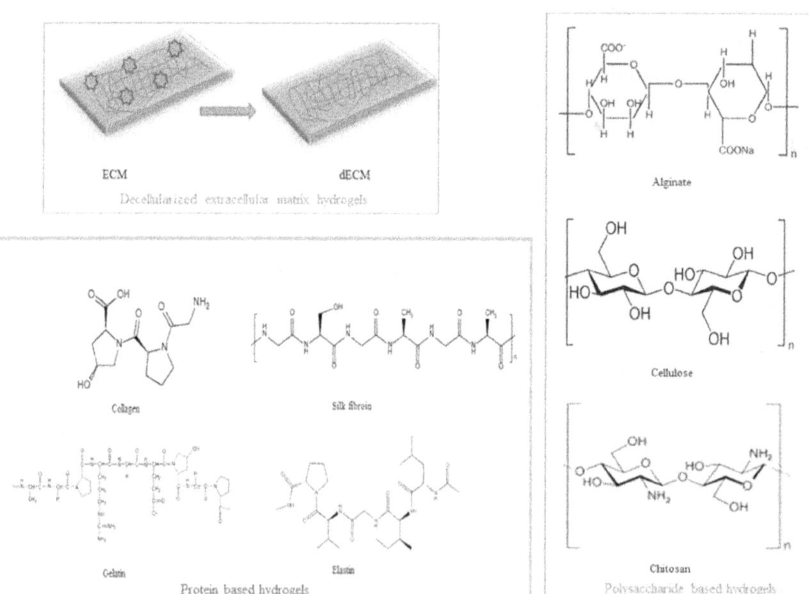

FIGURE 5.1 Natural hydrogel classification.

5.2.1.2.1 Collagen

Collagen (Col), which is found in connective tissues, is classified according to its 29-member structure consisting of at least 46 different polypeptide chains. More than 90% of the Col in the body is type I and most Col hydrogels are manufactured from type I, which under physiological conditions offers excellent flexibility, good tensile strength, and begins to self-organize into fibrils that can be further combined. However, Col-based bioinks offer low mechanical properties when they have low Col concentrations (Veiga et al., 2021). Col, one of the non-branched-chain fibrous proteins in the ECM component, plays a crucial role in sustaining tissue homeostasis, structural mechanics, and biological integrity. In general, Cols are composed of polypeptide chains composed of repeating triplet Glycine (Gly)-Proline (Pro)-Hydroxyproline (Hyp). Col, up to 25% of total proteins, is found in the bones, skin, and other connective tissues of animals (Li et al., 2018).

5.2.1.2.2 Elastin

Elastin is a fibrous protein that is an amphoteric polyelectrolyte and composed of various amino acids. There are studies in the literature on the recovery of elastin from byproducts. When Col and elastin are used together, they form connective tissue. Tropoelastin is produced in hybrid form with elastin-like polypeptides or other molecules by biosynthetic means, neither recombinant like *E. coli* nor by chemical synthesis (Ferraro et al., 2016; Li et al., 2020a; Mu et al., 2021).

5.2.1.2.3 Gelatin

Gelatin (Gel) has good biocompatibility, including arginine-glycine-aspartic acid (RGD) sequence obtained by hydrolysis of Col, which is conducive to cell adhesion, immunogenicity and cell migration (Xu et al., 2021). Gel is cheaper and has a relatively low antigenicity than Col. By selecting suitable photoinitiators with photocrosslinkable methacrylamide groups (GelMA), it is possible to obtain polymers with a high crosslinking degree in a short time at low concentrations, thus minimizing cytotoxicity (Zhao et al., 2016).

5.2.1.2.4 Silk Fibroin

Silk fibroin (SF) is a fibrous polymer manufactured by native silkworms which is biocompatible, has minimal inflammatory reactions, is biodegradable, and has excellent permeability. SF is able to be processed into various forms (i.e. gels, membranes, etc.). SF is used in TE, especially in SF-based products with suitable modified and adapted properties (Zhang et al., 2017).

5.2.1.3 Polysaccharide-Based Hydrogels

5.2.1.3.1 Alginate

Alginate, which is a linear polymer, consists of α-l-guluronic and β-d-mannuronic acid residues. Crosslinking of it can occur by formation of coordination bonds with divalent ions (Ca^{2+}, Mg^{2+}, Ba^{2+}, and Sr^{2+}) and guluronate blocks. As the alginate gels, its solubility decreases while the combination of conjugated carboxyl groups and water discharge increases (Fu et al., 2022).

5.2.1.3.2 Cellulose

Cellulose is the most abundant, biocompatible, and environmentally friendly material on earth. Cellulose with abundant hydroxyl groups can be easily used to arrange hydrogels with fascinating structures and properties (Chang and Zhang, 2011). Bacterial cellulose (BC) is an ideal scaffolding material to use for BTE due to its good air permeability, unique fiber network structure, good biocompatibility, high porosity, high elastic modulus, biodegradability, and water retention (Cao et al., 2022). Promogran® is a commercial dressing containing hydrophilic and relatively inexpensive cellulose (45% oxidized regenerated cellulose and 55% Col) (Madub et al., 2021).

5.2.1.3.3 Chitosan

Chitin is extracted from the shells of crustaceans and is able to be converted to chitosan (CS) during a deacetylation process. CS consists of glucosamine and *N*-acetylglucosamine units linked by β-1–4-glycosidic bonds, and it is positively charged at physiological pH. Hydrophilicity, biodegradability, and biocompatibility are prominent features of CS (Doustdar et al., 2022; Niu et al., 2020). It is known that the use of CS with chemical crosslinkers has a healing effect on its mechanical properties (Pitrolino et al., 2022). CS contains many -NH_2 and -OH active groups formed by the de-acetylation of natural chitin. It also has non-toxic properties, hemostasis ability, and broad-spectrum antibacterial activity (Badhe and Nipate, 2020; Xu et al., 2021).

5.2.2 Synthetic Hydrogels

5.2.2.1 Poly(Ethylene Glycol)

Poly(ethylene glycol) (PEG) is one of the most commonly used synthetic polymers in TE to obtain hydrogels. PEG can be linear, branched, or star-shaped after being synthesized by anionic polymerization of ethylene glycol. It is a very hydrophilic polymer with good biocompatibility and low immunogenicity. It is resistant to protein adsorption and is not hydrolytically degradable (Tamay and Hasirci, 2021; Zhu, 2010). PEG's two end hydroxyl groups allow for the creation of hydrogels with a wide range of mechanical and rheological properties by modifying them with azide, methoxyl, carboxyl, amine, acetylene, thiol, acrylate, and vinyl sulfone functional groups. Radiation, free radical polymerization, condensation, Michael-type addition, click chemistry, and enzymatic reactions could all be used to crosslink PEG hydrogels (Zhu, 2010). Photopolymerization is a common method for creating PEG hydrogels. This is accomplished by using PEG dimethacrylate, PEG diacrylate (PEGDA), and multiarm PEG acrylates (Zhu, 2010).

PEG molecules are not biodegradable, and PEGs with molecular weights of less than 10 (Spicer, 2020) or 30 kDa (Li et al., 2020a) are excreted by the kidneys. They can also be copolymerized with functional polymers like polyglycolic acid, polylactic acid (PLA), and polycaprolactone (PCL) to make them hydrolytically biodegradable, or they can be synthesized with enzyme-sensitive peptide sequences for proteolytic degradation (J. Zhu, 2010).

5.2.2.2 Poly(Vinyl Alcohol)

PVA is a hydrophilic polymer with high biocompatibility due to low cell and protein adhesion, low toxicity, and pendant hydroxyl groups that can be easily modified with various functional groups. PVA hydrogels could be formed by physical, chemical, and irradiation crosslinking techniques (Kumar and Han, 2017; Lim et al., 2018). Although PVA has high elasticity, because its mechanical characteristics are poor, it has been copolymerized with different monomers and incorporated with other synthetic or natural materials for use in hard TE applications (Spicer, 2020).

5.2.2.3 Poly(2-Hydroxyethyl Methacrylate)

Poly(2-hydroxyethyl methacrylate) (PHEMA), which can be a hydrogel due to pendant hydroxyl groups, can be synthesized utilizing the free radical reaction of acrylate groups under UV light. PHEMA is a biocompatible material used in contact lenses and TE. Because PHEMA has poor mechanical properties, it must be combined with other polymers before being used in hard tissue applications. PHEMA can be crosslinked with ethylene dimethacrylate (EDMA), ethylene glycol dimethacrylate (EGDMA), and dimethylol propionic acid (McCracken et al., 2016). Because the cell adhesion properties on the surface of PHEMA are poor, PHEMA can be modified by covalent binding of fibronectin (Patel and Mequanint, 2011), adsorption of cationic ε-poly (l-lysine) via hydroxyl groups (McCracken et al., 2016), or copolymerization of 2-aminoethyl methacrylate with the integrin-binding motifs (RGD or IKVAV) (Macková et al., 2016).

5.2.2.4 Polyacrylamides

Polyacrylamide hydrogels can be obtained using *N,N′*-methylenebisacrylamide as a crosslinker in the free radical polymerization of acrylamide monomers. Aside from free radical polymerization with ammonium persulfate, photoinitiators can be used to produce polyacrylamide gels under UV light. Polyacrylamide gel scaffolds can thus be 3D printed using stereolithographic techniques (Wang and Li, 2020). Hybrid structures with various natural polymers are established to improve cell compatibility and the mechanical properties of synthetic polymers. For example, since the resin prepared by mixing acrylamide with CS modified with methacrylate functional groups can be cured under UV light in the presence of photoinitiators and crosslinking agents, gels with good mechanical properties, and biocompatibility can be produced (He et al., 2021).

Poly(N-isopropylacrylamide) (PNIPAM) is a polymer with good biocompatibility and low immunogenicity that switches between solution and gel form depending on temperature. The lower critical solution temperature (LCST) of PNIPAM is around 32°C, making it interesting for various biomedical applications. When PNIPAM is copolymerized, its LCST value could alter. Furthermore, the mechanical characteristics of the produced copolymer could vary in a temperature-dependent manner, possibly resulting in an increase in stem cell differentiation with mechanical stimulation. Because *N*-isopropylacrylamide is cytotoxic, complete removal of the monomer after manufacture with these procedures should be required (Spicer, 2020).

5.2.2.5 Copolymeric Hydrogels

Copolymeric hydrogels generally consist of a temperature-sensitive hydrophobic segment and a hydrophilic segment that provide gelation. Such polymers pass from a solution state to a gel state at a certain critical concentration and temperature. One of the most widely researched of these polymers, poloxamers, contains hydrophobic poly(propylene glycol) (PPG) in the center and PEGs as end groups at various chain lengths. Poloxamers can be used as drug carriers, wound dressings, cell carriers, and sacrificial molds (Müller et al., 2015; Zarrintaj et al., 2020). Poloxamers can be modified with the methacrylate functional group to provide photocrosslinking to improve their mechanical properties (Fedorovich et al., 2009). Ionic crosslinking can be used to improve the mechanical properties of this hydrogel by immersing it in a solution containing Fe^{3+} ions that coordinate with the carboxylic acid groups of polyacrylic acid. Poly(3,4-ethylenedioxythiophene):polystyrene sulfonate (PEDOT:PSS) can be added to a poloxamer and acrylic acid mixture and 3D printed to construct an electrically conductive hydrogel structure (Imani et al., 2022).

Unlike poloxamers, triblock copolymers with a hydrophilic central group (PEG) and a hydrophobic group (PLA, PCL, poly(ε-caprolactone-co-l-lactide) (PCLA) (Cui et al., 2021), or poly(propylene fumarate) (Le Fer et al., 2021)) at both ends of the central group can be synthesized and 3D printed. Poly(2-methyl-2-oxazoline) can be used as a hydrophilic segment in addition to PEGs. Temperature-sensitive hydrogels made by synthesizing triblock copolymers with a hydrophobic segment in the center using poly(2-phenyl-2-oxazine) as a hydrophobic polymer can be printed using extrusion-based 3D printers (Hahn et al., 2021).

Polyurethane (PU) elastomers comprise a flexible soft segment composed of polyether or polyester polyols and a hard segment composed of isocyanate and a chain extender/crosslinker. Soft segments of PUs that can form hydrogels can be composed of diblock or triblock polymers formed by polyesters such as PCL, PDLLA, and PLLA with PEG (Tsai et al., 2015). By arranging the chemical composition of PUs, temperature-sensitive and/or pH-sensitive hydrogels can be generated. PUs that exhibit a sol-gel phase transition close to body temperature can be used to produce cell-laden bioinks. On the other hand, PUs carrying acrylic functional groups can also be photocrosslinked. Thus, a PU hydrogel with improved mechanical properties can be obtained (Hsiao and Hsu, 2018).

5.2.3 Composite Hydrogels

Heterogeneous biomaterials mimic the topological and mechanical properties of bone. In Zhu et al.'s study, multi-morphology porous scaffolds based on triple periodic minimal surfaces were designed and 3D printed with spatially varying pore patterns. According to the results, the multiple morphology structure allows a combination of relatively low elastic modulus and high yield strength to minimize bone damage and increase the stability of the bone-implant interface. As a result of the study, a 3D-printed multi-morphology porous Ti6AlV scaffold is an important and promising material for orthopedic applications (2018).

In Luo et al.'s studies, biomimetic composite scaffolds with high porosity, nano- to macro-scale properties, and high concentrations of alginate/GelMA were produced as bioinks. The proteins were loaded directly into the bioinks. *In vitro* cell assays have shown that scaffolds with excellent biocompatibility can promote cell adhesion and proliferation. *In vivo* studies showed that the biomimetic nano-apatite-coated hollow fiber scaffolds illustrated the ability to increase bone formation (2022).

Pal et al. made hydrogels by esterification of PVA and Gel, and membranes to which salicylic acid was added were characterized by Fourier transform infrared (FTIR) spectroscopy, differential scanning calorimetry (DSC), and X-ray diffraction (XRD). They stated that the hemocompatibility hydrogel can be used to obtain a wound dressing. Thus, it can also be used for various biomedical applications (2007).

Plant-based hydrogels are frequently used in biomedical fields because they are biocompatible, natural, sustainable, and convenient. Baniasadi et al. noted that cellulose nanofibrils (CNF) impart shape stability and proper porosity, mechanical strength, and water absorption capacity to objects after freeze-drying using bioinks composed of quince seed mucilage and CNF that are easily extruded into 3D lattice structures by direct ink writing. The compressive and elastic moduli of samples manufactured at the highest CNF content increased ~100%. The cell compatibility assay of the produced scaffolds was obtained using human liver cancer cells. Thus, they confirmed that non-cytotoxic 3D hydrogels show excellent proliferation of cells, cell attachment, and cell survival. As a result, these inks provided sustainable 3D biohydrogels for soft TE (2021).

5.3 HYDROGELS FOR BONE REGENERATION

Bones normally can renew themselves due to their highly vascularized structure; however, in the case of pathological and large bone fractures, the bones cannot repair themselves. Bone repair begins with an inflammatory response, followed by the formation of soft and hard calluses (Figure 5.2).

A hematoma is formed, which contains neutrophils, macrophages, and platelets and initiates an inflammatory response around the fracture and a temporary tissue scaffold. Because this temporary scaffold is not present in large bone fractures, bone implants should be used to fill this role (Xu et al., 2022b).

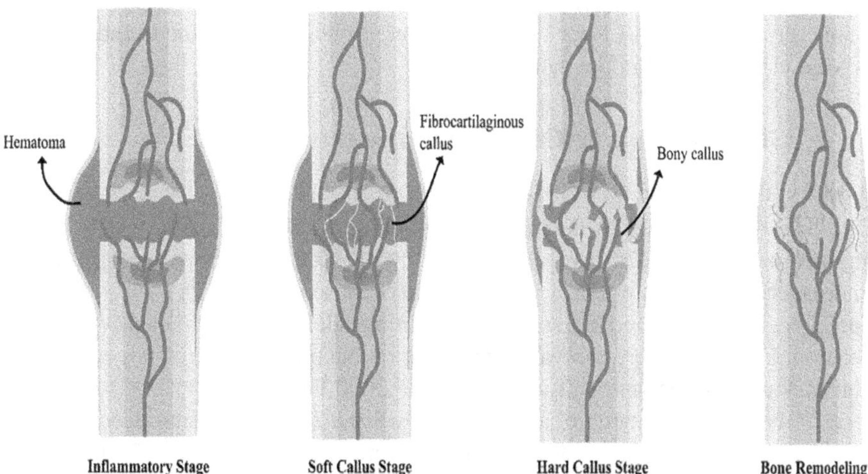

FIGURE 5.2 Repair process in bone fracture.

Although autologous bone grafting is the gold standard method for bone repair, it has limitations, such as limited donor sources and donor tissue damage. Other grafting methods, allograft and xenograft can result in conditions such as infection and disease transmission risk, as well as tissue rejection. Bone tissue can be created without these risks using 3D bioprinting techniques. 3D bioprinted polymeric hydrogels should be cytocompatible, biocompatible, and biodegradable; not produce an immune response; be reproducible with mechanical properties close to natural bone tissue and patient-specific; have an interconnected pore structure that allows vascularization, diffusion of nutrients and wastes, proliferation, migration, and differentiation of cells; and be able to release agents or drugs that accelerate tissue formation. Furthermore, the rate of degradation should be comparable to the rate of new tissue formation. These hydrogels should be osteoconductive and osteoinductive. The formation of bone tissue on the surface of polymeric hydrogels is referred to as osteoconductivity. The ability of polymeric hydrogels to differentiate stem cells into bone tissue is known as osteoinductivity (Tran et al., 2020).

Cell-laden or acellular hydrogels are usually generated using gel-forming natural or synthetic polymers. Pre-osteoblast cells and human osteogenic sarcoma cells are more typically employed as bone cell sources in cell-laden bioprinting studies. Furthermore, mesenchymal stem cells obtained from bone marrow or adipose tissue are utilized in the formation of bone tissue in an osteogenic environment. Human nasal inferior turbinate tissue-derived mesenchymal stem cells and dental pulp stem cells with higher osteogenic differentiation capacity have been evaluated (Yazdanpanah et al., 2022). Bone morphogenetic protein-2 (BMP-2) is commonly utilized in BTE to differentiate stem cells. Experiments with other bone morphogenetic proteins, vascular endothelial growth factor, and some others have also been conducted (Tran et al., 2020). Various ceramic structures, such as calcium phosphates, silicates, and polyphosphates, could also be added to these hydrogel structures to provide mechanical properties and osteogenic stimulation. This type of hydrogel was generally printed using pneumatic- or piston-driven extrusion-based printing technologies, which enable 3D printing in a wide range of viscosities (Heid and Boccaccini, 2020). Apart from these printing technologies, research has also been carried out with DLP- or LCD-based stereolithographic methods and thermal- or piezoelectric-based inkjet methods.

5.3.1 3D Bioprinting of Cell-Laden Hydrogels

5.3.1.1 Polymer-Based Cell-Laden Hydrogels

One of the first studies of cell-laden 3D bioprinting of bone tissue was based on alginate or Lutrol F127 hydrogels (a PEO-PPO-PEO triblock copolymer). Printing multilayer scaffolds is possible with alginate because it ($\eta = 11$ Pas, 2% w/v, 23°C) quickly gels when printed in a solution containing calcium ions, which provides ionic gelation. Fiber diameters can vary depending on the pneumatic pressure and needle diameter used. For example, Lutrol F127 ($\eta = 3600$ Pas, 25% w/v, 23°C) hydrogels form a fiber with a diameter of about 430 μm when a 210 μm diameter needle is used at a pressure of 0.2 MPa and fiber with a diameter of approximately 1280 μm when a 610 μm diameter needle is used at a pressure of 0.02 MPa. For consistent printing, as the needle diameter decreases, higher pneumatic pressure and a slower deposition rate should be selected (Fedorovich et al., 2008).

A sufficient supply of oxygen and nutrients in the tissue scaffold during culture is required for cell proliferation and differentiation in cell-laden hydrogels. In a study examining the effect of oxygen on cell proliferation and osteogenic differentiation in cell-laden porous and non-porous hydrogels prepared with 10% w/v alginate solution, with an average porosity of 48%, cell viability was found to be 85% at the end of the seventh day, while 41% of the cells were viable in solid hydrogels. Furthermore, viable cells in solid hydrogels were only found at the periphery of the hydrogels. While alkaline phosphatase (ALP)-positive cells, one of the early osteogenic differentiation markers of cells, were 20% in porous hydrogels, it was only 5% in solid hydrogels. Moreover, similar results were observed when the deposition of Col type I, one of the late osteogenic markers, was examined. Furthermore, when tissue development in hydrogels was studied *in vivo*, blood vessel and fibrous tissue formation were seen in porous structures, whereas partial tissue formation was seen without blood vessel formation in degraded regions of solid hydrogels (Fedorovich et al., 2011).

Since alginate lacks the ability to be recognized and adhered to by cells, their surfaces should be modified or mixed with polymers containing the RGD sequence (i.e. Gel and Col) (Neufurth et al., 2014) and dECM (Lee et al., 2020a). The addition of Gel to alginate hydrogels also improves the mechanical properties of the scaffold (Neufurth et al., 2014). Gel has limited mechanical properties; it can be methacrylated for photocrosslinking, resulting in stable hydrogel synthesis (Buyuksungur et al., 2021). When dECM is modified with methacrylate functional groups and crosslinked under UV light, it improves the printability and mechanical properties of hydrogel structures (Lee et al., 2020a). Human osteogenic sarcoma cell (SaOS-2) is one of the cell sources in BTE applications due to its strong response to osteogenic compounds such as β-glycerophosphate, ascorbic acid, and dexamethasone by forming calcium carbonate and phosphate deposits. Polyphosphates, a polymer known to be synthesized by osteoblasts, have a significant positive effect on cell proliferation and differentiation when complexed with calcium ions and exposed to SaOS-2 cells (Neufurth et al., 2014). 3D-printed hydrogels with a core-shell structure have been developed to enhance the mechanical properties of hydrogels. While the shell of these struts is composed of cell-laden alginate hydrogel, the core is made of α-tricalcium phosphate (α-TCP), which forms calcium-deficient hydroxyl apatite with a crystal structure similar to that of natural bone. After printing, the scaffold was immersed in a 2.5% calcium chloride solution for ionic crosslinking of the alginate and kept for 30 minutes. Then, for cementation of the α-TCP core tissue scaffold, it was immersed in PBS solution and kept for 6 hours. The scaffold was then immersed in a culture medium to ensure cell proliferation and differentiation (Raja and Yun, 2016). Methylcellulose can be incorporated to improve alginate hydrogels' printability and mechanical properties. Since these polymers do not contain binding motifs, human plasma can be added for cell attachment, proliferation, and differentiation. α-TCP can be added to the structure further to improve both mechanical properties and bone tissue formation (Ahlfeld et al., 2020). In another study, carboxymethylated

CS molecules were added to alginate hydrogels. The water solubility of CS has been improved by modifying it with carboxymethyl groups. The mechanical properties of the cell-laden hydrogels were improved by ionic bonding between the amine groups in the carboxymethyl CS molecules and the carboxyl groups in the alginate molecules (Huang et al., 2016). Since inflammatory compounds can inhibit cell proliferation and differentiation in the hydrogel, an anti-inflammatory agent can be added to the CS solution, allowing it to be absorbed into scaffolds and released in a controlled manner (Lin et al., 2018). Cell-laden hydrogels can be prepared using modified PEG polymers. Modification is usually carried out by adding methacrylate or acrylate groups. Similarly, to increase the degree of crosslinking of ionic crosslinked alginate molecules, they can be modified with acrylate or methacrylate groups and photo-crosslinked with a photoinitiator (Kamaraj et al., 2021).

5.3.1.2 Composite Cell-Laden Hydrogels

Composite bioinks are produced by combining cell-laden polymeric hydrogels with bioactive inorganic fillers. Inorganic fillers are able to be added to enhance the printability and mechanical properties of hydrogels, cell differentiation, adhesion, and proliferation. Composite bioinks have been produced in 3D bioprinters for BTE applications by adding calcium phosphates, bioactive glasses, metal nanoparticles, and graphene oxide to cell-laden hydrogels.

Hydroxyapatite (HAp) ($Ca_{10}(PO_4)_6(OH)_2$) makes up approximately 60% of bone. Calcium phosphates, primarily HAp, were used as inorganic filler materials in the production of composite bioinks. Adding HAp to CS and alginate-based hydrogels increased their mechanical characteristics and lowered their pore sizes. HAp-added hydrogels can improve cell adherence to the surface and provide osteogenic differentiation compared to alginate and CS-based hydrogels (Demirtaş et al., 2017). HAp and PVA can be added to alginate hydrogels to improve the viscosity and printability of the gel, as well as the biocompatibility, mechanical properties, and osteoconductivity of the scaffold. The effect of printing conditions in cell-laden alginate-PVA-HAp hydrogels and immersing time in a calcium-containing solution to increase the degree of crosslinking of the alginate on the viability of the cells in the hydrogel was investigated, and it was observed that approximately 96% of the cells were alive after printing. On the other side, the relatively high concentration of calcium ions in the environment and the shrinkage of the alginate hydrogel after crosslinking may have caused cell death by putting the cells under additional stress (Bendtsen et al., 2017). The inclusion of nano HAp in alginate-Gel-based hydrogels had little influence on cell survival or proliferation but had a substantial effect on osteogenic differentiation. Osteogenic differentiation of cells was more pronounced when cultured in an osteogenic medium than when cultured in a proliferation medium. Bone formation was observed only on the periphery of the porous structures in alginate–Gel hydrogels, while in scaffolds containing HAp, bone formation was generated both inside and outside the porous structures (Wang et al., 2016). A similar effect of HAps on cell viability and proliferation was observed in GelMA-Gel hydrogel scaffolds. Furthermore, the scaffold has become more resistant to enzymatic degradation due to the addition of HAp (Nicholas et al., 2022).

Another bioceramic, β-TCP (β-$Ca_3(PO_4)_2$), provides differentiation of cells and formation of bone tissue without the need for an osteogenic medium. The addition of β-TCP to Col hydrogels decreased the degree of gelation of the hydrogel. Thus, the structural stability of hydrogels printed with increasing amounts of bioceramic decreased. In addition, a decrease in pore size was observed with the addition of β-TCP, as seen in HAp-doped hydrogels. When more than 20 wt. % of β-TCP is added, the viscosity of the composite hydrogel rises even further, and cell viability decreases significantly owing to the high shear stress during printing (Kim and Kim, 2019).

Composite hydrogels can be obtained by using silicate-based ceramics other than calcium phosphate. In a study, biocompatible, bioactive, and osteoinductive bioactive glass (BaG), composed of 47.12% SiO_2, 6.73% B_2O_3, 6.77% CaO, 22.66% Na_2O, 1.72% P_2O_5, 5% MgO, and a 10% SrO molar ratio, was incorporated into hydrogels containing alginate, Gel, and CNF. A HAp layer forms on the surface of BaGs, and ions released from BaGs accelerate bone tissue formation. Also, ALP activity levels obtained by normalizing to the cell population were greater in hydrogels containing bioactive glass. However, with the addition of BaGs to alginate–Gel-based hydrogels at a rate of 1% w/w, the viscosity of the hydrogel increased approximately five times, and the cells were destroyed by shear stress during extrusion (Ojansivu et al., 2019). Another BaG composed of SiO_2:CaO:P_2O_5 with a molar ratio of 55:40:5 was used by mixing with alginate/Gel-based hydrogels. In addition, various osteoinductive silica structures and osteoinductive and osteoconductive polyphosphate·Ca^{2+} (polyP·Ca^{2+}) complexes were added to hydrogel structures, and their effects on cell proliferation and bone tissue formation were investigated. PolyP enables cells to synthesize mineral deposits and increase the expression of ALP and Col type I. Cell proliferation was significantly increased when BaG was added to hydrogels containing PolyP·Ca^{2+} or PolyP·Ca^{2+} and biosilica (Wang et al., 2014).

Laponite is a two-dimensional synthetic nanosilicate material approved by the FDA, whose degradation products enable osteogenic differentiation of stem cells, and whose surface is negatively and positively charged. Less heavy metal-containing Laponite XLG nanosilicate ($Na_{0.7}[(Mg_{5.5}Li_{0.3})Si_8O_{20}\ (OH)_4]_{0.7}$) can be mixed with polyampholite Gel or anionic alginate to form strong physical bonds and improve the printability and mechanical properties of the hydrogel. It has been observed that 3D-printed hydrogels stimulate osteogenic differentiation of stem cells after 21 days of incubation, regardless of whether the culture medium is osteogenic. The Ca/P ratio of the nodules formed on the cells was close to the ratio of HAp. Significant bone formation was observed at 12 weeks after *in vivo* implantation in μCT analysis (Liu et al., 2020). A similar study was carried out on hydrogels based on gellan gum, an anionic polysaccharide. The addition of laponite did not have a negative effect on cell viability, and cell proliferation was found to be significantly higher. Laponite nanosilicates can also be loaded with growth factors or drugs for controlled release (Cidonio et al., 2019).

CNF, which is used to increase the printability of alginate, is produced from natural cellulose using high mechanical shear after the defibrillation process. CNFs can be oxidized with 2,2,6,6-tetramethylpiperidine-1-oxyl, 2,2,6,6-tetramethyl-1-piperidinyloxy (TEMPO) to form carboxyl groups on their surfaces for crosslinking with alginate. For the formation of mineralization on the alginate surface, HAp can be incorporated into the hydrogel structure or immersed in a solution containing phosphate ions to form HAp by interacting with calcium ions during crosslinking, or HAp can be formed on the surface by immersing it in simulated body fluid. Carboxylate groups in TEMPO-oxidized CNFs also play an important role in the nucleation of HAps (Abouzeid et al., 2018). After the periodate oxidation of TEMPO-oxidized CNFs, dialdehyde structures are formed in the molecule. Thus, hydrogels with high mechanical properties can be obtained by crosslinking with polymers containing hydroxyl groups, such as PVA (Abouzeid et al., 2020).

5.3.2 3D Bioprinting of Acellular Hydrogels

5.3.2.1 Polymer-Based Acellular Hydrogels

Lutrol F127, a poloxamer, can be methacrylated and crosslinked with photoinitiators under UV light to improve the mechanical properties of the scaffold. The modified Lutrol F127 inks prepared at a 25% w/v concentration in a culture medium were 3D printed using a nozzle with an inner diameter of 210 µm at 0.2 MPa pressure and 16 mm/s printing speed, and photocrosslinking was performed under UV light. Multiple stromal cells (MSC) were seeded on tissue scaffolds to investigate cell differentiation and proliferation. The hydrogels showed low cell viability (60%) at 2 and 3 weeks. After 1 week of incubation in osteogenic cell media, ALP activity in around 10% of MSCs and Col type I synthesis, a late osteogenic marker, were detected (Fedorovich et al., 2009).

BMP-7 is one of the growth factors involved in new bone formation by stimulating osteogenesis. Bone formation peptide-1 (BFP1, GQGFSYPYKAVFSTQ) derived from BMP-7 was used instead since BMP-7 has a short biological half-life. The hydrogel was prepared by binding the peptide sequence to the alginate surface, which was then 3D bioprinted, and its influence on bone tissue formation from stem cells was studied. The cells showed a rounded, clustered morphology in alginate hydrogels, whereas they showed a uniformly dispersed and diffused morphology in BFP1-modified hydrogels. BFP1 did not show a toxic effect on cell viability but increased cell proliferation compared to those without BFP1 (Heo et al., 2017).

Alginate molecules were sulfated and combined with pure alginate to create BMP-2-loaded hydrogels to slow the release of BMP-2 from the alginate-based hydrogel. While sulfation of alginate did not change the printability of the hydrogel, higher values of ALP activity and calcium deposition were obtained after 7 days of incubation (Park et al., 2018). The osteoinductive properties of hydrogels prepared by loading 14-3-3ε, another protein that can enable the differentiation of stem cells, on GelMA-alginate hydrogels were examined, and the ALP activity value was found to be higher in protein-loaded hydrogels (Aldana et al., 2020). Micro-RNAs, which are involved in post-transcriptional control of gene expression and have osteoinductive properties, can also be attached to hydrogels (Pan et al., 2022).

Lactoferrin is a globular protein involved in organ morphogenesis, wound healing, and bone formation. Lactoferrin can be added to carboxymethyl cellulose and CS-based hydrogels to improve cell adhesion and proliferation (Janarthanan et al., 2020). Cellulose nanocrystals (CNCs) can be produced through the acid hydrolysis reaction of cellulose. The addition of CNC to alginate–Gel hydrogels improved gelation and mechanical characteristics. CNC also improved cell differentiation, proliferation, and mineralization (Dutta et al., 2021).

5.3.2.2 Composite Acellular Hydrogels

The inclusion of glycerol can improve the printability of Gel-HAp-based composite hydrogels. Glycerol is a non-toxic viscous liquid used as a plasticizer and to avoid microscale structural deformation during the freeze-drying process. The inclusion of glycerol improves the 3D printability of hydrogels with a high HAp content (16.2% w/w) (Kim et al., 2020).

Using a high concentration of β-TCP in the bioink formulations may have a negative effect on cell viability. When the cells were seeded on scaffolds after printing, there was no significant negative effect on cell proliferation up to around 40% w/w β-TCP concentrations. Electrostatic interaction between Ca^{2+} in β-TCP and COO^- groups in Gel ensures the stability of the hydrogel structure. After printing, crosslinking with glutaraldehyde can be performed to improve the mechanical properties of Gel/β-TCP scaffolds further. However, since it is toxic, the unreacted aldehyde groups should be blocked by immersing the scaffolds in a 0.1 M glycine solution (Jeong et al., 2020; Kalkandelen et al., 2019).

Prevascularization of bone replacement materials has been studied using different growth factors or endothelial cells to promote adequate bone healing in large bone defects. As illustrated in Figure 5.3, such a structure can be created by printing a cell-laden hydrogel for vascularization and a composite hydrogel for bone tissue formation around the cell-laden hydrogel with DLP-based 3D printers.

Composite hydrogels can be produced using GelMA hydrogels incorporating octacalcium phosphates, which are biodegradable as β-TCP and promote bone tissue formation by supporting osteoblast differentiation. Increasing the concentration of octacalcium phosphate up to 20% w/v increased ALP activity, whereas a decrease in cell proliferation was observed (Anada et al., 2019).

Alginate-based hydrogels can be produced to form a double network (DN) to increase their mechanical properties. Hard and soft networks of DN hydrogels can be generated by UV crosslinking of PEGDA and ionic crosslinking of sodium alginate, respectively. When PolyP, which can bind to alginate molecules via divalent cations such as Ca^{2+}, is added to DN hydrogels, they can show strong osteogenic activity (Zhang et al., 2021a).

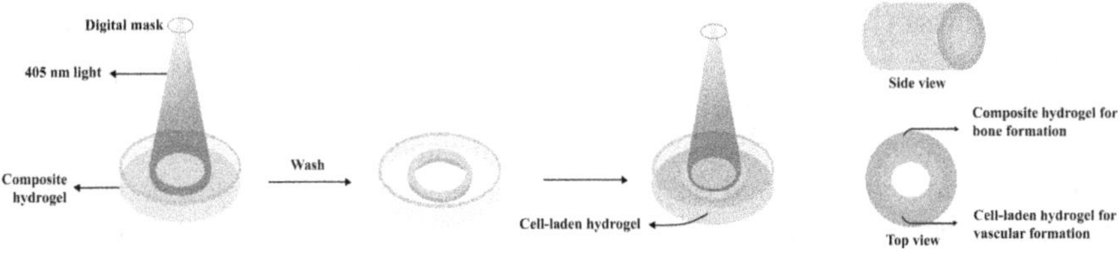

FIGURE 5.3 Schematic illustration of the DLP-based fabrication process for hollow core-shell 3D hydrogel constructs.

Bioceramics, such as osteoinductive and osteoconductive SiO_2, can be introduced to polymeric structures to improve the mechanical characteristics of hydrogels. Hydrogen bonds can occur between -OH groups on SiO_2 nanoparticles and -COOH groups on biopolymers such as sodium alginate, Gel, and Col. Furthermore, Si^{4+} ions released from SiO_2 can enhance bone tissue regeneration by stimulating vascularization (Roopavath et al., 2019). Mesoporous SiO_2 structures can be used as carriers for the controlled release of drugs. Anti-inflammatory drugs, such as curcumin, can be loaded into these carriers to promote the tissue healing process (Liu et al., 2019). Curcumin can also increase osteoblast cell growth and eliminate osteosarcoma cells. Curcumin can be loaded into gellan gum-graphene oxide hydrogels and applied after a bone cancer surgery to stimulate bone growth and destroy potential remaining tumor cells (Zhu et al., 2021).

Composite hydrogels were produced by mixing alginate, water-soluble modified CS, methyl cellulose, silicate glass (SiO_2), or bioactive glass (CaO-SiO_2; 3:7 mol/mol) as the ceramic phase. Although cell viability can be decreased in cell-laden BaG-containing hydrogels even at low BaG ratios, acellular composite hydrogels can attain good cell viability (Fermani et al., 2021). Mesoporous SiO_2-CaO BaG can also be used as a carrier for the controlled release of icariin, which has an osteogenic effect (Monavari et al., 2021). Doxycycline, another drug with osteogenic activity, can be loaded into HAp and PCL structures (El-Habashy et al., 2021).

SiP nanosheets, which are biodegradable and have highly biocompatible degradation products, can be used to make composite hydrogels. These structures can be modified with acryloyl chloride to contain ethylene groups for crosslinking with polymeric structures such as GelMA-PEGDA. In addition, the sustainable release of Si and P ions from modified SiP nanosheets promotes the formation of blood vessels and biomineralization, respectively (Xu et al., 2022a).

Composite hydrogels consisting of osteogenic and osteoinductive silicate-based nanoclays such as laponite (Dong et al., 2021; Man et al., 2022), attapulgite (Liu et al., 2021), and montmorillonite (Leu Alexa et al., 2021) can also be 3D printable for BTE applications.

5.4 HYDROGELS FOR SKIN TISSUE REGENERATION

The skin (Figure 5.4) is the largest organ in terms of surface area and has many functions such as protection from the environment, temperature regulation, and adaptation to body contours during movement (Joodaki and Panzer, 2018).

The skin has a surface area of about $2\,m^2$ and a mass equal to about 15% of the total body mass (Dąbrowska et al., 2018). The epidermis, which does not contain blood vessels, is composed of keratinocytes (KCs), Merkel cells, melanocytes, and Langerhans cells. Blood vessels and nerves are located in the dermis (the middle layer). The innermost layer consists of adipocytes and Col (Weng et al., 2021). The variety of skin properties and the complex relationships between skin permeability and other properties must be taken into account in the design of treatments based on neither skin modeling nor transdermal application (Dąbrowska et al., 2018). Skin appendages contain sweat glands, hair follicles, and sebaceous glands. Hair follicles,

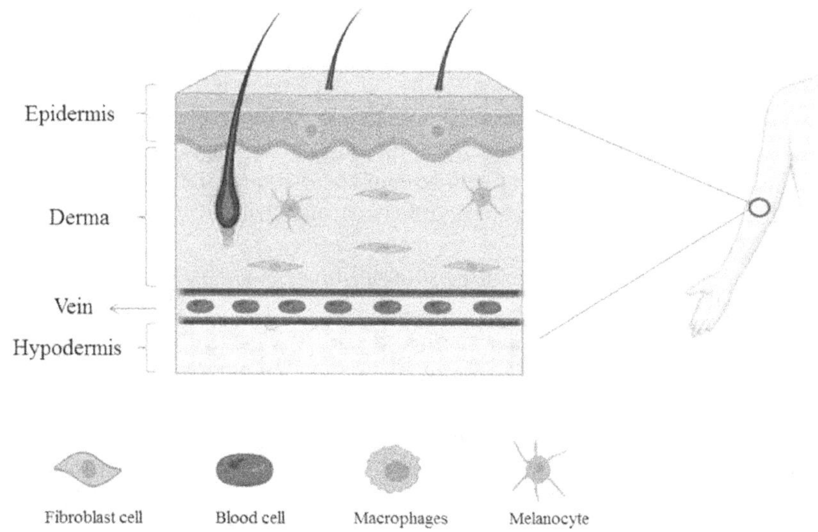

FIGURE 5.4 Illustration of skin tissue.

which form a physical barrier, can show antibacterial ability and prevent scar formation. Eccrine sweat glands manufacture urea, lactic acid, and creatine while regulating body temperature, thus preventing bacterial growth on the skin surface. Skin color is mainly related to MCs located in the basal layer of the epidermis and capable of producing melanin. Adding MCs to the 3D skin bioprinting process can solve the non-pigment problem (Weng et al., 2021).

The skin is damaged by diabetes, acute trauma, and chronic ulcers. Millions of people are in pain from non-self-healing skin wounds each year and incur significant healthcare costs. Serious skin wounds, particularly full-thickness injuries involving damage to the epidermal and dermal layers, appendages, and underlying subcutaneous tissues, often result in dysfunctional scarring. Effectively renewing these skin extensions is difficult (Qi et al., 2018). Skin wounds are classified into two types: acute and chronic, and are heterogeneous with different levels of penetration through the skin. Different strategies are used to meet various biological requirements for the development of wound healing treatments (Madub et al., 2021). Skin defects from external injuries or diseases often lead to loss of bodily fluids and bacterial infections (Xu et al., 2021).

Creating blood vessels with physiologically similar sizes to capillaries is one of the limitations of 3D bioprinting skin structures. The lowest reported diameter of a 3D bioprinted perfused vessel in a skin structure was 80 μm compared to the physiological measurement of <26 μm in the superficial horizontal plexus and <50 μm in the dermal-subcutaneous plexus (Chen et al., 2021). In the literature, a solution was developed for this constraint by promoting vascular self-assembly in human skin-like structures. First, they bioprinted the vascularized dermal compartment, dermal fibroblasts, human endothelial cells, and human placental pericytes suspended in Col type I. They promoted vascular self-assembly by culturing them in Lonza EGM-2 endothelial cell growth medium. Second, the epidermal compartment containing KCs was bioprinted on day 4. Thus, reaching the pre-clinical stage, the patch allowed epidermal keratinization as well as self-assembly of endothelial networks in the dermis. In their *in vitro* study, they reported that vascular structures were formed after 4 weeks (Baltazar et al., 2020).

In the future, an ideal 3D bioprinting skin substitute should include the epidermis and dermis, as well as some key skin attachments such as blood vessels, hair follicles, and sweat glands. New materials should also be considered in the selection of the ideal bioink for this target. Currently, many groups are conducting bioprinting skin studies to meet the requirement for skin tissues convenient for transplantation. 3D-printed ECM facilitates the isochronous and highly specific deposition of multiple types of skin cells and biomaterials, a process lacking in traditional skin TE approaches (Wang et al., 2019). While the advancement of technologies is not yet sufficient in temperature control and sensory formation while reproducing the structural totality and functionality of natural skin to allow for wound repair, 3D bioprinting is expected to overcome these barriers thanks to new approaches evolving over time (Weng et al., 2021). Hydrogels used for skin regeneration are summarized in Table 5.1.

Lee et al. developed a new 3D bioprinter using a high cell viability electromechanical microvalve to produce human fibroblasts (FB) and KCs cultured on a Col hydrogel scaffold with on-demand 3D multilayer printing in order to improve skin tissue regeneration. It is made using a layer-by-layer distribution of skin cells and hydrogels. In addition, this is the first study to print both FB and KC with the formation of dermal/epidermal-like distinctive layers on the scaffold (2009).

In Zhu et al.'s study, the critical role of macrophages in bioactive glass/sodium alginate (BG/NaAlg) hydrogel-enhanced skin wound healing was elucidated using *in vitro* and *in vivo*. Their results illustrated that when BG/NaAlg hydrogel was used, macrophages were required, as the non-existence of macrophages in macrophage-depleted mice significantly inhibited BG/NaAlg hydrogel-mediated skin regeneration (2020). Lee et al. did preliminary work on the production of human skin using a 3D bioprinter. Through further optimization, it could simplify the fabrication of a complex model of human skin (2014).

Repairing massive rotator cuff tendon defects remains challenging because of the high rate of retear after surgical intervention. The 3D printing has shown itself as a promising method for tendon regeneration, enabling the production of engineered tissues. Jiang et al. combined the 3D-printed polylactic-co-glycolic acid (PLGA) scaffold with cell-loaded Col-fibrin hydrogels for rotator cuff tendon repair in two ways: one with a separate layer-by-layer structure and the other with a three-layer structure type of scaffolding as a whole. The imprinted scaffold with Col-fibrin hydrogels beneficially promoted the growth, tenogenic differentiation, and proliferation of MSCs. Implantation of multilayer scaffolds demonstrated their good *in vivo* biocompatibility (2020).

TABLE 5.1
Hydrogels That Are Used for Skin Regeneration

Materials	Crosslinking	Cells	Characterization	Result	References
Col type I (rat tail)	Nebulized aqueous sodium bicarbonate	hFBs and hKCs	Live/dead assay kit (Molecular Probes, MA) and immuno-histochemistry for immunostaining	A new 3D bioprinter using a high cell viability electromechanical microvalve produced a human FB and KC cultured Col hydrogel scaffold with on-demand 3D multilayer printing. The method is able to be used to a various applications from creating tissue engineered materials to drug screening.	Lee et al. (2009)
BG/NaAlg	-	-	The Transwell migration assay, immune-histochemical staining, and in vivo analysis	They state that macrophages are necessary to treat skin wound, as BG/NaAlg significantly inhibits hydrogel-mediated skin regeneration.	Zhu et al. (2020)
Col type I (rat tail)	Nebulized or aerosolized sodium bicarbonate	hFBs and hKCs	Live/dead staining, hemotoxylin and eosin (H&E) staifning	These models could lead to important advances in understanding of the human skin as an organ by engineering superior wound grafts.	Lee et al. (2014)
PLGA/Gel	-	Human adipose-derived MSCs (hADMSCs)	SEM, tensile strength tester, and *in vitro* cell culture test	It is stated that multilayer scaffolds show excellent *in vivo* biocompatibility.	Jiang et al. (2020)
GelMA/ SPn	UV light irradiation	-	FTIR, SEM, H^1-NMR, rheometer, electronic universal testing machine, degradation test, and *in vitro* tests (CCK-8 cell)	It is stated that they provide an artificial dermal substitute with pro-angiogenic capabilities for skin regeneration, thanks to the scaffold they have designed.	Chu et al. (2021)

(Continued)

TABLE 5.1 (*Continued*)
Hydrogels That Are Used for Skin Regeneration

Materials	Crosslinking	Cells	Characterization	Result	References
DT/CA	Oxidative crosslinking chemistry by conjugating catechol moieties	-	UV–Vis spectroscopy, dialysis, FTIR, SEM, H^1-NMR, rotating rheometer, *in vitro* cell tests, and *in vivo* analysis (mouse)	This system is the first report of a catechol or gallol-conjugated DT hydrogel form as an alternative to the limitations of conventional DT hydrogels for tissue regeneration.	Lee et al. (2021)
HA-NB/DDM	Photo-triggered imine crosslinking	Adipose-derived stem cells (ASCs)	Flow cytometry, multipotent differentiation assay, *in vivo* analysis, and H&E staining	HA-NB/DDM hydrogel can serve as a structure that gels quickly *in situ*, adheres to tissues, and accelerates wound healing.	Bo et al. (2020)
p(NIPAAm-AA) and fibrin hydrogel + PVA scaffold	Magnesium chloride	Human umbilical vein endothelial cells (HUVECs)	SEM and *in vitro* cell tests	The prepared hydrogel to be used as potential implants for effective wound.	Zhang et al. (2020)

Lee et al. used catechol chemistry for oxidative crosslinking of a decellularized tissue (DT) hydrogel. Thus, they created the 3D hydrogel structure that was used to cause osteogenesis in human stem cells, long-term stability, and advanced mechanical properties. The existence of oxidized catechol fragments has been noted to provide outstanding tissue adhesion to the DT hydrogel. The DT/CA hydrogel combined with growth factors made possible skin regeneration. Finally, they demonstrated that another phenolic adhesive moiety (pyrogallol, PG) is used to modify the DT hydrogel, resulting in a DT/PG hydrogel that exhibits improved regenerative activity. This is the first report of a neither catechol nor gallol-conjugated DT hydrogel form in order to accomplish the disadvantages (2021).

Zhang et al. prepared a thermo-sensitive poly (*N*-isopropylacrylamide-co-acrylic acid) (P(NIPAAm-AA)) hydrogel to be used as potential implants for effective wound healing and different types of single-nozzle extrusion presses, coaxial needles, and double syringes. They have successfully used it for 3D printing methods. KCs, fibroblasts, and endothelial cells have stated that the hybrid bioink (as P(NIPAAm-AA) and fibrin) has relatively high cell viability when 3D hybrid printing with cells. The hybrid bioink they developed is biocompatible with customized patterns and thicknesses. They reported that by pressing on a porous supporting PVA scaffold. The superficial cornification of the epidermis layer and the sprouting and separation of subcutaneous endothelial cells were demonstrated by histology and immunofluorescence imaging (2020).

5.5 CONCLUSION AND FUTURE PERSPECTIVES

3D printers are used in the process of producing a virtual object designed. Hydrogels are water-insoluble and crosslinked polymers used in various areas, such as artificial organ construction and TE. Hydrogels, with their moisturizing effect, help autolytic debridement while increasing collagenase production and moisture content of necrotic wounds. Large and deep non-healing chronic wounds continue to be difficult for clinicians to heal completely. Ideal skin coverage should not only preserve the wound and stimulate tissue regeneration but also improve patients' aesthetics, satisfaction, and well-being. So far, various bioengineering products have been developed based on synthetic or natural scaffolds (Tavakoli and Klar, 2021). 3D printing technologies are more applicable and effective in research laboratories than typical and traditional manufacturing techniques; therefore, their use is increasing. In the future, it will be developed enough to print human organs such as a damaged finger, heart, and liver, which can be placed on 3D/4D printers and printed in a few minutes (Mallakpour et al., 2022). In TE applications, microporous structures play a crucial role in providing adequate transport for embedded cells. Despite the advances in advanced 3D bioprinting technologies, it is difficult to design micropores of 100 μm or smaller in cell-loaded structures. Studies are ongoing to eliminate this disadvantage in the literature (Ouyang et al., 2022). The 3D bioprinting technology has been a viable method to fabricate bone and skin substitutes using patients' own cells. Nevertheless, this technology is still in its infancy and will be further developed in the near future.

REFERENCES

Abouzeid, R. E., Khiari, R., Beneventi, D., & Dufresne, A. (2018). Biomimetic mineralization of three-dimensional printed alginate/TEMPO-oxidized cellulose nanofibril scaffolds for bone tissue engineering [Research-article]. *Biomacromolecules*, *19*(11), 4442–4452. doi: 10.1021/acs.biomac.8b01325.

Abouzeid, R. E., Khiari, R., Salama, A., Diab, M., Beneventi, D., & Dufresne, A. (2020). In situ mineralization of nano-hydroxyapatite on bifunctional cellulose nanofiber/polyvinyl alcohol/sodium alginate hydrogel using 3D printing. *International Journal of Biological Macromolecules*, *160*, 538–547. doi: 10.1016/j.ijbiomac.2020.05.181.

Ahlfeld, T., Cubo-Mateo, N., Cometta, S., Guduric, V., Vater, C., Bernhardt, A., Akkineni, A. R., Lode, A., & Gelinsky, M. (2020). A novel plasma-based bioink stimulates cell proliferation and differentiation in bioprinted, mineralized constructs. *ACS Applied Materials & Interfaces*, *12*(11), 12557–12572. doi: 10.1021/acsami.0c00710.

Aimar, A., Palermo, A., & Innocenti, B. (2019). The role of 3D printing in medical applications: A state of the art. *Journal of Healthcare Engineering*. doi: 10.1155/2019/5340616.

Aldana, A. A., Uhart, M., Abraham, G. A., Bustos, D. M., & Boccaccini, A. R. (2020). 14-3-3ε protein-loaded 3D hydrogels favor osteogenesis. *Journal of Materials Science: Materials in Medicine*, *31*(11), 105. doi: 10.1007/s10856-020-06434-1.

Anada, T., Pan, C.-C., Stahl, A., Mori, S., Fukuda, J., Suzuki, O., & Yang, Y. (2019). Vascularized bone-mimetic hydrogel constructs by 3D bioprinting to promote osteogenesis and angiogenesis. *International Journal of Molecular Sciences*, *20*(5), 1096. doi: 10.3390/ijms20051096.

Badhe, R. V., & Nipate, S. S. (2020). Cellulosic materials as bioinks for 3D printing applications. In *Advanced 3D-Printed Systems and Nanosystems for Drug Delivery and Tissue Engineering*. doi: 10.1016/b978-0-12-818471-4.00005-4.

Baltazar, T., Merola, J., Catarino, C., Xie, C. B., Kirkiles-Smith, N. C., Lee, V., Hotta, S., Dai, G., Xu, X., Ferreira, F. C., Saltzman, W. M., Pober, J. S., & Karande, P. (2020). Three dimensional bioprinting of a vascularized and perfusable skin graft using human keratinocytes, fibroblasts, pericytes, and endothelial cells. *Tissue Engineering - Part A*. doi: 10.1089/ten.tea.2019.0201.

Baniasadi, H., Polez, R. T., Kimiaei, E., Madani, Z., Rojas, O. J., Österberg, M., & Seppälä, J. (2021). 3D printing and properties of cellulose nanofibrils-reinforced quince seed mucilage bio-inks. *International Journal of Biological Macromolecules*. doi: 10.1016/j.ijbiomac.2021.10.078.

Bendtsen, S. T., Quinnell, S. P., & Wei, M. (2017). Development of a novel alginate-polyvinyl alcohol-hydroxyapatite hydrogel for 3D bioprinting bone tissue engineered scaffolds. *Journal of Biomedical Materials Research Part A*, *105A*(5), 1457–1468. doi: 10.1002/jbm.a.36036.

Bo, Q., Yan, L., Li, H., Jia, Z., Zhan, A., Chen, J., Yuan, Z., Zhang, W., Gao, B., & Chen, R. (2020). Decellularized dermal matrix-based photo-crosslinking hydrogels as a platform for delivery of adipose derived stem cells to accelerate cutaneous wound healing. *Materials and Design*. doi: 10.1016/j.matdes.2020.109152.

Buyuksungur, S., Hasirci, V., & Hasirci, N. (2021). 3D printed hybrid bone constructs of PCL and dental pulp stem cells loaded GelMA. *Journal of Biomedical Materials Research Part A*, *109*(12), 2425–2437. doi: 10.1002/jbm.a.37235.

Cao, S., Li, Q., Zhang, S., Liu, K., Yang, Y., & Chen, J. (2022). Oxidized bacterial cellulose reinforced nanocomposite scaffolds for bone repair. *Colloids and Surfaces B: Biointerfaces*, *211*, 112316. doi: 10.1016/j.colsurfb.2021.112316.

Catoira, M. C., Fusaro, L., Di Francesco, D., Ramella, M., & Boccafoschi, F. (2019). Overview of natural hydrogels for regenerative medicine applications. *Journal of Materials Science: Materials in Medicine*. doi: 10.1007/s10856-019-6318-7.

Chang, C., & Zhang, L. (2011). Cellulose-based hydrogels: Present status and application prospects. *Carbohydrate Polymers*. doi: 10.1016/j.carbpol.2010.12.023.

Chen, E. P., Toksoy, Z., Davis, B. A., & Geibel, J. P. (2021). 3D bioprinting of vascularized tissues for in vitro and in vivo applications. *Frontiers in Bioengineering and Biotechnology*. doi: 10.3389/fbioe.2021.664188.

Choi, Y., Kim, C., Kim, H. S., Moon, C., & Lee, K. Y. (2021). 3D Printing of dynamic tissue scaffold by combining self-healing hydrogel and self-healing ferrogel. *Colloids and Surfaces B: Biointerfaces*. doi: 10.1016/j.colsurfb.2021.112108.

Chu, B., He, J., Wang, Z., Liu, L., Li, X., Wu, C. X., Chen, C., & Tu, M. (2021). Proangiogenic peptide nanofiber hydrogel/3D printed scaffold for dermal regeneration. *Chemical Engineering Journal*. doi: 10.1016/j.cej.2020.128146.

Cidonio, G., Cooke, M., Glinka, M., Dawson, J. I., Grover, L., & Oreffo, R. O. C. (2019). Printing bone in a gel: using nanocomposite bioink to print functionalised bone scaffolds. *Materials Today Bio*, *4*, 100028. doi: 10.1016/j.mtbio.2019.100028.

Cui, H., Nowicki, M., Fisher, J. P., & Zhang, L. G. (2017). 3D bioprinting for organ regeneration. *Advanced Healthcare Materials*. doi: 10.1002/adhm.201601118.

Cui, Y., Jin, R., Zhou, Y., Yu, M., Ling, Y., & Wang, L.-Q. (2021). Crystallization enhanced thermal-sensitive hydrogels of PCL-PEG-PCL triblock copolymer for 3D printing. *Biomedical Materials*, *16*(3), 035006. doi: 10.1088/1748-605X/abc38e.

Dąbrowska, A. K., Spano, F., Derler, S., Adlhart, C., Spencer, N. D., & Rossi, R. M. (2018). The relationship between skin function, barrier properties, and body-dependent factors. *Skin Research and Technology*. doi: 10.1111/srt.12424.

Decante, G., Costa, J. B., Silva-Correia, J., Collins, M. N., Reis, R. L., & Oliveira, J. M. (2021). Engineering bioinks for 3D bioprinting. *Biofabrication*. doi: 10.1088/1758-5090/abec2c.

Demirtaş, T. T., Irmak, G., & Gümüşderelioğlu, M. (2017). A bioprintable form of chitosan hydrogel for bone tissue engineering. *Biofabrication*, *9*(3), 035003. doi: 10.1088/1758-5090/aa7b1d.

Derby, B. (2012). Printing and prototyping of tissues and scaffolds. *Science*. doi: 10.1126/science.1226340.

Dong, L., Bu, Z., Xiong, Y., Zhang, H., Fang, J., Hu, H., Liu, Z., & Li, X. (2021). Facile extrusion 3D printing of gelatine methacrylate/Laponite nanocomposite hydrogel with high concentration nanoclay for bone tissue regeneration. *International Journal of Biological Macromolecules*, *188*, 72–81. doi: 10.1016/j.ijbiomac.2021.07.199.

Doustdar, F., Olad, A., & Ghorbani, M. (2022). Development of a novel reinforced scaffold based on chitosan/cellulose nanocrystals/halloysite nanotubes for curcumin delivery. *Carbohydrate Polymers*, *282*, 119127. doi: 10.1016/j.carbpol.2022.119127.

Dutta, S. D., Hexiu, J., Patel, D. K., Ganguly, K., & Lim, K.-T. (2021). 3D-printed bioactive and biodegradable hydrogel scaffolds of alginate/gelatin/cellulose nanocrystals for tissue engineering. *International Journal of Biological Macromolecules*, *167*, 644–658. doi: 10.1016/j.ijbiomac.2020.12.011.

El-Habashy, S. E., El-Kamel, A. H., Essawy, M. M., Abdelfattah, E.-Z. A., & Eltaher, H. M. (2021). 3D printed bioinspired scaffolds integrating doxycycline nanoparticles: Customizable implants for in vivo osteoregeneration. *International Journal of Pharmaceutics*, *607*, 121002. doi: 10.1016/j.ijpharm.2021.121002.

Ergul, N. M., Unal, S., Kartal, I., Kalkandelen, C., Ekren, N., Kilic, O., Chi-Chang, L., & Gunduz, O. (2019). 3D printing of chitosan/ poly(vinyl alcohol) hydrogel containing synthesized hydroxyapatite scaffolds for hard-tissue engineering. *Polymer Testing*, *79*, 106006. doi: 10.1016/j.polymertesting.2019.106006.

Fang, Y., Guo, Y., Liu, T., Xu, R., Mao, S., Mo, X., Zhang, T., Ouyang, L., Xiong, Z., & Sun, W. (2022). Advances in 3D Bioprinting. *Chinese Journal of Mechanical Engineering: Additive Manufacturing Frontiers*, 100011. doi: 10.1016/j.cjmeam.2022.100011.

Fedorovich, N. E., De Wijn, J. R., Verbout, A. J., Alblas, J., & Dhert, W. J. A. (2008). Three-dimensional fiber deposition of cell-laden, viable, patterned constructs for bone tissue printing. *Tissue Engineering - Part A.*, *14*(1), 127–133. doi: 10.1089/ten.a.2007.0158.

Fedorovich, N. E., Kuipers, E., Gawlitta, D., Dhert, W. J. A., & Alblas, J. (2011). Scaffold porosity and oxygenation of printed hydrogel constructs affect functionality of embedded osteogenic progenitors. *Tissue Engineering Part A*, *17*(19–20), 2473–2486. doi: 10.1089/ten.tea.2011.0001.

Fedorovich, N. E., Swennen, I., Girones, J., Moroni, L., Van Blitterswijk, C. A., Schacht, E., Alblas, J., & Dhert, W. J. A. (2009). Evaluation of photocrosslinked lutrol hydrogel for tissue printing applications. *Biomacromolecules*, *10*(7), 1689–1696. doi: 10.1021/bm801463q.

Fermani, M., Platania, V., Kavasi, R., Karavasili, C., Zgouro, P., Fatouros, D., Chatzinikolaidou, M., & Bouropoulos, N. (2021). 3D-printed scaffolds from alginate/methyl cellulose/trimethyl chitosan/silicate glasses for bone tissue engineering. *Applied Sciences*, *11*(18), 8677. doi: 10.3390/app11188677.

Ferraro, V., Anton, M., & Santé-Lhoutellier, V. (2016). The "sisters" α-helices of collagen, elastin and keratin recovered from animal by-products: Functionality, bioactivity and trends of application. *Trends in Food Science and Technology*. doi: 10.1016/j.tifs.2016.03.006.

Fu, Z., Ouyang, L., Xu, R., Yang, Y., & Sun, W. (2022). Responsive biomaterials for 3D bioprinting: A review. *Materials Today*. doi: 10.1016/j.mattod.2022.01.001.

Gopinathan, J., & Noh, I. (2018). Recent trends in bioinks for 3D printing. *Biomaterials Research*. doi: 10.1186/s40824-018-0122-1.

Ha, D. H., Chae, S., Lee, J. Y., Kim, J. Y., Yoon, J., Sen, T., Lee, S. W., Kim, H. J., Cho, J. H., & Cho, D. W. (2021). Therapeutic effect of decellularized extracellular matrix-based hydrogel for radiation esophagitis by 3D printed esophageal stent. *Biomaterials*. doi: 10.1016/j.biomaterials.2020.120477.

Hahn, L., Karakaya, E., Zorn, T., Sochor, B., Maier, M., Stahlhut, P., Forster, S., Fischer, K., Seiffert, S., Pöppler, A.-C., Detsch, R., & Luxenhofer, R. (2021). An inverse thermogelling bioink based on an ABA-type poly(2-oxazoline) amphiphile. *Biomacromolecules*, *22*(7), 3017–3027. doi: 10.1021/acs.biomac.1c00427.

He, Y., Wang, F., Wang, X., Zhang, J., Wang, D., & Huang, X. (2021). A photocurable hybrid chitosan/acrylamide bioink for DLP based 3D bioprinting. *Materials & Design*, *202*, 109588. doi: 10.1016/j.matdes.2021.109588.

Heid, S., & Boccaccini, A. R. (2020). Advancing bioinks for 3D bioprinting using reactive fillers: A review. *Acta Biomaterialia*, *113*, 1–22. doi: 10.1016/j.actbio.2020.06.040.

Heo, E. Y., Ko, N. R., Bae, M. S., Lee, S. J., Choi, B.-J., Kim, J. H., Kim, H. K., Park, S. A., & Kwon, I. K. (2017). Novel 3D printed alginate–BFP1 hybrid scaffolds for enhanced bone regeneration. *Journal of Industrial and Engineering Chemistry*, *45*, 61–67. doi: 10.1016/j.jiec.2016.09.003.

Hernandez, M. J., Yakutis, G. E., Zelus, E. I., Hill, R. C., Dzieciatkowska, M., Hansen, K. C., & Christman, K. L. (2020). Manufacturing considerations for producing and assessing decellularized extracellular matrix hydrogels. *Methods*. doi: 10.1016/j.ymeth.2019.09.015.

Hsiao, S.-H., & Hsu, S. (2018). Synthesis and characterization of dual stimuli-sensitive biodegradable polyurethane soft hydrogels for 3D cell-laden bioprinting. *ACS Applied Materials & Interfaces*, *10*(35), 29273–29287. doi: 10.1021/acsami.8b08362.

Huang, J., Fu, H., Wang, Z., Meng, Q., Liu, S., Wang, H., Zheng, X., Dai, J., & Zhang, Z. (2016). BMSCs-laden gelatin/sodium alginate/carboxymethyl chitosan hydrogel for 3D bioprinting. *RSC Advances*, *6*(110), 108423–108430. doi: 10.1039/C6RA24231F.

Hussein, K. H., Park, K. M., Yu, L., Kwak, H. H., & Woo, H. M. (2020). Decellularized hepatic extracellular matrix hydrogel attenuates hepatic stellate cell activation and liver fibrosis. *Materials Science and Engineering C*. doi: 10.1016/j.msec.2020.111160.

Imani, K. B. C., Jo, A., Choi, G. M., Kim, B., Chung, J., Lee, H. S., & Yoon, J. (2022). High-resolution 3D printing of mechanically tough hydrogels prepared by thermo-responsive poloxamer ink platform. *Macromolecular Rapid Communications*, *43*(2), 2100579. doi: 10.1002/marc.202100579.

Janarthanan, G., Tran, H. N., Cha, E., Lee, C., Das, D., & Noh, I. (2020). 3D printable and injectable lactoferrin-loaded carboxymethyl cellulose-glycol chitosan hydrogels for tissue engineering applications. *Materials Science and Engineering: C*, *113*, 111008. doi: 10.1016/j.msec.2020.111008.

Jeong, J. E., Park, S. Y., Shin, J. Y., Seok, J. M., Byun, J. H., Oh, S. H., Kim, W. D., Lee, J. H., Park, W. H., & Park, S. A. (2020). 3D printing of bone-mimetic scaffold composed of gelatin/β-tri-calcium phosphate for bone tissue engineering. *Macromolecular Bioscience*, *20*(12), 2000256. doi: 10.1002/mabi.202000256.

Jiang, X., Wu, S., Kuss, M., Kong, Y., Shi, W., Streubel, P. N., Li, T., & Duan, B. (2020). 3D printing of multilayered scaffolds for rotator cuff tendon regeneration. *Bioactive Materials*. doi: 10.1016/j.bioactmat.2020.04.017.

Joodaki, H., & Panzer, M. B. (2018). Skin mechanical properties and modeling: A review. *Proceedings of the Institution of Mechanical Engineers, Part H: Journal of Engineering in Medicine*. doi: 10.1177/0954411918759801.

Kalkandelen, C., Ulag, S., Ozbek, B., Eroglu, G. O., Ozerkan, D., Kuruca, S. E., Oktar, F. N., Sengor, M., & Gunduz, O. (2019). 3D printing of gelatine/alginate/β-tricalcium phosphate composite constructs for bone tissue engineering. *ChemistrySelect*, *4*(41), 12032–12036. doi: 10.1002/slct.201902878.

Kamaraj, M., Sreevani, G., Prabusankar, G., & Rath, S. N. (2021). Mechanically tunable photo-cross-linkable bioinks for osteogenic differentiation of MSCs in 3D bioprinted constructs. *Materials Science and Engineering: C*, *131*, 112478. doi: 10.1016/j.msec.2021.112478.

Karoyo, A. H., & Wilson, L. D. (2021). A review on the design and hydration properties of natural polymer-based hydrogels. *Materials*. doi: 10.3390/ma14051095.

Kim, D., Lee, J. U., & Kim, G. H. (2020). Biomimetic gelatin/HA biocomposites with effective elastic properties and 3D-structural flexibility using a 3D-printing process. *Additive Manufacturing*, *36*, 101616. doi: 10.1016/j.addma.2020.101616.

Kim, W., & Kim, G. (2019). Collagen/bioceramic-based composite bioink to fabricate a porous 3D hASCs-laden structure for bone tissue regeneration. *Biofabrication*, *12*(1), 015007. doi: 10.1088/1758-5090/ab436d.

Kumar, A., & Han, S. S. (2017). PVA-based hydrogels for tissue engineering: A review. *International Journal of Polymeric Materials and Polymeric Biomaterials*, *66*(4), 159–182. doi: 10.1080/00914037.2016.1190930.

Le Fer, G., Dilla, R. A., Wang, Z., King, J., Chuang, S. S. C., & Becker, M. L. (2021). Clustering and hierarchical organization of 3D printed poly(propylene fumarate)- block -PEG-block -poly(propylene fumarate) ABA triblock copolymer hydrogels. *Macromolecules*, *54*(7), 3458–3468. doi: 10.1021/acs.macromol.1c00132.

Lee, J., Hong, J., Kim, W., & Kim, G. H. (2020a). Bone-derived dECM/alginate bioink for fabricating a 3D cell-laden mesh structure for bone tissue engineering. *Carbohydrate Polymers*, *250*, 116914. doi: 10.1016/j.carbpol.2020.116914.

Lee, J. S., Choi, Y. S., Lee, J. S., Jeon, E. J., An, S., Lee, M. S., Yang, H. S., & Cho, S. W. (2021). Mechanically-reinforced and highly adhesive decellularized tissue-derived hydrogel for efficient tissue repair. *Chemical Engineering Journal*. doi: 10.1016/j.cej.2021.130926.

Lee, V., Singh, G., Trasatti, J. P., Bjornsson, C., Xu, X., Tran, T. N., Yoo, S. S., Dai, G., & Karande, P. (2014). Design and fabrication of human skin by three-dimensional bioprinting. *Tissue Engineering - Part C: Methods*. doi: 10.1089/ten.tec.2013.0335.

Lee, W., Debasitis, J. C., Lee, V. K., Lee, J. H., Fischer, K., Edminster, K., Park, J. K., & Yoo, S. S. (2009). Multi-layered culture of human skin fibroblasts and keratinocytes through three-dimensional freeform fabrication. *Biomaterials*. doi: 10.1016/j.biomaterials.2008.12.009.

Leu Alexa, R., Ianchis, R., Savu, D., Temelie, M., Trica, B., Serafim, A., Vlasceanu, G. M., Alexandrescu, E., Preda, S., & Iovu, H. (2021). 3D printing of alginate-natural clay hydrogel-based nanocomposites. *Gels*, *7*(4), 211. doi: 10.3390/gels7040211.

Li, J., Wang, M., Qiao, Y., Tian, Y., Liu, J., Qin, S., & Wu, W. (2018). Extraction and characterization of type I collagen from skin of tilapia (Oreochromis niloticus) and its potential application in biomedical scaffold material for tissue engineering. *Process Biochemistry*. doi: 10.1016/j.procbio.2018.07.009.

Li, J., Wu, C., Chu, P. K., & Gelinsky, M. (2020a). 3D printing of hydrogels: Rational design strategies and emerging biomedical applications. *Materials Science and Engineering: R*, *140*, 100543. doi: 10.1016/j.mser.2020.100543.

Li, J., Rao, Z., Zhao, Y., Xu, Y., Chen, L., Shen, Z., Bai, Y., Lin, Z., & Huang, Q. (2020b). A decellularized matrix hydrogel derived from human dental pulp promotes dental pulp stem cell proliferation, migration, and induced multidirectional differentiation in vitro. *Journal of Endodontics*. doi: 10.1016/j.joen.2020.07.008.

Li, L., Yu, F., Zheng, L., Wang, R., Yan, W., Wang, Z., Xu, J., Wu, J., Shi, D., Zhu, L., Wang, X., & Jiang, Q. (2019). Natural hydrogels for cartilage regeneration: Modification, preparation and application. *Journal of Orthopaedic Translation*. doi: 10.1016/j.jot.2018.09.003.

Lim, K. S., Levato, R., Costa, P. F., Castilho, M. D., Alcala-Orozco, C. R., van Dorenmalen, K. M. A., Melchels, F. P. W., Gawlitta, D., Hooper, G. J., Malda, J., & Woodfield, T. B. F. (2018). Bio-resin for high resolution lithography-based biofabrication of complex cell-laden constructs. *Biofabrication*, *10*(3), 034101. doi: 10.1088/1758-5090/aac00c.

Lin, H.-Y., Chang, T.-W., & Peng, T.-K. (2018). Three-dimensional plotted alginate fibers embedded with diclofenac and bone cells coated with chitosan for bone regeneration during inflammation. *Journal of Biomedical Materials Research Part A*, *106*(6), 1511–1521. doi: 10.1002/jbm.a.36357.

Liu, B., Li, J., Lei, X., Cheng, P., Song, Y., Gao, Y., Hu, J., Wang, C., Zhang, S., Li, D., Wu, H., Sang, H., Bi, L., & Pei, G. (2020). 3D-bioprinted functional and biomimetic hydrogel scaffolds incorporated with nanosilicates to promote bone healing in rat calvarial defect model. *Materials Science and Engineering: C*, *112*, 110905. doi: 10.1016/j.msec.2020.110905.

Liu, C., Qin, W., Wang, Y., Ma, J., Liu, J., Wu, S., & Zhao, H. (2021). 3D printed gelatin/sodium alginate hydrogel scaffolds doped with nano-attapulgite for bone tissue repair. *International Journal of Nanomedicine*, *16*, 8417–8432. doi: 10.2147/IJN.S339500.

Liu, S., Hu, Y., Zhang, J., Bao, S., Xian, L., Dong, X., Zheng, W., Li, Y., Gao, H., & Zhou, W. (2019). Bioactive and biocompatible macroporous scaffolds with tunable performances prepared based on 3D printing of the pre-crosslinked sodium alginate/hydroxyapatite hydrogel ink. *Macromolecular Materials and Engineering*, *304*(4), 1800698. doi: 10.1002/mame.201800698.

Luo, Y., Chen, B., Zhang, X., Huang, S., & Wa, Q. (2022). 3D printed concentrated alginate/GelMA hollow-fibers-packed scaffolds with nano apatite coatings for bone tissue engineering. *International Journal of Biological Macromolecules*, *202*, 366–374. doi: 10.1016/j.ijbiomac.2022.01.096.

Macková, H., Plichta, Z., Proks, V., Kotelnikov, I., Kučka, J., Hlídková, H., Horák, D., Kubinová, Š., & Jiráková, K. (2016). RGDS- and SIKVAVS-modified superporous poly(2-hydroxyethyl methacrylate) scaffolds for tissue engineering applications. *Macromolecular Bioscience*, *16*(11), 1621–1631. doi: 10.1002/mabi.201600159.

Madub, K., Goonoo, N., Gimié, F., Ait Arsa, I., Schönherr, H., & Bhaw-Luximon, A. (2021). Green seaweeds ulvan-cellulose scaffolds enhance in vitro cell growth and in vivo angiogenesis for skin tissue engineering. *Carbohydrate Polymers*. doi: 10.1016/j.carbpol.2020.117025.

Mallakpour, S., Tabesh, F., & Hussain, C. M. (2022). A new trend of using poly(vinyl alcohol) in 3D and 4D printing technologies: Process and applications. *Advances in Colloid and Interface Science*, *301*, 102605. doi: 10.1016/j.cis.2022.102605.

Man, K., Barroso, I. A., Brunet, M. Y., Peacock, B., Federici, A. S., Hoey, D. A., & Cox, S. C. (2022). Controlled release of epigenetically-enhanced extracellular vesicles from a GelMA/nanoclay composite hydrogel to promote bone repair. *International Journal of Molecular Sciences*, *23*(2), 832. doi: 10.3390/ijms23020832.

Mao, H., Yang, L., Zhu, H., Wu, L., Ji, P., Yang, J., & Gu, Z. (2020). Recent advances and challenges in materials for 3D bioprinting. *Progress in Natural Science: Materials International*. doi: 10.1016/j.pnsc.2020.09.015.

Masri, S., Zawani, M., Zulkiflee, I., Salleh, A., Fadilah, N. I. M., Maarof, M., Wen, A. P. Y., Duman, F., Tabata, Y., Aziz, I. A., Idrus, R. B. H., & Fauzi, M. B. (2022). Cellular interaction of human skin cells towards natural bioink via 3d-bioprinting technologies for chronic wound: A comprehensive review. *International Journal of Molecular Sciences*. doi: 10.3390/ijms23010476.

McCracken, J. M., Badea, A., Kandel, M. E., Gladman, A. S., Wetzel, D. J., Popescu, G., Lewis, J. A., & Nuzzo, R. G. (2016). Programming mechanical and physicochemical properties of 3D hydrogel cellular microcultures via direct ink writing. *Advanced Healthcare Materials*, *5*(9), 1025–1039. doi: 10.1002/adhm.201500888.

Monavari, M., Homaeigohar, S., Fuentes-Chandía, M., Nawaz, Q., Monavari, M., Venkatraman, A., & Boccaccini, A. R. (2021). 3D printing of alginate dialdehyde-gelatin (ADA-GEL) hydrogels incorporating phytotherapeutic icariin loaded mesoporous SiO_2-CaO nanoparticles for bone tissue engineering. *Materials Science and Engineering C*, *131*, 112470. doi: 10.1016/j.msec.2021.112470.

Mu, X., Agostinacchio, F., Xiang, N., Pei, Y., Khan, Y., Guo, C., Cebe, P., Motta, A., & Kaplan, D. L. (2021). Recent advances in 3D printing with protein-based inks. *Progress in Polymer Science*. doi: 10.1016/j.progpolymsci.2021.101375.

Müller, M., Becher, J., Schnabelrauch, M., & Zenobi-Wong, M. (2015). Nanostructured Pluronic hydrogels as bioinks for 3D bioprinting. *Biofabrication*, *7*(3), 035006. doi: 10.1088/1758–5090/7/3/035006.

Neufurth, M., Wang, X., Schröder, H. C., Feng, Q., Diehl-Seifert, B., Ziebart, T., Steffen, R., Wang, S., & Müller, W. E. G. (2014). Engineering a morphogenetically active hydrogel for bioprinting of bioartificial tissue derived from human osteoblast-like SaOS-2 cells. *Biomaterials*, *35*(31), 8810–8819. doi: 10.1016/j.biomaterials.2014.07.002.

Nicholas, B. A., Abar, B., Johnson, L., Burbano, J., Danilkowicz, R. M., & Adams, S. B. (2022). 3D-bioprinted GelMA-gelatin-hydroxyapatite osteoblast-laden composite hydrogels for bone tissue engineering. *Bioprinting*, *26*, e00196. doi: 10.1016/j.bprint.2022.e00196.

Niu, X., Wei, Y., Liu, Q., Yang, B., Ma, N., Li, Z., Zhao, L., Chen, W., & Huang, D. (2020). Silver-loaded microspheres reinforced chitosan scaffolds for skin tissue engineering. *European Polymer Journal*. doi: 10.1016/j.eurpolymj.2020.109861.

Ojansivu, M., Rashad, A., Ahlinder, A., Massera, J., Mishra, A., Syverud, K., Finne-Wistrand, A., Miettinen, S., & Mustafa, K. (2019). Wood-based nanocellulose and bioactive glass modified gelatin–alginate bioinks for 3D bioprinting of bone cells. *Biofabrication*, *11*(3), 035010. doi: 10.1088/1758-5090/ab0692.

Ouyang, L., Wojciechowski, J. P., Tang, J., Guo, Y., & Stevens, M. M. (2022). Tunable microgel-templated porogel (MTP) bioink for 3D bioprinting applications. *Advanced Healthcare Materials*, e2200027. doi: 10.1002/adhm.202200027.

Pal, K., Banthia, A. K., & Majumdar, D. K. (2007). Preparation and characterization of polyvinyl alcohol-gelatin hydrogel membranes for biomedical applications. *AAPS PharmSciTech*. doi: 10.1208/pt080121.

Pan, T., Song, W., Xin, H., Yu, H., Wang, H., Ma, D., Cao, X., & Wang, Y. (2022). MicroRNA-activated hydrogel scaffold generated by 3D printing accelerates bone regeneration. *Bioactive Materials*, *10*, 1–14. doi: 10.1016/j.bioactmat.2021.08.034.

Park, J., Lee, S. J., Lee, H., Park, S. A., & Lee, J. Y. (2018). Three dimensional cell printing with sulfated alginate for improved bone morphogenetic protein-2 delivery and osteogenesis in bone tissue engineering. *Carbohydrate Polymers*, *196*, 217–224. doi: 10.1016/j.carbpol.2018.05.048.

Patel, A., & Mequanint, K. (2011). Synthesis and characterization of polyurethane- block -poly(2-hydroxyethyl methacrylate) hydrogels and their surface modification to promote cell affinity. *Journal of Bioactive and Compatible Polymers*, *26*(2), 114–129. doi: 10.1177/0883911511398713.

Peng, Y., Qing, X., Lin, H., Huang, D., Li, J., Tian, S., Liu, S., Lv, X., Ma, K., Li, R., Rao, Z., Bai, Y., Chen, S., Lei, M., Quan, D., & Shao, Z. (2021). Decellularized Disc Hydrogels for hBMSCs tissue-specific differentiation and tissue regeneration. *Bioactive Materials*. doi: 10.1016/j.bioactmat.2021.03.014.

Pitrolino, K. A., Felfel, R. M., Pellizzeri, L. M., MLaren, J., Popov, A. A., Sottile, V., Scotchford, C. A., Scammell, B. E., Roberts, G. A. F., & Grant, D. M. (2022). Development and in vitro assessment of a bi-layered chitosan-nano-hydroxyapatite osteochondral scaffold. *Carbohydrate Polymers*, *282*, 119126. doi: 10.1016/j.carbpol.2022.119126.

Qi, C., Xu, L., Deng, Y., Wang, G., Wang, Z., & Wang, L. (2018). Sericin hydrogels promote skin wound healing with effective regeneration of hair follicles and sebaceous glands after complete loss of epidermis and dermis. *Biomaterials Science*. doi: 10.1039/c8bm00934a.

Raja, N., & Yun, H. (2016). A simultaneous 3D printing process for the fabrication of bioceramic and cell-laden hydrogel core/shell scaffolds with potential application in bone tissue regeneration. *Journal of Materials Chemistry B*, *4*(27), 4707–4716. doi: 10.1039/C6TB00849F.

Rao, Z., Lin, T., Qiu, S., Zhou, J., Liu, S., Chen, S., Wang, T., Liu, X., Zhu, Q., Bai, Y., & Quan, D. (2021). Decellularized nerve matrix hydrogel scaffolds with longitudinally oriented and size-tunable microchannels for peripheral nerve regeneration. *Materials Science and Engineering C*. doi: 10.1016/j.msec.2020.111791.

Roopavath, U. K., Soni, R., Mahanta, U., Deshpande, A. S., & Rath, S. N. (2019). 3D printable SiO_2 nanoparticle ink for patient specific bone regeneration. *RSC Advances*, *9*(41), 23832–23842. doi: 10.1039/C9RA03641E.

Rosiak, J. M., & Yoshii, F. (1999). Hydrogels and their medical applications. *Nuclear Instruments and Methods in Physics Research, Section B: Beam Interactions with Materials and Atoms*. doi: 10.1016/S0168-583X(99)00118-4.

Saunders, R. E., Gough, J. E., & Derby, B. (2008). Delivery of human fibroblast cells by piezoelectric drop-on-demand inkjet printing. *Biomaterials*. doi: 10.1016/j.biomaterials.2007.09.032.

Shahrubudin, N., Lee, T. C., & Ramlan, R. (2019). An overview on 3D printing technology: Technological, materials, and applications. *Procedia Manufacturing*, *35*, 1286–1296. doi: 10.1016/j.promfg.2019.06.089.

Spicer, C. D. (2020). Hydrogel scaffolds for tissue engineering: The importance of polymer choice. *Polymer Chemistry*, *11*(2), 184–219. doi: 10.1039/C9PY01021A.

Tamay, D. G., & Hasirci, N. (2021). Bioinks—materials used in printing cells in designed 3D forms. *Journal of Biomaterials Science, Polymer Edition*, *32*(8), 1072–1106. doi: 10.1080/09205063.2021.1892470.

Tavakoli, S., & Klar, A. S. (2021). Bioengineered skin substitutes: Advances and future trends. *Applied Sciences (Switzerland)*. doi: 10.3390/app11041493.

Tran, H. D. N., Park, K. D., Ching, Y. C., Huynh, C., & Nguyen, D. H. (2020). A comprehensive review on polymeric hydrogel and its composite: Matrices of choice for bone and cartilage tissue engineering. *Journal of Industrial and Engineering Chemistry*, *89*, 58–82. doi: 10.1016/j.jiec.2020.06.017.

Tsai, Y.-C., Li, S., Hu, S.-G., Chang, W.-C., Jeng, U.-S., & Hsu, S. (2015). Synthesis of thermoresponsive amphiphilic polyurethane gel as a new cell printing material near body temperature. *ACS Applied Materials & Interfaces*, *7*(50), 27613–27623. doi: 10.1021/acsami.5b10697.

Tsui, J. H., Leonard, A., Camp, N. D., Long, J. T., Nawas, Z. Y., Chavanachat, R., Smith, A. S. T., Choi, J. S., Dong, Z., Ahn, E. H., Wolf-Yadlin, A., Murry, C. E., Sniadecki, N. J., & Kim, D. H. (2021). Tunable electroconductive decellularized extracellular matrix hydrogels for engineering human cardiac microphysiological systems. *Biomaterials*. doi: 10.1016/j.biomaterials.2021.120764.

Ulusoy, A., & Dikmen, N. (2020). Hidrojellerin Tıpta Uygulamaları. *Arşiv Kaynak Tarama Dergisi*. doi: 10.17827/aktd.603432.

Veiga, A., Silva, I. V., Duarte, M. M., & Oliveira, A. L. (2021). Current trends on protein driven bioinks for 3d printing. *Pharmaceutics*. doi: 10.3390/pharmaceutics13091444.

Vrana, N. E., Gupta, S., Mitra, K., Rizvanov, A. A., Solovyeva, V. V., Antmen, E., Salehi, M., Ehterami, A., Pourchet, L., Barthes, J., Marquette, C. A., von Unge, M., Wang, C.-Y., Lai, P.-L., & Bit, A. (2022). From 3D printing to 3D bioprinting: The material properties of polymeric material and its derived bioink for achieving tissue specific architectures. *Cell and Tissue Banking*. doi: 10.1007/s10561-021-09975-z.

Wang, R., Wang, Y., Yao, B., Hu, T., Li, Z., Huang, S., & Fu, X. (2019). Beyond 2D: 3D bioprinting for skin regeneration. *International Wound Journal*. doi: 10.1111/iwj.13003.

Wang, X. F., Lu, P. J., Song, Y., Sun, Y. C., Wang, Y. G., & Wang, Y. (2016). Nano hydroxyapatite particles promote osteogenesis in a three-dimensional bio-printing construct consisting of alginate/gelatin/hASCs. *RSC Advances*, *6*(8), 6832–6842. doi: 10.1039/c5ra21527g.

Wang, X., Tolba, E., Schröder, H. C., Neufurth, M., Feng, Q., Diehl-Seifert, B., & Müller, W. E. G. (2014). Effect of Bioglass on Growth and Biomineralization of SaOS-2 Cells in Hydrogel after 3D Cell Bioprinting. *PLoS ONE*, *9*(11), e112497. doi: 10.1371/journal.pone.0112497.

Wang, Y., & Li, D. (2020). Creating complex polyacrylamide hydrogel structures using 3D printing with applications to mechanobiology. *Macromolecular Bioscience*, *20*(7), 2000082. doi: 10.1002/mabi.202000082.

Weng, T., Zhang, W., Xia, Y., Wu, P., Yang, M., Jin, R., Xia, S., Wang, J., You, C., Han, C., & Wang, X. (2021). 3D bioprinting for skin tissue engineering: Current status and perspectives. *Journal of Tissue Engineering*. doi: 10.1177/20417314211028574.

Xin, S., Chimene, D., Garza, J. E., Gaharwar, A. K., & Alge, D. L. (2019). Clickable PEG hydrogel microspheres as building blocks for 3D bioprinting. *Biomaterials Science*, *7*(3), 1179–1187. doi: 10.1039/C8BM01286E.

Xu, C., Chang, Y., Xu, Y., Wu, P., Mu, C., Nie, A., Qu, Y., Duan, D., Guo, X., Liu, Z., Wang, J., & Luo, Z. (2022a). Silicon-phosphorus-nanosheets-integrated 3D-printable hydrogel as a bioactive and biodegradable scaffold for vascularized bone regeneration. *Advanced Healthcare Materials*, *11*(6), 2101911. doi: 10.1002/adhm.202101911.

Xu, J., Fang, H., Zheng, S., Li, L., Jiao, Z., Wang, H., Nie, Y., Liu, T., & Song, K. (2021). A biological functional hybrid scaffold based on decellularized extracellular matrix/gelatin/chitosan with high biocompatibility and antibacterial activity for skin tissue engineering. *International Journal of Biological Macromolecules*. doi: 10.1016/j.ijbiomac.2021.07.162.

Xu, T., Zhao, W., Zhu, J. M., Albanna, M. Z., Yoo, J. J., & Atala, A. (2013). Complex heterogeneous tissue constructs containing multiple cell types prepared by inkjet printing technology. *Biomaterials*. doi: 10.1016/j.biomaterials.2012.09.035.

Xu, Y., Zhang, F., Zhai, W., Cheng, S., Li, J., & Wang, Y. (2022b). Unraveling of advances in 3D-printed polymer-based bone scaffolds. *Polymers*, *14*(3), 566. doi: 10.3390/polym14030566.

Yan, Q., Dong, H., Su, J., Han, J., Song, B., Wei, Q., & Shi, Y. (2018). A review of 3D printing technology for medical applications. *Engineering*. doi: 10.1016/j.eng.2018.07.021.

Yazdanpanah, Z., Johnston, J. D., Cooper, D. M. L., & Chen, X. (2022). 3D bioprinted scaffolds for bone tissue engineering: State-of-the-art and emerging technologies. *Frontiers in Bioengineering and Biotechnology*, 10, 824156. doi: 10.3389/fbioe.2022.824156.

Yuk, H., Lu, B., Lin, S., Qu, K., Xu, J., Luo, J., & Zhao, X. (2020). 3D printing of conducting polymers. *Nature Communications*. doi: 10.1038/s41467-020-15316-7.

Zarrintaj, P., Ramsey, J. D., Samadi, A., Atoufi, Z., Yazdi, M. K., Ganjali, M. R., Amirabad, L. M., Zangene, E., Farokhi, M., Formela, K., Saeb, M. R., Mozafari, M., & Thomas, S. (2020). Poloxamer: A versatile tri-block copolymer for biomedical applications. *Acta Biomaterialia*, *110*, 37–67. doi: 10.1016/j.actbio.2020.04.028.

Zhang, J., Yun, S., Karami, A., Jing, B., Zannettino, A., Du, Y., & Zhang, H. (2020). 3D printing of a thermosensitive hydrogel for skin tissue engineering: A proof of concept study. *Bioprinting*. doi: 10.1016/j.bprint.2020.e00089.

Zhang, M., Qian, T., Deng, Z., & Hang, F. (2021a). 3D printed double-network alginate hydrogels containing polyphosphate for bioenergetics and bone regeneration. *International Journal of Biological Macromolecules*, *188*, 639–648. doi: 10.1016/j.ijbiomac.2021.08.066.

Zhang, W., Du, A., Liu, S., Lv, M., & Chen, S. (2021b). Research progress in decellularized extracellular matrix-derived hydrogels. *Regenerative Therapy*. doi: 10.1016/j.reth.2021.04.002.

Zhang, X., Jia, C., Qiao, X., Liu, T., & Sun, K. (2017). Silk fibroin microfibers and chitosan modified poly (glycerol sebacate) composite scaffolds for skin tissue engineering. *Polymer Testing*. doi: 10.1016/j.polymertesting.2017.06.012.

Zhao, X., Lang, Q., Yildirimer, L., Lin, Z. Y., Cui, W., Annabi, N., Ng, K. W., Dokmeci, M. R., Ghaemmaghami, A. M., & Khademhosseini, A. (2016). Photocrosslinkable gelatin hydrogel for epidermal tissue engineering. *Advanced Healthcare Materials*. doi: 10.1002/adhm.201500005.

Zhu, J. (2010). Bioactive modification of poly(ethylene glycol) hydrogels for tissue engineering. *Biomaterials*, *31*(17), 4639–4656. doi: 10.1016/j.biomaterials.2010.02.044.

Zhu, L. Y., Li, L., Shi, J. P., Li, Z. A., & Yang, J. Q. (2018). Mechanical characterization of 3D printed multi-morphology porous Ti6AL4V scaffolds based on triply periodic minimal surface architectures. *American Journal of Translational Research, 10*, 3443–3454.

Zhu, S., Yao, L., Pan, C., Tian, J., Li, L., Luo, B., Zhou, C., & Lu, L. (2021). 3D printed gellan gum/graphene oxide scaffold for tumor therapy and bone reconstruction. *Composites Science and Technology*, *208*, 108763. doi: 10.1016/j.compscitech.2021.108763.

Zhu, Y., Ma, Z., Kong, L., He, Y., Chan, H. F., & Li, H. (2020). Modulation of macrophages by bioactive glass/sodium alginate hydrogel is crucial in skin regeneration enhancement. *Biomaterials*. doi: 10.1016/j.biomaterials.2020.120216.

Zhou, F., Hong, Y., Liang, R., Zhang, X., Liao, Y., Jiang, D., Zhang, J., Sheng, Z., Xie, C., Peng, Z., Zhuang, X., Bunpetch, V., Zou, Y., Huang, W., Zhang, Q., Alakpa, E. V., Zhang, S., & Ouyang, H. (2020). Rapid printing of bio-inspired 3D tissue constructs for skin regeneration. *Biomaterials*. doi: 10.1016/j.biomaterials.2020.120287.

6 Design and Development of Biopolymers-Based Gene Delivery Applications

S. Sajeesh
Lehigh University

A.K. Dipin Das, and M.R. Rekha
SCTIMST

CONTENTS

6.1 Introduction 131
6.2 Natural Polymers for Gene Therapy 133
  6.2.1 Chitosan-Based Gene Delivery Systems 133
  6.2.2 Dextran 137
    6.2.2.1 Dextran and Derivatives for Gene Delivery Application 138
  6.2.3 Pullulan 139
    6.2.3.1 Pullulan and Its Derivatives in Gene Delivery 140
6.3 Conclusion 143
References 144

6.1 INTRODUCTION

Gene therapy has gained attention as potential solution for treating several chronic diseases and genetically acquired disorders [1]. Gene therapy has also been considered as a suitable substitute for conventional small-molecule or antibody-based therapy [2,3]. The two essential components of gene therapy are an effective therapeutic gene that can be expressed at the target site and a carrier system that transfers the therapeutic genes to a specific target tissue or organ [4]. Therefore, the primary role of gene delivery systems is to protect the genetic materials from premature degradation in the blood stream and to efficiently transfer the therapeutic genes to tissues [4,5]. Additionally, advanced gene carrier systems should also facilitate delivery specifically to the target organ and enable the release of therapeutic agents from the endosomal compartment after cellular internalization [5].

DOI: 10.1201/9781003251767-6

The most successful gene therapy systems available as of now are viral vectors [6]. This includes retroviruses, adenoviruses, adeno-associated viruses and lentiviruses. These viral carriers have been modified by deleting some areas of their genomes to disrupt their replication. However, viral vectors have some limitations, such as immunogenicity, insertional mutagenesis and limitations in transgenic capacity size [7,8]. Although non-viral vectors have limitations in terms of gene transfer efficiency, they have an advantage over their viral counterparts in terms of safety and cargo carrying capacity [9,10]. Non-viral vectors have low immunogenicity and production costs compared to viral vectors and pose no risk of endogenous virus recombination. Non-viral carriers offer the possibility of modification with ligands for tissue- or cell-specific gene delivery [10]. Thus, non-viral vectors constructed with biocompatible materials (polymers/lipids) using innovative fabrication approaches offer a promising solution for safe and efficient gene therapy [11–14].

Among various non-viral gene carriers, cationic lipid-based systems are the most ideal platform for the delivery of nucleic acid therapeutics [14]. Liposomes represent an extremely versatile nanocarrier platform for drug delivery [15], and cationic lipid-based liposomes have been extensively investigated for nucleic acid delivery [16]. Lipid nanoparticles (LNPs), an advanced version of liposomes, represent the most efficient non-viral gene delivery platforms, especially for RNA-based therapeutics [17]. LNPs offer advantages over other existing delivery vehicles not only in terms of ease of preparation and versatility but also in terms of their biocompatibility and biodegradability [17]. The basic principle of LNP formation is via self-assembly, through a combination of cationic lipids with so-called helper lipids, comprising fusogenic phospholipids, polyethylene glycol (PEG) lipids and cholesterol [18]. The LNP platform has been successfully used in the clinic for the delivery of mRNA vaccines against COVID-19 and also for the delivery of siRNAs (Onpattro) for the treatment of hereditary amyloidogenic transthyretin (TTR) amyloidosis [19,20]. Both of these mark major milestones for nucleic acid therapeutics. However, these lipid-based carriers have limitations in terms of toxicity and immune responses, and this might be an obstacle in clinical application, particularly if higher doses are required or if frequent, repetitive application is mandatory [21].

Cationic polymers are among the most commonly utilized non-viral vectors for gene transfer owing to their ability to condense and protect the genetic material and transfer it into target cells [12,22]. Cationic polymers bind electrostatically with nucleic acids (DNA/RNA) to form particles (polyplexes) of a few tens to a few hundred nanometers in hydrodynamic diameter (D_H) [22]. A wide variety of commercially sourced synthetic polymers such as poly(ethylenimines) (PEI), poly-l-lysine (PLL), poly-β-amino acids and polyamidoamine dendrimers have been used for gene delivery applications [23–26]. Even though cationic polymers offer several advantages over other categories of non-viral gene carriers, they suffer major drawbacks due to difficulties in formulation, in vivo stabilization, toxicity and low transfection efficiency [27,28]. Lack of biodegradation of polymeric gene delivery vehicles poses significant toxicity due to their accumulation in tissues. Several modification strategies, such as PEGylation, multifunctional modification, etc., have been adopted to reduce the toxicity and improve the gene delivery efficiency of cationic polymer-based systems [29,30]. However, their overall gene transfer efficacy is much lower than that of viral vectors or even lipid-based carriers [31].

Natural polymers have been extensively utilized for formulating gene delivery systems, and they avoid several safety concerns raised by other categories of non-viral gene carriers [32]. Unlike synthetic polymers, natural polymers often lack a well-defined structure and finely tunable degradation kinetic and mechanical properties. However, these natural polymers have advantages in terms of their biocompatibility, biodegradability and low immunogenicity [33–35]. Additionally, most biopolymers contain reactive sites suitable for the attachment of ligands, cross-linking and other modifications that render the polymer tailored for a range of clinical applications [36]. Several natural polymers, such as chitosan and its derivatives, pullulan, collagen, etc. have been used for delivering genetic materials and offer several distinct advantages over existing gene delivery platforms [37–40]. Despite their benefits, choosing a suitable biopolymer and formulating the polymer with genetic material to achieve desired bio-distribution and effective transfer into the target gene remains a major challenge.

6.2 NATURAL POLYMERS FOR GENE THERAPY

6.2.1 Chitosan-Based Gene Delivery Systems

Chitosan is one of the most explored polymers for biomedical and pharmaceutical applications due to its biodegradability, biocompatibility and mucoadhesive properties [34,41–43]. Being cationic in nature, chitosan is being investigated as a non-toxic alternative to other cationic polymer-based gene delivery systems [37]. Chitosan is a cationic polysaccharide composed of randomly distributed β-(1–4)-linked d-glucosamines and *N*-acetyl-d-glucosamines obtained through partial deacetylation of chitin, with molecular weights ranging from 50 to 200 kDa and varying degrees of deacetylation (40%–98%) [44].

Due to its cationic characteristics, chitosan forms complexes with negatively charged nucleic acids through electrostatic interactions, leading to the formation of polymer-nucleic acid complexes (polyplexes) that condense and protect nucleic acids [37,45]. The negative charge on the cellular and nuclear membranes enables their interaction with these polyplexes, resulting in the cellular uptake and nuclear relocation of the complex [44]. The primary amines in the chitosan backbone get protonated at a slightly acidic pH (<pH 6.5), resulting in the availability of positive charges for the interaction with nucleic acids via electrostatic forces. However, chitosan gets deprotonated at pH above 6.5, losing its polycationic characteristics, and this limits its interaction with anionic nucleic acid residues at physiological pH. Therefore, the practical use of chitosan for gene therapy applications has been largely limited to its modified forms [46]. Chitosan was initially used for plasmid DNA (pDNA) delivery initially [47] and was later used for mucosal gene delivery applications owing to its mucoadhesive properties [37,42,48]. Chitosan-based delivery systems were also used to deliver shorter versions of nucleic acids, such as siRNAs, miRNAs, etc. [49,50] (Figure 6.1).

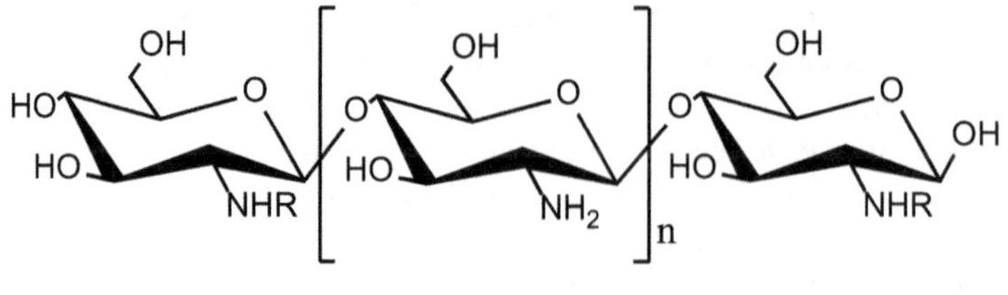

Where R = H, $COCH_3$

FIGURE 6.1 Chemical structure of chitosan.

Chitosan–DNA interaction resulted in the formation of polyplexes with a diameter of several hundred nanometers; however, the relatively low cationic density on the chitosan backbone made the complexes less compact [51]. This is a major disadvantage for chitosan-based gene therapy systems compared to other cationic polymers such as PEI and PLL, which possess high cationic densities [11,12,37]. Low molecular weight versions of chitosan were found to be more effective carriers than their high molecular weight versions in terms of complex stability and toxicity [52,53]. Low molecular weight (>10 kDa) chitosan formulated with pDNA produced homogenous, stable polyplexes of diameter approximately 50–100 nm and efficiently transfected cells [52]. Chitosan oligomers with a well-defined molecular weight (1.2–10 kDa) were found to be more effective for in vivo gene delivery applications compared to high molecular weight ultra-purified chitosan [53]. A water-soluble version of low molecular weight chitosan (5 kDa) with 99% deactylated degree was complexed with DNA at varied charged ratios [54]. However, at higher charge ratios (8:1 chitosan/DNA), the strong interaction of chitosan with DNA prevented gene unpacking from the chitosan vector, which consequently reduced target gene expression. Even though several studies tried to correlate the physicochemical properties of chitosan (molecular weight, degree of deactylation, etc.) with their transfection efficiency, the criteria and strategies for the design of efficient chitosan-based gene delivery systems remain inconclusive [55–58]. Nevertheless, the gene transfer efficiency of unmodified chitosan is reported to be low compared to other cationic polymers used for gene therapy [37,59].

To overcome the issues associated with chitosan-based gene delivery systems, chemically modified chitosan with increased solubility was investigated for gene delivery applications [60]. Chemical modification was achieved through the attachment of small molecules or polymer chains onto the chitosan backbone or via quaternization of the amino groups (Figure 6.2). Chitosan chains possess three reactive sites suitable for chemical modification: two hydroxyl groups (primary or secondary) and one primary amine from the glucosamine units [44]. A quaternized derivative of chitosan possessing a net cationic charge and solubility over a wide range of pH seems to be a good candidate for gene delivery applications [61]. Trimethyl chitosan (TMC) proved to be an effective derivative of chitosan for gene delivery applications [62–64]. *N*-(4-(*N*,*N*,*N*-trimethylammonium)benzyl)chitosan chloride (TMAB-CS) also demonstrated pronounced transfection efficiency even with a low degree of substitution (DS) [65]. Chitosan modification with oligoamine polymers, arginine, etc. was also an effective method for improving the transfection efficiency of native chitosan [66,67]. Ampholytical chitosan derivative, *N*-imidazolyl-*O*-carboxymethyl chitosan (IOCMCS) enhanced the solubility of chitosan in a wide pH range (4–10) without inducing cytotoxicity, and this modification demonstrated high transfection efficiency depending on the degree of imidazolyl substitution [68]. Solubility of chitosan was increased through the introduction of carboxyl groups as well, and the succinated version of chitosan demonstrated enhanced transfection efficiency compared to nascent chitosan [69]. These studies have clearly demonstrated that the gene transfer efficiency of chitosan is highly dependent on its solubility, and the retention of cationic charge at physiological pH might enhance its efficacy.

Self-assembled polymeric amphiphiles of chitosan generated through hydrophobic modification were also utilized for gene delivery applications. Chitosan modified with deoxycholic acid, 5β-cholanic acid, stearic acid, etc. formed self-aggregates in aqueous media, and their complex with pDNA significantly improved the transfection efficacy compared to unmodified chitosan [70–72]. The transfection efficiency of chitosan was also enhanced through the attachment of specific ligands, facilitating receptor mediated endocytosis [73]. Modification of chitosan with galactose,

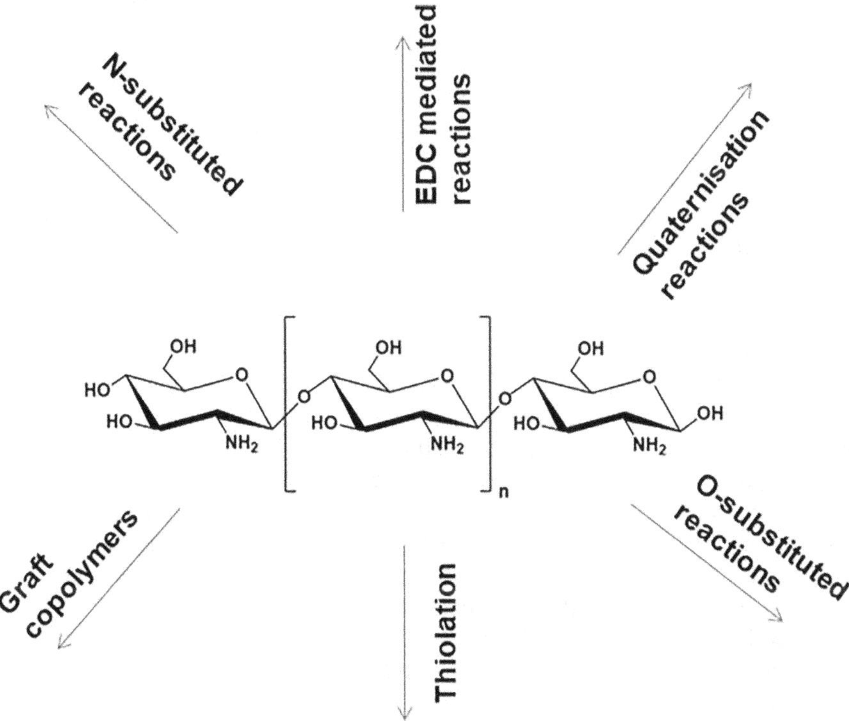

FIGURE 6.2 Most prominent reactions for developing modified chitosan with appropriate functional groups for various biomedical applications.

lactose and lactobionic acid (LA) was an effective strategy for hepatocyte-specific gene therapy [74,75], while mannose-modified chitosan was used as an efficient gene carrier for antigen presenting cells (APCs), such as macrophages and dendritic cells [76]. Folate-based modification of chitosan improved the targeted delivery of pDNA to the folate receptor-bearing tumor cells [77].

Combination of chitosan with lipids or other synthetic polymers was also an effective strategy for enhancing gene delivery. Liposome-encapsulated chitosan nanoparticles, or lipochitoplexes (LCPs) entrapped with pDNA, offered improved DNA protection, reduced cytotoxicity and enhanced transfection efficiency under physiological conditions [78]. Grafting of synthetic cationic polymers, such as PEI, was also an effective approach to enhancing the transfection efficiency of chitosan [79].

Even though chitosan-based delivery systems have much lower gene transfer efficacy than viral-based or non-viral synthetic cationic lipid/polymer carriers, their mucoadhesive properties can make chitosan a suitable candidate for mucosal gene delivery applications [48,80]. Oral administration of chitosan–DNA nanoparticles resulted in transduced gene expression in the intestinal epithelium of mice, and the results from this study possibly suggest oral allergen-gene immunization with chitosan–DNA nanoparticles is an effective strategy in modulating anaphylactic responses [48]. Chitosan and depolymerized oligomers have been successfully used to deliver a reporter gene to the intestinal tract [80]. Oral delivery of chitosan–DNA microparticles in mice resulted in the expression of the Lac Z gene and the activity of α-galactosidase enzyme in stomach and small intestine tissues [81]. Similarly, oral delivery of chitosan-pmEo nanoparticles efficiently delivered genes to enterocytes, suggesting their utility as an oral gene delivery platform [82]. Thiol modification appears to enhance the mucoadhesive and cell penetration properties of chitosan, and thiol-modified chitosan derivatives were used for oral and intranasal delivery of pDNA [83,84]. Thiolated chitosans condensed pDNA to form nanocomplexes and exhibited significantly higher gene transfer potential and sustained gene expression, indicating their great potential for gene therapy via alternative routes [83,84].

Chitosan has also received attention in the formulation of small-interfering RNAs (siRNA) and other shorter RNA versions [85]. Unlike pDNA, which is often several kilobase pairs long and can be efficiently condensed into small nanometric particles through complexation with cationic polymers, siRNAs are much shorter in size (21 bp) and are quite stiff in nature [86,87]. siRNA interaction with cationic polymers may often result in the formation of large, unstable polyplexes, leading to poor intracellular uptake of the complex [86]. Moreover, siRNAs need an efficient endocytic vesicle to release them into the cytoplasm to trigger an RNA interference-based gene silencing mechanism [88]. Several studies have indicated that chitosan alone is not efficient enough to promote endosomal rupture and facilitate siRNA release in the cytoplasm [85,89]. Chitosan/siRNA formulations prepared with low molecular weight chitosan (~10 kDa) showed almost no knockdown of endogenous gene expression, whereas one prepared with higher molecular weight (64.8–170 kDa) showed greater gene silencing [89]. Chitosan nanoparticles prepared by the ionic gelation method using tripolyphosphate (TPP) with entrapped siRNAs demonstrated high siRNA binding capacity and loading efficiency compared to chitosan–siRNA complexes; however, their gene silencing efficacy needs to be further elevated [90]. Several chitosan derivatives, including trimethylated, PEGylated and guandinylated versions, have emerged for siRNA delivery applications, and these modification strategies resulted in improved solubility, transfection efficiency and reduced toxicity [91–95].

Studies have helped researchers understand the limitations of using chitosan-based gene delivery platforms, including their poor water solubility at physiological pH, inadequate complex stability and low buffering capacity, which affect overall gene silencing efficiency. Several modification and combination strategies have helped improve the efficacy of chitosan-based gene delivery systems. Even with several limitations, chitosan is a unique natural polymer with great potential for developing multifunctional nanocarrier systems to deliver large varieties of therapeutic agents administered in multiple ways with reduced side effects.

6.2.2 Dextran

Dextran is a bacterial polysaccharide synthesized from sucrose by certain lactic-acid bacteria and consists of main chains from α-(1–6)-linked d-glucose units with different ratios of linkages and branches, depending on the bacterial strains. The chemical structure of dextran (Figure 6.3) includes α-(1–6) linkages that can vary from 97% to 50% of total glucosidic bonds. The branching is made in positions α-(1–2), α-(1–3) or α-(1–4). The majority of derivatization is favored for the hydroxyl groups in dextran. The C-2 hydroxyl groups appear to be the first to react because the hydroxyl groups of C-6 are concerned in α-1,6 linkages. Different types of dextrans of varying size and structure are synthesized depending on the dextran–sucrase produced by the strain. As a plasma expander, dextrans' low molecular weight fractions are employed. Furthermore, dextrans are widely under investigation as polymeric carriers in novel drug and gene delivery systems [96].

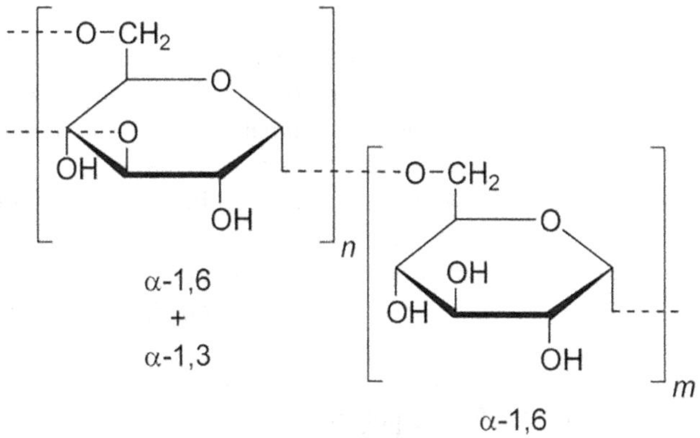

FIGURE 6.3 Chemical structure of dextran.

6.2.2.1 Dextran and Derivatives for Gene Delivery Application

Due to its biodegradability, non-specific cell adhesion, resistance to protein adsorption, low cost and simplicity of structural modification, dextran has been a popular study subject in gene delivery. The degree of branching and molecular weight of dextran are correlated. It may be easily chemically altered, and other glycoconjugates can be produced by etherification, esterification, amidation, oxidation and other processes. These benefits offer a solid foundation for the creation of new material delivery systems [96]. According to studies, dextran modification can significantly lessen biological toxicity and increase the stability of a cationic gene carrier in blood serum.

Cationic polymer gene carriers, which make up the majority of non-viral gene carriers, may introduce genes into cells by creating polyplexes with negatively charged genes through electrostatic interactions [97]. However, the majority of commonly used cationic polymer-based gene carriers, including polyethyleneimine (PEI), polyamidoamine (PAMAM) and polypropyleneimine (PPI), exhibit severe cytotoxicity and offer low transfection efficacy, with the exception of fewer cationic gene carriers like chitosan-based gene carriers [98]. These cationic polymer gene carriers can combine with negatively charged cells when they are injected into the circulatory system, increasing the danger of blood clotting. The reticuloendothelial system may easily remove cationic polymer gene carriers during systemic circulation. The clinical and therapeutic usefulness of cationic polymer gene carriers has been constrained by these drawbacks. As a result, methods to carry genes effectively and securely are still lacking. This problem can only be solved by enhancing the biocompatibility and security of gene carriers. A successful approach has involved the modification of cationic polymers with charge neutral hydrophilic macromolecules, such as polyethylene glycol (PEG) and dextran, to significantly increase the safety and biocompatibility of gene carriers, as well as lengthen the circulating time and improve the stability of the polyplex [99].

Based on the dextran backbone, Hu et al. created five distinct dextran-peptide vectors (DRxHy). In terms of gene delivery, D-R3H7 stood out from the competition due to its superior DNA-binding capability, low toxicity, high luciferase expression and superior buffering ability. Additionally, comparable to D-R3H7, D-R5H5 demonstrated the maximum cell absorption at a low N/P ratio of 2. Due to possessing the most ionizable groups, D-R3H7 exhibited the maximum buffering capacity [100]. An effective transfection reagent, polyethyleneimine (PEI), was reported to be coupled with dextran to lessen PEI's toxicity and enhance its stability in the presence of serum [101]. The micro-RNA-145 (miR-145) was transferred utilizing polyelectrolyte complexes of chitosan and carboxymethyl dextran, improving chitosan-mediated gene delivery [102].

As a multifunctional gene delivery vector for targeted gene delivery to ovarian cancer SKOV-3 cells in vitro and in vivo, a folate-decorated, disulfide-based cationic dextran conjugate with dextran as the main chain and disulfide-linked 1,4-bis(3-aminopropyl)piperazine (BAP) residues as the grafts was designed and successfully prepared. One of the most effective polymeric vectors for intravenous gene delivery in vivo, Dex-SSBAP30-FA, was found to be effective for targeted gene delivery to SKOV-3 tumor xenografts in a nude mouse model by intravenous injection.

It caused a higher level of gene expression in the tumor than Dex-SSBAP30 lacking FA and comparable gene expression to linear polyethylenimine. Thus, the disulfide-based cationic dextran method offers significant promise for intravenous gene therapy [103].

For the purpose of delivering epidermal growth factor receptor (EGFR) siRNA for the treatment of head and neck cancer, a nano-sized polyelectrolyte complex (nano complex) based on poly-l-arginine (PLR) and dextran sulfate (DEX) was created. Following intratumoral injection, the anti-tumor effectiveness of PLR-DEX/siRNA was discovered in a tumor xenografted mouse model [104].

To facilitate effective in vitro gene transfection, Kuo Sun and colleagues created cationic biodegradable DEX-ADM-PEI nanoparticles based on low molecular weight PEI and dextran. Additionally, they demonstrated that their nanoparticles could carry adriamycin into osteosarcoma cells with great efficiency, leading to an increase in therapeutic effectiveness compared to free adriamycin. Both pEGFP-N1 and an anti-cancer medication were effectively and selectively delivered into osteosarcoma cells via their nanoplatform. These nanoparticles have important properties such as regulated molecular features, biodegradability and minimal cytotoxicity. They are also simple to manufacture [105].

The chemical modification of dextran by the click conjugation of poly(amidoamine) (PAMAM) dendrons for the transport of plasmid pEGFP-N3 to human embryonic kidney (HEK293) cells was developed in 2015 by Kaijin Mai and colleagues [106]. Dextran polysaccharide now has an excellent capacity for buffering and a great affinity for binding to pDNA, according to the report's chemical alteration. The compound (Dex-D4) with a larger formation of poly(amidoamine) dendrons was discovered to have a greater gene transfection in the presence of serum, demonstrating a considerable application potential for effective gene delivery.

A dextran-based coacervate gene carrier was developed by Wang et al. by combining a gene directly with a cationic dextran graft copolymer. They added disulfide bonds to the junction locations of the dextran-based coacervate in order to successfully release the gene into target cells. This dextran-based coacervate nanocarrier was formed by the self-assembly of cationic dextran-based graft copolymers and was used as a gene delivery platform that combines high efficiency with low toxicity [107].

6.2.3 Pullulan

Maltotriose units make up the polysaccharide polymer known as pullulan, often referred to as 1,4-; 1,6-glucan (Figure 6.4). Maltotriose has three glucose units linked by a 1,4-glycosidic bonds, whereas the units of sugar are joined by a 1,6-glycosidic bond. Pullulan's biocompatible and non-toxic nature make it a strong candidate for biological applications such as delivering vaccines, molecular chaperoning, tissue engineering, gene delivery, medication administration, etc., and as a plasma expander.

Pullulan is highly biocompatible in nature; however, it cannot be used as such for gene delivery owing to its non-ionic nature. However, pullulan is a versatile molecule that can be easily modified under mild reaction conditions and can be conjugated with any functional group of choice that can render it suitable for gene delivery applications.

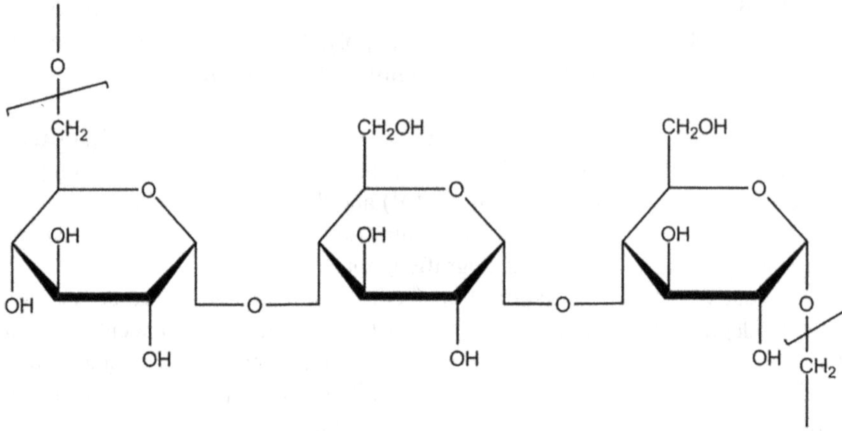

FIGURE 6.4 Chemical structure of pullulan.

6.2.3.1 Pullulan and Its Derivatives in Gene Delivery

The modified pullulan formulations make it simple to entrap the genes, shielding them from DNase cleavage while they are delivered to the targeted cells or organs. Modified pullulan hydrogels show sustained DNA release into cancer cells and strong plasmid DNA loading efficiency [108]. For the treatment of Parkinson's disease, pullulan spermine is said to enhance the release of dopamine and convey the notch intracellular gene [109]. For the transfer of genes to nearby arteries or muscle cells and to shield them from DNase destruction, diethylaminoethylamine pullulan can be synthesized in tubular or three-dimensional matrices [110]. The efficacy of gene transfection is increased, and gene silencing is improved by modification with folate [111]. Pullulan derivative formulations, such as succinylated pullulan [112], pullulan-g-poly(l-lysine) [113] and pullulan–protamine [114–116], are effective for targeted gene delivery with fewer side effects. In cancer cell lines (C6 and HeLa), dextran and pullulan coated with PEI were shown to have high cytocompatibility, excellent cellular internalization and transfection effectiveness, but L929 cells, which are non-cancerous, did not exhibit any transfection efficiency.

It has previously been demonstrated that pullulan–spermine complexed with plasmid DNA is a powerful carrier system for non-viral gene therapy [117–119]. Although it is known that pullulan–spermine may enter cells by clathrin- or raft/caveolae-dependent endocytosis, the processes behind its cellular absorption and subsequent internalization remain unknown. Using both cationic and anionic pullulan–spermine, complexes of plasmid DNA containing cDNA for the reporter gene HcRed fluorescent protein were developed, and it was shown that the cationic complexes can transfect immortalized human brain microvascular endothelial cells (HBMECs) and rat brain endothelial cells (RBE4s). Release of human growth hormone 1 (hGH1) was demonstrated upon transfection of HBMECs, supporting the use of BCECs as a new carrier for non-viral gene therapy [120].

Gupta et al. synthesized highly monodisperse pullulan nanoparticles encasing plasmids inside the aqueous core of AOT/n-hexane reverse micelles [121]. Due to

TABLE 6.1
Modified Biopolymers for Gene Delivery Applications

Biopolymer	Target Cell/ Tissue	In Vitro/In Vivo Evaluation	Major Findings	References
Lactose and galactosylated modified chitosan	Intracellular delivery relating to gene expression and targeting gene delivery system to liver	HepG2 cells	Increased physico-chemical stability and high transfection efficiency	[74]
Mannose-modified chitosan	Antigen presenting cells (APCs), especially dendritic cells having mannose receptors	Dendritic cells	Mannose–chitosan was successfully prepared and targeted gene delivery system to DCs was evaluated	[76]
Thiolated chitosans	Oral delivery of therapeutic genes to targeted sites	HEK293 cells and in vivo evaluation in mice	Thiolated chitosan supports significantly enhanced transfection in cells, higher than a commercial transfection reagent lipofectin	[83,84]
A folate-decorated, disulfide-based cationic dextran conjugate with dextran as the main chain and disulfide-linked 1,4-bis(3-aminopropyl) piperazine (BAP) residues as the grafts	Targeted to SKOV-3 xenograft tumor model in nude mice	SKOV-3 cells and MCF-7	Folate conjugate bioreducible dextran conjugate was found to be an efficient gene delivery system for targeted gene delivery to SKOV-3 xenograft tumor in nude mouse model when administered intravenously. The DexSSBAP30-FA was found to have transfection efficiency than the carrier without FA and comparable efficiency with that of linear PEI 22KDa	[103]

(*Continued*)

TABLE 6.1 *(Continued)*
Modified Biopolymers for Gene Delivery Applications

Biopolymer	Target Cell/ Tissue	In Vitro/In Vivo Evaluation	Major Findings	References
DEX-ADM-PEI nanoparticles based on low molecular weight PEI for drug and gene delivery	Osteosarcoma cells	MG-63 and Saos-2 cells	Highly efficient in delivering both drug and gene into osteosarcoma cells	[105]
Modification of dextran by the click conjugation of poly (amidoamine) (PAMAM) dendrons	Plasmid pEGFP-N3 to human embryonic kidney cells	In vitro evaluation in HEK293	Dextran modified with PAMAM dendrons exhibited low cytotoxicity and good transfection efficiency	[106]
Ethyl amine of diethyl aminoethylamine modified pullulan tubular gels	Implantable local reservoirs for plasmid DNA for arterial gene therapy	Vascular smooth muscle cells (VMSC)	This material can be used in any form as an implantable local reservoir to mediate gene therapy	[110]
pH and redox sensitive charge-reversible pullulan derivative (CAPL) containing β-carboxylic amide bond and disulfide-containing poly(-amino ester) (ssPBAE) nanoparticles for gene and drug delivery	Hepatoma	HepG2 cells	CAPL/ssPBAE-MTX/TAMRA-DNA nanoparticles showed excellent redox- and pH response behavior and these particles significantly inhibited the cell growth	[123]
Disulphide cross-linked cationic pullulan–PEI for gene and drug delivery as well as efflux pump inhibition	Cancer cells	C6, A549 and HeLa cells	Pullulan conjugation considerably decreased toxicity and subsequent functionalization thiol compounds, significantly increased transfection effectiveness, drug retention in cells and enhanced cell death	[127,129]

their excellent biocompatibility, controlled release features, high transfection potential, non-toxicity and great stability against DNase degradation, the synthesized pullulan–DNA nanoparticles constitute a flexible vector for gene therapy. These nanoparticles provide the potential for alternative targeting techniques since particular targeting ligands may be attached to the surface of the particles. Pullulan nanoparticles are being developed as a means of delivering medications and genes inside cells, and the study's findings are hopeful in that regard.

Pullulan was modified with quaternized ammonium groups by reacting glycidyltrimethylammonium chloride (GTMAC) and was used for developing nanoplexes with miRNA, which provided a simple and adaptable approach as well as a novel and promising platform for gene delivery [122].

A unique pH- and redox-responsive nanoparticle system was developed by Zhang et al. based on charge-reversible pullulan derivative (CAPL) and disulfide-containing poly(-amino ester) (ssPBAE) for the simultaneous delivery of a gene and a chemotherapeutic drug that targets hepatoma. Significant pH- and redox-responsive behavior was seen in vitro in CAPL/ssPBAE-MTX/pDNA nanoparticles. The endo/lysosomes of HepG2 cells may effectively internalize and release CAPL/ssPBAE-MTX/TAMRA-DNA nanoparticles. Additionally, in a concentration- and time-dependent way, the nanoparticles greatly slowed down the proliferation of cells. For combined gene/chemotherapy in hepatoma, this innovative nanoparticle method showed a great deal of promise [123].

Any cationic polymer used for gene transport must strike a balance between cytotoxicity and transfection efficiency. However, due to the strong positive surface charge of these cationic polymers, an increase in transfection efficiency is typically accompanied by an increase in toxicity. In our group, we have developed various conjugates based on pullulan–PEI. Pullulan, being a highly water-soluble and flexible molecule, reduced the toxicity of polyethyleneimine on conjugation. Polyethyleneimine of both molecular weights 10 and 25 KDa was conjugated and analyzed for its transfection efficiency. Although pullulan conjugation significantly reduced the toxicity, further functionalization with other molecules, such as vinyl monomers of thiol molecules, significantly improved the transfection efficiency and improved cytocompatibility [124–129]. Table 6.1 cites a few examples of biopolymer modifications for gene delivery applications.

6.3 CONCLUSION

The non-viral vectors started gaining attention following the adverse events associated with the clinical trials using viral vectors for gene delivery. Although non-viral vectors have evolved significantly since their inception, the number of vectors reaching clinical trials is still very limited. The understanding of the various diseases and absent or mutated genes, along with the exponential growth in the development of various gene delivery systems, have opened up new possibilities. The biopolymers can be easily modified, and being relatively more biocompatible and biodegradable, they are widely explored as gene delivery vectors and have resulted in many successful studies. However, taking it to a translational level is challenging and still requires constant efforts to materialize it.

REFERENCES

1. Mulligan R. C. 1993. The basic science of gene therapy. *Science* 260, 926–932.
2. Cring M. R., and Val C. S. 2022. Gene therapy and gene correction—targets, progress, and challenges for treating human diseases. *Gene Therapy* 29, 3–12.
3. Cavazzana-Calvo M., Adrian T., and Fulvio M. 2004. The future of gene therapy. *Nature* 427, 779–781.
4. Kamimura K., Takeshi S., Guisheng Z., and Dexi L. 2011. Advances in gene delivery systems. *Pharmaceutical Medicine* 25, 293–306.
5. Gao X., Keun-Sik K., and Dexi L. 2007. Nonviral gene delivery—what we know and what is next. *The AAPS Journal* 9, E92–E104.
6. Kootstra N. A., and Inder M. V. 2003. Gene therapy with viral vectors. *Annual Review of Pharmacology and Toxicology* 43, 413–439.
7. Nayak S., and Roland W. H. Progress and prospects—immune responses to viral vectors. *Gene Therapy* 17, 295–304.
8. Thomas C. E., Anja E., and Mark A. K. 2003. Progress and problems with the use of viral vectors for gene therapy. *Nature Reviews Genetics* 4, 346–358.
9. Al-Dosari M. S., Xiang G. 2009. Nonviral gene delivery—principle, limitations, and recent progress. *The AAPS Journal* 11, 671–681.
10. Guo X., Leaf H. 2012. Recent advances in nonviral vectors for gene delivery. *Accounts of Chemical Research* 45, 971–979.
11. Wong S. Y., Jeisa M. P., David P. 2007. Polymer systems for gene delivery—past, present, and future. *Progress in Polymer Science* 32, 799–837.
12. De Smedt, S. C., Joseph D., Hennink W. E. 2000. Cationic polymer based gene delivery systems. *Pharmaceutical Research* 17, 113–126.
13. de Ilarduya, C. T., Yan S., and Nejat D. 2010. Gene delivery by lipoplexes and polyplexes. *European Journal of Pharmaceutical Sciences* 40, 159–170.
14. Cullis, P. R., Michael J. H. 2017. Lipid nanoparticle systems for enabling gene therapies. *Molecular Therapy* 25, 1467–1475.
15. Bozzuto G., Agnese M. 2015. Liposomes as nanomedical devices. *International Journal of Nanomedicine* 10, 975.
16. Liu C., Ligang Z., Wenhui Z., Raoqing G., Huamin S., Xi C., and Ning D. 2020. Barriers and strategies of cationic liposomes for cancer gene therapy. *Molecular Therapy-Methods & Clinical Development* 18, 751–764.
17. Kulkarni J. A., Pieter R. C., Roy V. D. M. 2018. Lipid nanoparticles enabling gene therapies—from concepts to clinical utility. *Nucleic Acid Therapeutics* 28, 146–157.
18. Wang C., Yuebao Z., Yizhou D. 2021. Lipid nanoparticle–mRNA formulations for therapeutic applications. *Accounts of Chemical Research* 54, 4283–4293.
19. Hou X., Tal Z., Robert L., Yizhou D. 2021. Lipid nanoparticles for mRNA delivery. *Nature Reviews Materials* 6, 1078–1094.
20. Akinc A., Martin A. M., Muthiah M., Kevin F., Muthusamy J., Scott B., Ansell S. et al. 2019. The Onpattro story and the clinical translation of nanomedicines containing nucleic acid-based drugs. *Nature Nanotechnology* 14, 1084–1087.
21. Tenchov R., Robert B., Allison E. C., Qiongqiong Z. 2021. Lipid nanoparticles—from liposomes to mRNA vaccine delivery, a landscape of research diversity and advancement. *ACS Nano* 15, 16982–17015.
22. Hwang S. J., Davis M. E. 2001. Cationic polymers for gene delivery—designs for overcoming barriers to systemic administration. *Current Opinion in Molecular Therapeutics* 3, 183–191.
23. Lemkine G. F., Demeneix B. A. 2001. Polyethylenimines for in vivo gene delivery. *Current Opinion in Molecular Therapeutics* 3, 178–182.

24. Pandey A. P., Krutika K. S. 2016. Polyethylenimine—A versatile, multifunctional non-viral vector for nucleic acid delivery. *Materials Science and Engineering—C* 68, 904–918.
25. Anderson D. G., David M. L., Robert L. 2003. Semi-automated synthesis and screening of a large library of degradable cationic polymers for gene delivery. *Angewandte Chemie* 115, 3261–3266.
26. Byrne M., Danielle V., Alan H., Martin L., Andreas H., Sally-Ann C. 2013. Molecular weight and architectural dependence of well-defined star-shaped poly (lysine) as a gene delivery vector. *Biomaterials Science* 1, 1223–1234.
27. Lv H., Shubiao Z., Bing W., Shaohui C., Jie Y. 2006. Toxicity of cationic lipids and cationic polymers in gene delivery." *Journal of Controlled Release* 114, 100–109.
28. Breunig M., Uta L., Renate L., Achim G. 2007. Breaking up the correlation between efficacy and toxicity for nonviral gene delivery. *Proceedings of the National Academy of Sciences* 104, 14454–14459.
29. Nelson C. E., Kintzing J. R., Hanna A., Shannon J. M., Gupta M. K., and Duvall C. L. 2013. Balancing cationic and hydrophobic content of PEGylated siRNA polyplexes enhances endosome escape, stability, blood circulation time, and bioactivity in vivo. *ACS Nano* 7, 8870–8880.
30. Kim W. J., Sung W. K. 2007. Targeted polymeric gene delivery for anti-angiogenic tumor therapy." *Macromolecular Research* 15, 100–108.
31. Wahane A., Akaash W., Alexander K., Karishma D., Anisha G., Raman B. 2020. Role of lipid-based and polymer-based non-viral vectors in nucleic acid delivery for next-generation gene therapy. *Molecules* 25, 2866.
32. Dang, J. M., Kam W. L. Natural polymers for gene delivery and tissue engineering. *Advanced Drug Delivery Reviews* 58, 487–499.
33. Anwunobi A. P., Emeje M. O. 2011. Recent applications of natural polymers in nano-drug delivery. *J Nanomedic Nanotechnol* S4. doi: 10.4172/2157-7439.S4-002.
34. Choi C., Joung-Pyo N., Nah J.-W. 2016. Application of chitosan and chitosan derivatives as biomaterials. *Journal of Industrial and Engineering Chemistry* 33, 1–10.
35. Kulkarni V. S., Butte K. D., Sudha S. R. 2012. Natural polymers–A comprehensive review." *International Journal of Research In Pharmaceutical And Biomedical Sciences* 3, 1597–1613.
36. Aravamudhan A., Daisy M. R., Ahmed A. N., Sangamesh G. K. 2014. Natural polymers—polysaccharides and their derivatives for biomedical applications. In *Natural and Synthetic Biomedical Polymers*, pp. 67–89. Elsevier. doi: 10.1016/B978-0-12-396983-5.00004-1.
37. Borchard G. 2001. Chitosans for gene delivery. *Advanced Drug Delivery Reviews* 52, 145–150.
38. Sarvari R., Mohammad N., Ag S., Laila R., Amirhouman S., Alexander M. S., Peyman K. 2022. A summary on non-viral systems for gene delivery based on natural and synthetic polymers. *International Journal of Polymeric Materials and Polymeric Biomaterials* 71, 246–265.
39. Rekha M. R., Sharma C. P. 2009. Blood compatibility and in vitro transfection studies on cationically modified pullulan for liver cell targeted gene delivery. *Biomaterials* 30, 6655–6664.
40. Sano A., Miho M., Shunji N., Takahiro O., Kimi H., Hiroshi I., Teruo M., Keiji F. 2003. Atelocollagen for protein and gene delivery. *Advanced Drug Delivery Reviews* 55, 1651–1677.
41. Chandy T., Sharma C. P. 1990. Chitosan-as a biomaterial. *Biomaterials, Artificial Cells And Artificial Organs* 18, 1–24.
42. Bowman K., Kam W. L. 2006. Chitosan nanoparticles for oral drug and gene delivery." *International Journal of Nanomedicine* 1, 117.

43. Andreas B.-S., Sarah D. 2012. Chitosan-based drug delivery systems. *European Journal of Pharmaceutics and Biopharmaceutics* 81, 463–469.
44. Ravikumar M. N. V., Muzzarelli R. A. A., Muzzarelli C., Sashiwa H., Domb A. J. 2004. Chitosan chemistry and pharmaceutical perspectives. *Chemical Reviews* 104, 6017–6084.
45. Kritchenkov A. S., Stanislav A., Yury A.S. 2017. Chitosan and its derivatives—Vectors in gene therapy. *Russian Chemical Reviews* 86, 231.
46. Tong H., Qin S., Julio C. F., Liu L. I., Kerong D., Xiaoling Z. 2009. Progress and prospects of chitosan and its derivatives as non-viral gene vectors in gene therapy. *Current Gene Therapy* 9, 495–502.
47. Mumper, R. J. 1995. Novel polymeric condensing carriers for gene transfer. In *Proc Natl Symp Control Rel Bioact Mater*, vol. 22, pp. 178–179.
48. Roy K., Hai-Quan M., Shau-Ku H., and Kam W. L. 1999. Oral gene delivery with chitosan–DNA nanoparticles generates immunologic protection in a murine model of peanut allergy. *Nature Medicine* 5, 387–391.
49. Rudzinski W. E., Tejraj M. A. 2010. Chitosan as a carrier for targeted delivery of small interfering RNA. *International Journal of Pharmaceutics* 399, 1–11.
50. Santos-Carballal B., Aaldering L. J., Markus R., Pereira S., Norbert S., Moerschbacher B. M., Martin G., Francisco M. G. 2015. Physicochemical and biological characterization of chitosan-microRNA nanocomplexes for gene delivery to MCF-7 breast cancer cells. *Scientific Reports* 5, 1–15.
51. Erbacher P., Shaomin Z., Thierry B., Anne-Marie S., Jean-Serge R. 1998. Chitosan-based vector/DNA complexes for gene delivery—biophysical characteristics and transfection ability. *Pharmaceutical Research* 15, 1332–1339.
52. Richardson, S. C. W., Hanno V. J. K., Ruth D. 1999. Potential of low molecular mass chitosan as a DNA delivery system—biocompatibility, body distribution and ability to complex and protect DNA. *International Journal of Pharmaceutics* 178, 231–243.
53. Köping-Höggård M., Vårum K. M., Issa M., Danielsen S., Christensen B. E., Stokke B. T., Artursson P. 2004. Improved chitosan-mediated gene delivery based on easily dissociated chitosan polyplexes of highly defined chitosan oligomers. *Gene Therapy* 11, 1441–1452.
54. Liu W., Shujun S., Zhiqiang C., Xin Z., Kangde Y., William W. L., Luk K. D. K. 2005. An investigation on the physicochemical properties of chitosan/DNA polyelectrolyte complexes. *Biomaterials* 26, 2705–2711.
55. Sato T., Tsuyoshi I., Yoshio O. 2001. In vitro gene delivery mediated by chitosan. Effect of pH, serum, and molecular mass of chitosan on the transfection efficiency. *Biomaterials* 22, 2075–2080.
56. Bordi F., Laura C., Cleofe P., Francesca B., Antonio D. M., Noemi C., Barbara P., Fiorentina A., Simona S. 2014. Chitosan–DNA complexes—Effect of molecular parameters on the efficiency of delivery. *Colloids and Surfaces A—Physicochemical and Engineering Aspects* 460, 184–190.
57. Strand S. P., Sylvie L., Nina K. R., de Lange Davies C., Per A., Kjell M. V. 2010. Molecular design of chitosan gene delivery systems with an optimized balance between polyplex stability and polyplex unpacking. *Biomaterials* 31, 975–987.
58. Kiang T., Jie W., Huay W. L., Kam W. L. 2004. The effect of the degree of chitosan deacetylation on the efficiency of gene transfection. *Biomaterials* 25, 5293–5301.
59. Cao Y., Yang F. T., Yee S. W., Melvin W. J. L., Subbu V. 2019. Recent advances in chitosan-based carriers for gene delivery. *Marine Drugs* 17, 381.
60. Jaiswal A., Arun C., Siddhartha S. G. 2012. Functional chitosan nanocarriers for potential applications in gene therapy. *Materials Letters* 68, 261–264.
61. Thanou M., Florea B. I., Geldof M., Junginger H. E., Borchard G. 2002. Quaternized chitosan oligomers as novel gene delivery vectors in epithelial cell lines. *Biomaterials* 23, 153–159.

62. Mourya V. K., Nazma N. I. 2009. Trimethyl chitosan and its applications in drug delivery. *Journal of Materials Science—Materials in Medicine* 20, 1057–1079.
63. Zhao X., Lichen Y., Jieying D., Cui T., Shaohua G., Chunhua Y., Yumin M. 2010. Thiolated trimethyl chitosan nanocomplexes as gene carriers with high in vitro and in vivo transfection efficiency. *Journal of Controlled Release* 144, 46–54.
64. Kean T., Susanne R., Maya T. 2005. Trimethylated chitosans as non-viral gene delivery vectors—cytotoxicity and transfection efficiency. *Journal of Controlled Release* 103, 643–653.
65. Raik S. V., Daria N. P., Tatiana A. L., Dmitry S. P., Vasilyev V. B., Andreii S. K., Yury A. S. 2018. N-(4-(N, N, N-trimethylammonium) benzyl) chitosan chloride—Synthesis, interaction with DNA and evaluation of transfection efficiency. *Carbohydrate polymers* 181, 693–700.
66. Lu B., Chang-Fang W., De-Qun W., Cao L., Xian-Zheng Z., Ren-Xi Z. 2009. Chitosan based oligoamine polymers—Synthesis, characterization, and gene delivery. *Journal of Controlled Release* 137, 54–62.
67. Gao Y., Zhenghong X., Shangwei C., Wangwen G., Lingli C., Yaping L. 2008. Arginine-chitosan/DNA self-assemble nanoparticles for gene delivery—In vitro characteristics and transfection efficiency. *International Journal of Pharmaceutics* 359, 241–246.
68. Shi B., Zheyu S., Hu Z., Jingxiu B., Sheng D. 2012. Exploring N-imidazolyl-O-carboxymethyl chitosan for high performance gene delivery. *Biomacromolecules* 13, 146–153.
69. Toh E. K.-W., Hsing-Yin C., Yu-Lun L., Shih-Jer H., Li-Fang W. 2011. Succinated chitosan as a gene carrier for improved chitosan solubility and gene transfection. *Nanomedicine—Nanotechnology, Biology and Medicine* 7, 174–183.
70. Kim Y. H., Se H. G., Chong R. P., Kuen Y. L., Tae W. K., Ick C. K., Hesson C., Seo Y. J. 2001. Structural characteristics of size-controlled self-aggregates of deoxycholic acid-modified chitosan and their application as a DNA delivery carrier. *Bioconjugate Chemistry* 12, 932–938.
71. Yoo H. S., Jung E. L., Hesson C., Ick C. K., Seo Y. J. 2005. Self-assembled nanoparticles containing hydrophobically modified glycol chitosan for gene delivery. *Journal of Controlled Release* 103, 235–243.
72. Hu F.-Q., Meng-Dan Z., Hong Y., Jian Y., Yong-Zhong D., Su Z. 2006. A novel chitosan oligosaccharide–stearic acid micelles for gene delivery—Properties and in vitro transfection studies. *International Journal of Pharmaceutics* 315, 158–166.
73. Guy J., Dubravka D., Michael A. 1995. Delivery of DNA into mammalian cells by receptor-mediated endocytosis and gene therapy. *Molecular Biotechnology* 3, 237–248.
74. Kim T. H., In K. P., Jae W. N., Yun J. C., Chong S. C. 2004. Galactosylated chitosan/DNA nanoparticles prepared using water-soluble chitosan as a gene carrier. *Biomaterials* 25, 3783–3792.
75. Hashimoto M., Minoru M., Hiroyuki S., Yoshihiro S., Toshinori S. 2006. Lactosylated chitosan for DNA delivery into hepatocytes—the effect of lactosylation on the physicochemical properties and intracellular trafficking of pDNA/chitosan complexes. *Bioconjugate Chemistry* 17, 309–316.
76. Kim, T. H., Jae W. N., Myung-Haing C., Tae G. P., Chong S. C. 2006. Receptor-mediated gene delivery into antigen presenting cells using mannosylated chitosan/DNA nanoparticles. *Journal of Nanoscience and Nanotechnology* 6, 2796–2803.
77. Mansouri S., Yan C., Francoise W., Qin S., Patrick L., Mohamed B., Eric B., Julio C. F. Characterization of folate-chitosan-DNA nanoparticles for gene therapy. *Biomaterials* 27, 2060–2065.
78. Baghdan E., Shashank R. P., Boris S., Konrad H. E., Jens S., Udo B. 2018. Lipid coated chitosan-DNA nanoparticles for enhanced gene delivery. *International Journal of Pharmaceutics* 535, 473–479.

79. Wong K., Guobin S., Xueqing Z., Hui D., Ye L., Chaobin H., Kam W. L. 2006. PEI-g-chitosan, a novel gene delivery system with transfection efficiency comparable to polyethylenimine in vitro and after liver administration in vivo. *Bioconjugate Chemistry* 17, 152–158.
80. MacLaughlin F. C., Russell J. M., Jijun W., Jenna M. T., Inder G., Mike H., Alain P. R. Chitosan and depolymerized chitosan oligomers as condensing carriers for in vivo plasmid delivery. *Journal of Controlled Release* 56, 259–272.
81. Guliyeva Ü, Filiz Ö, Şule Ö, Rıfkı H. 2006. Chitosan microparticles containing plasmid DNA as potential oral gene delivery system. *European Journal of Pharmaceutics and Biopharmaceutics* 62, 17–25.
82. Chen J., Wu-Li Y., Ge L., Ji Q., Jing-Lun X., Shou-Kuan F., Da-Ru L. 2004. Transfection of mEpo gene to intestinal epithelium in vivo mediated by oral delivery of chitosan-DNA nanoparticles. *World Journal of Gastroenterology* 10, 112.
83. Lee D., Weidong Z., Shawna A. S., Xiaoyuan K., Gary R. H., Richard F. L., Shyam S. M. 2007. Thiolated chitosan/DNA nanocomplexes exhibit enhanced and sustained gene delivery. *Pharmaceutical Research* 24, 157–167.
84. Martien R., Brigitta L., Marlene T., Sayeh M., Andreas B.-S. Chitosan–thioglycolic acid conjugate—an alternative carrier for oral nonviral gene delivery? *Journal of Biomedical Materials Research Part A* 82, 1–9.
85. Ragelle H., Gaëlle V., Véronique P. Chitosan-based siRNA delivery systems. *Journal of Controlled Release* 172, 207–218.
86. Gary D. J., Nitin P., You-Yeon W. 2007. Polymer-based siRNA delivery—perspectives on the fundamental and phenomenological distinctions from polymer-based DNA delivery. *Journal of Controlled Release* 121, 64–73.
87. Scholz C., Ernst W. 2012. Therapeutic plasmid DNA versus siRNA delivery—common and different tasks for synthetic carriers. *Journal of Controlled Release* 161, 554–565.
88. Shuey D. J., McCallus D. E., Tony G. 2002. RNAi—gene-silencing in therapeutic intervention. *Drug Discovery Today* 7, 1040–1046.
89. Liu X., Kenneth A. H., Mingdong D., Morten Ø. A., Ulrik L. R., Mads G. J., Ole C. H., Flemming B., Jørgen K. 2007. The influence of polymeric properties on chitosan/siRNA nanoparticle formulation and gene silencing. *Biomaterials* 28, 1280–1288.
90. Katas H., Alpar O. H. 2006. Development and characterisation of chitosan nanoparticles for siRNA delivery. *Journal of Controlled Release* 115, 216–225.
91. Dehousse V., Nancy G., Alain C., Brigitte E. 2010. Development of pH–responsive nanocarriers using trimethylchitosans and methacrylic acid copolymer for siRNA delivery. *Biomaterials* 31, 1839–1849.
92. Varkouhi A. K., Rolf J. V., Raymond M. S., Twan L., Gert S., Wim E. H. 2010. Gene silencing activity of siRNA polyplexes based on thiolated N, N, N-trimethylated chitosan. *Bioconjugate Chemistry* 21, 2339–2346.
93. Malhotra M., Tomaro-Duchesneau C., Prakash S. 2013. Synthesis of TAT peptide-tagged PEGylated chitosan nanoparticles for siRNA delivery targeting neurodegenerative diseases. *Biomaterials* 34, 1270–1280.
94. Zhang J., Cui T., Chunhua Y. Galactosylated trimethyl chitosan–cysteine nanoparticles loaded with Map4k4 siRNA for targeting activated macrophages. *Biomaterials* 34, 3667–3677.
95. Ni S., Yuwen X., Yue T., Yun L., Jing C., Siyan Z. 2017. Nebulized anionic guanidinylated O-carboxymethyl chitosan/N-2-hydroxypropyltimehyl ammonium chloride chitosan nanoparticles for siRNA pulmonary delivery—preparation, characterization and in vitro evaluation. *Journal of Drug Targeting* 25, 451–462.
96. Huang S., Huang G. 2019. The dextrans as vehicles for gene and drug delivery. *Future Med Chem* 11, 1659–1667.

97. Verma I. M., Somia N. 1997. Gene therapy - promises, problems and prospects. *Nature* 389, 239–242.
98. Rui D., Yanan Y., Fan J., Yangchao C., Hsiang-Fu K., Marie C. M., Lin C. W. 2009. Revisit the complexation of PEI and DNA — How to make low cytotoxic and highly efficient PEI gene transfection non-viral vectors with a controllable chain length and structure. *Journal of Controlled Release* 140, 40–46.
99. Fu-Wei H., Hui-Yuan W., Cao L., Hua-Fen W., Yun-Xia S., Jun F., Xian-Zheng Z., Ren-Xi Z. 2010. PEGylated PEI-based biodegradable polymers as non-viral gene vectors. *Acta Biomaterialia* 6, 4285–4295.
100. Hu Y., Wang H., Song H., et al. 2019. Peptide-grafted dextran vectors for efficient and high-loading gene delivery. *Biomaterials Science* 7, 1543–1553.
101. Jiang D., Salem A. 2012. Optimized dextran-polyethylenimine conjugates are efficient non-viral vectors with reduced cytotoxicity when used in serum containing environments. *International Journal of Pharmaceutics* 427, 71–79.
102. Tekie F., Kiani M., Zakerian A., Pilevarian F., et al. 2017. Nano polyelectrolyte complexes of carboxymethyl dextran and chitosan to improve chitosan-mediated delivery of MiR-145. *Carbohydrate Polymers* 159, 66–75.
103. Song Y., Lou B., Zhao P., Lin C. 2014. Multifunctional disulfide-based cationic dextran conjugates for intravenous gene delivery targeting ovarian cancer cells. *Molecular Pharmaceutics* 11, 2250–2261.
104. Cho H. J., Chong S., Chung S. J., Shim C. K., Kim D. D. 2012. Poly-L-arginine and dextran sulfate-based nanocomplex for epidermal growth factor receptor (EGFR) siRNA delivery—Its application for head and neck cancer treatment. *Pharmaceutical Research* 29, 1007–1019.
105. Sun K., Wang J., Zhang J., Hua M., Liu C. and Chen T. 2011. Dextran–g–PEI nanoparticles as a carrier for co-delivery of adriamycin and plasmid into osteosarcoma cells. *International Journal of Biological Macromolecules* 49, 173–180.
106. Mai K., Zhang S., Liang B., Gao C., Du W., Zhang L. M. 2015. Water soluble cationic dextran derivatives containing poly(amidoamine) dendrons for efficient gene delivery. *Carbohydrate Polymers* 123, 237–245.
107. Wang C., Xiong S., You J., Guan W., Xu G., Dou H. 2020. Dextran-based coacervate nanodroplets as potential gene carriers for efficient cancer therapy. *Carbohydrate Polymers* 231, 115687.
108. Gupta M., Gupta A. K. 2004. Hydrogel pullulan nanoparticles encapsulating pBUD-LacZ plasmid as an efficient gene delivery carrier. *Journal of Controlled Release* 99, 157–166.
109. Nagane K., Kitada M., Wakao S., Dezawa M., Tabata Y. 2009. Practical induction system for dopamine-producing cells from bone marrow stromal cells using spermine-pullulan mediated reverse transfection method. *Tissue Engineering Part A* 15, 1655–1665.
110. Juan A. S., Ducrocq G., Hlawaty H., Bataille I., Guenin E., Letourneur D., Feldman L. J. 2007. Tubular cationized pullulan hydrogels as local reservoirs for plasmid DNA. *Journal of Biomedical Materials Research Part A* 83A, 819–827.
111. Wang J., Dou B., Bao Y. 2014. Efficient targeted pDNA/siRNA delivery with folate-low molecular-weight polyethyleneimine-modified pullulan as non-viral carrier. *Materials Science & Engineering—C* 34, 98–109.
112. Kim H., Na K. 2010. Evaluation of succinylated pullulan for long-term protein delivery in poly(lactide-co-glycolide) microspheres. *Macromolecular Research* 18, 812–819.
113. Park J. S., Park J. K., Nam J. P., Kim W. S., Choi C., Kim M. Y., Jang M. K., Nah J. W. 2012. Preparation of pullulan-g-poly(L-lysine) and its evaluation as a gene carrier. *Macromolecular Research* 20, 667–672.

114. Liu Y., Wang Y., Zhang C., Zhou P., Liu Y., An T., Sun D., Zhang N., Wang Y. 2014. Coreshell nanoparticles based on pullulan and poly(β-amino) ester for hepatoma-targeted codelivery of gene and chemotherapy agent. *Applied Materials & Interfaces* 6, 18712–18720.
115. Priya S. S., Rekha M. R., Sharma C. P. 2014. Pullulan-protamine as efficient haemocompatible gene delivery vector—Synthesis and in vitro characterization. *Carbohydrate Polymers* 102, 207–215.
116. Yang X. C., Niu Y. L., Zhao N. N., Mao C., Xu F. J. 2014. A biocleavable pullulan-based vector via ATRP for liver cell-targeting gene delivery. *Biomaterials* 35, 3873–3884.
117. Thakor D. K., Teng Y. D., Tabata Y. 2009. Neuronal gene delivery by negatively charged pullulan–spermine/DNA anioplexes. *Biomaterials* 30, 1815–1826.
118. Kanatani I., Ikai T., Okazak A., Jo J., Yamamoto M., Imamura M., Kanematsu A., Yamamoto S., Ito N., Ogawa O., Tabata Y. 2006. Efficient gene transfer by pullulan–spermine occurs through both clathrin- and raft/caveolae-dependent mechanisms. *Journal of Controlled Release* 116, 75–82.
119. Jo J. I., Ikai T., Okazaki A., Nagane K., Yamamoto M., Hirano Y., Tabata Y. 2007. Expression profile of plasmid DNA obtained using spermine derivatives of pullulan with different molecular weights. *Journal of Biomaterials Science, Polymer Edition* 18, 883–899.
120. Louiza B. T., Jacek L., Kwang S. K., Torben M. 2011. Gene delivery by pullulan derivatives in brain capillary endothelial cells for protein secretion. *Journal of Controlled Release* 5, 45–50.
121. Gupta M., Gupta A. K. 2004. Hydrogel pullulan nanoparticles encapsulating pBUD-LacZ plasmid as an efficient gene delivery carrier. *Journal of Controlled Release* 99, 157–166.
122. Moraes F. C., Antunes J. C., Marcela F. R. L., Aprile P., Franck G., Chauvierre C., Chaubet F., Letourneur D. 2020. Synthesis of cationic quaternized pullulan derivatives for miRNA delivery. *International Journal of Pharmaceutics* 577, 119041.
123. Zhang S., Wang D., Li Y., Li L., Chen H., Xiong Q., Liu Y., Wang Y. 2018. pH- and redox-responsive nanoparticles composed of charge-reversible pullulan-based shells and disulfide-containing poly (ß-amino ester) cores for co-delivery of a gene and chemotherapeutic agent. *Nanotechnology* 29, 325101.
124. Priya S. S., Rekha M. R. 2022. Intracellular delivery of p53 gene and drug using cationised pullulan thiomer lowers the effective therapeutic doses of chemotherapeutic drug in cancer cells. *Materials Today Communications* 30, 103129.
125. Caroline D. S. M. , Rekha M. R. 2022. Exploring the efficacy of ethylene glycol dimethacrylate crosslinked cationised pullulan for gene delivery in cancer cell. *Journal of Drug Delivery Science and Technology* 68, 103129.
126. Caroline D. S. M., Rekha M. R. and Harikrishnan V. S. 2020. Cationised dextran and pullulan modified with diethyl aminoethyl methacrylate for gene delivery in cancer cell. *Carbohydrate Polymers* 242, 116426.
127. Priya S. S. and Rekha M. R. 2017. Redox sensitive cationic pullulan for efficient gene transfection and drug retention in C6 glioma cells. *International Journal of Pharmaceutics* 530, 401–414.
128. Caroline D. S. and Rekha M. R. 2017. Efficacy of vinyl imidazole grafted cationized pullulan and dextran as gene delivery vectors—A comparative study. *International Journal of Biological Macromolecules* 105, 947–955.
129. Priya S. S., Rekha M. R. 2016. Disulphide cross linked pullulan based cationic polymer for improved gene delivery and efflux pump inhibition. *Colloids and Surfaces B—Biointerfaces* 146, 879–887.

7 Stimuli-Responsive Microgels as Drug Carriers and Theranostics

Aastha Gupta, Ankita Dhiman
Indian Institute of Technology Mandi

Sangram K. Samal
Indian Institute of Science

Garima Agrawal
Indian Institute of Technology Mandi

CONTENTS

7.1 Introduction 151
7.2 Synthesis of Smart Microgels 153
7.3 Stimuli-Responsive Microgels for Drug Delivery 155
  7.3.1 Microgels with Degradable Crosslinking Points 155
  7.3.2 Active and Passive Targeting for Drug Delivery 157
  7.3.3 Stimuli-Responsive Drug Release in Biological Environment 158
  7.3.4 Remotely Controlled Drug Release 162
7.4 Stimuli-Responsive Microgels as Theranostics 165
7.5 Conclusions 167
Acknowledgments 167
References 168

7.1 INTRODUCTION

In recent years, significant research has been performed on advanced nano/microscopic materials such as nanoparticles, liposomes, micelles, microgels, etc. to explore them for a variety of applications, including drug delivery and bioimaging (Sauraj et al. 2020; Agrawal and Agrawal 2019; Sood et al. 2021; Agarwal et al. 2021; Sood, Gupta, and Agrawal 2021; Doermbach et al. 2014; Wang et al. 2013a; Gupta et al. 2022a,b; Sood et al. 2022). However, successful clinical use of microgels is still hampered owing to various issues such as lack of cytotoxic specificity, insufficient biodistribution, premature drug release, and so on (Sauraj et al. 2020). Among various nanostructured biomaterials, microgels exhibit immense promise for achieving difficult targets in complex biological environments (Agrawal, Agrawal,

DOI: 10.1201/9781003251767-7

and Pich 2017). Microgels are aqueous, polymeric, crosslinked particles exhibiting tunable size, functionality, a large surface area, superior colloidal stability, and biocompatibility (Kwok, Sun, and Ngai 2019). The most attractive feature exhibited by microgels is their stimuli responsiveness (e.g. sensitivity to temperature, pH, reducing environment, etc.), which renders them suitable for drug delivery and bioimaging (Agrawal et al. 2012; Mutharani, Ranganathan, and Chen 2020; Wei, Li, and Serpe 2019). Readers are referred to different review articles available in the literature that describe different physicochemical aspects of microgels (Feng et al. 2022; Agrawal and Agrawal 2018a, b; Plamper and Richtering 2017) (Figure 7.1).

Microgels are soft, polymeric, crosslinked materials that exhibit a faster response to stimuli as compared to bulk materials (Agrawal and Agrawal 2018b). The fusion of soft and porous characteristics with self-standing structure achieved by an intramolecularly crosslinked network of polymer chains allows the design of microgels with different architectures while still maintaining the same chemical composition. Microgels are able to exhibit higher accumulation at cancer sites, facilitated by the enhanced permeation and retention (EPR) effect (Lei et al. 2020; Yan et al. 2021). This is further supported by the flexibility of polymer chains, which helps the microgels pass through various barriers (Martin-Molina and Quesada-Pérez 2019; Beningo, and Wang 2002). Once the drug carrier reaches the tumor site, it releases the payload in response to changes in temperature (Agrawal et al. 2013b), pH (Agrawal, Agrawal, and Pich 2017), reducing conditions (Mackiewicz et al. 2021), magnetism (Wiemer et al. 2017), and the degraded byproducts can be subjected to renal clearance.

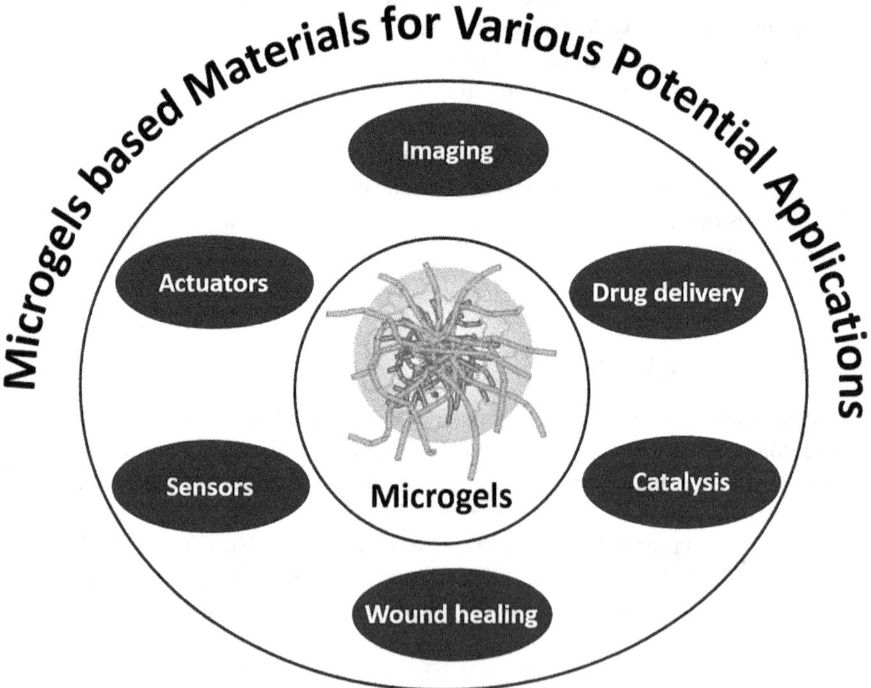

FIGURE 7.1 Schematic representation of various applications of microgels.

Furthermore, an ideal biomaterial for bioimaging of cancer cells requires easy handling, excellent biocompatibility, suitable interaction with adjacent tissue, higher sensitivity, high bioimaging times, noninvasive nature, and high spatial resolution (Agrawal and Agrawal 2018a; Fan et al. 2021). In recent years, scientists all over the world have made significant efforts to exploit microgels for cell bioimaging applications. Here, using drug-loaded microgels further facilitates the simultaneous diagnostic bioimaging and treatment processes (Van Elk et al. 2015).

A precise control of microgel size, chemical functionality, stability, and degradability is the prime requisite to move further in the direction of widespread clinical use. Herein, we will discuss the fundamentals of various synthetic approaches to fabricating the microgels, along with their advantages and disadvantages. Additionally, we will also summarize the progress made in the last few years in using these microgels for drug delivery and bioimaging.

7.2 SYNTHESIS OF SMART MICROGELS

The choice of an appropriate synthetic approach is of prime importance for synthesizing the microgels with the required dimensions, polydispersity, and physicochemical properties (Agrawal et al. 2013a). Various synthetic methods can be generally classified into the following categories: (i) in homogeneous phase by physical self-assembly of prepolymers/biopolymers and crosslinking; (ii) in heterogeneous phase by precipitation polymerization or miniemulsion polymerization; (iii) photolithographic methods; (iv) microfluidic technique; and (v) membrane emulsification (Agrawal and Agrawal 2018a,b; Agrawal et al. 2013b; Xu et al. 2020; Farjami and Madadlou 2017).

Microgel synthesis in homogeneous phase is performed by coacervation and desolvation techniques, where polymer chains are phase separated followed by crosslinking. Maeda et al. (2009) prepared coacervate droplets by heating the aqueous mixture of nonionic poly(*N*-isopropylacrylamide) (PNIPAM)-co-2-hydroxyisopropylacrylamide and ionic PNIPAM-co-2-carboxyisopropylacrylamide. The obtained coacervate droplets were further crosslinked by using divinyl sulfone, and thus semi-interpenetrating thermoresponsive microgels were synthesized. Yin et al. (2003) reported microgel formation by fabricating complex coacervates of PEG modified poly(styrene-alt-maleic anhydride) with poly(diallyldimethylammonium chloride) (PDADMAC). These coacervates were further crosslinked with polyethylenimine to generate stable microgels. On the other hand, gelatin and modified starch-based microgels were synthesized by Wu et al. (2015) based on acidic pH-induced coacervation for improving the texture and sensory quality of low-calorie food products. Fettis et al. (2016) developed peptide-based microgels via desolvation of peptide nanofibers for controlled delivery of proteins. Here, ethanol was added to the aqueous solution of peptide nanofibers under stirring, which resulted in physically crosslinked peptide-based microgels due to the desolvating effect of ethanol.

Among heterogeneous phase methods, precipitation polymerization is a widely used method for fabricating monodisperse microgels of poly(*N*-isopropylacrylamide) (PNIPAM), poly(*N*-isopropylmethacrylamide) (PNIPMAM), poly(*N*,*N*-diethylacrylamide) (PDEAAM), poly(*N*-vinylcaprolactam) (PVCL), etc. (Birkholz et al. 2016). This method involves dissolving all the reaction components, including the monomer, initiator, and crosslinker, in water, followed by increasing the temperature to 50°C–70°C (Agrawal et al. 2014, 2019), The reaction temperature is generally higher as compared to the volume phase transition temperature (VPTT) of temperature-responsive polymers. This results in the collapse of the polymer chains once they reach a critical number of repeating units, and thus precursor particles are formed. These precursor particles grow further either by precipitation of newly formed polymer chains or by absorption and polymerization of monomers, resulting in the formation of shrunken, crosslinked microgels (Figure 7.2) (Klinger and Landfester 2012). Once the reaction mixture is cooled down after the completion of polymerization, the microgel particles achieve a swollen state. Here, microgel size can be adjusted by changing various parameters like solvent composition and temperature, along with crosslinker, surfactant, initiator, and comonomer ratios in the reaction mixture (Agrawal and Agrawal 2018a, b). In the literature, microgels functionalized with various small molecules, polymers, metal nanoparticles, and numerous comonomers (e.g. acrylic acid (AA), methacrylic acid (MAA), vinyl imidazole (Vim), and glycidyl methacrylate (GMA)) have been reported for targeted applications (Agrawal, Agrawal, and Pich 2017; Agrawal et al. 2012, 2013a, 2014; Giussi et al. 2020). Apart from homogeneously functionalized microgels, Xu et al. (2020) have taken a step further to develop Janus microgels using PNIPAM, itaconic acid, and Vim. Here, microgels with interesting Janus features were formed based on the self-assembly and coacervation of growing polymer chains, having opposite charges from itaconic acid and Vim, in precipitation polymerization.

The precipitation polymerization method allows fabrication in parts or in a continuous way, producing microgels having tunable size, monodispersity, and layered shell architecture with different chemical compositions (Agrawal and Agrawal 2018b). However, this method cannot be used for temperature-sensitive biological molecules. Additionally, this process also requires the removal of sol the fraction later (Agrawal and Agrawal 2018a). Several reviews and books existing in the literature can be referred to for understanding various aspects and features of the precipitation polymerization technique (Agrawal and Agrawal 2018a,b; Plamper and Richtering 2017; Richtering and Saunders 2014; Meyer-Kirschner et al. 2016).

The miniemulsion method is emerging as a promising technology for developing highly charged microgels using various synthetic and natural polymers (Huang et al. 2018). In this method, kinetically stable small droplets (50–500 nm) are developed by applying high shear stress, which act as reactors for the polymerization

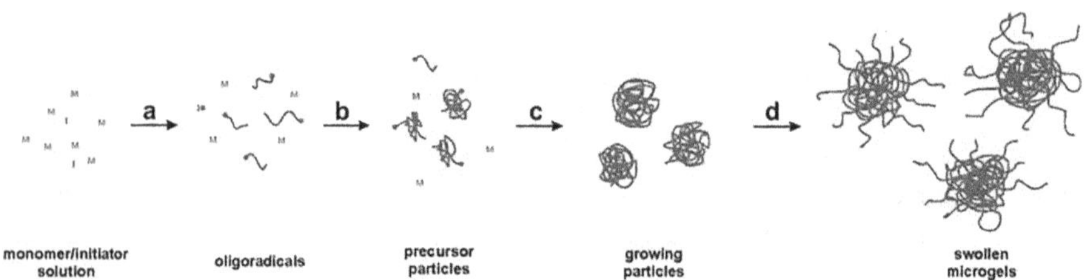

FIGURE 7.2 Synthesis of microgels via precipitation polymerization. Reproduced from Klinger, and Landfester 2012, with permission.

using crosslinkers like *N,N'*-methylene-bis-acrylamide (BIS), resulting in microgels. Numerous polyacrylic acid (PAA) and PNIPAM- based microgels functionalized with redox active units and light-sensitive units have been developed by this method (Agrawal and Agrawal 2018a, b). Furthermore, hydrophilic monomer-based microgels and highly charged microgels can be prepared by this method. However, in comparison to precipitation polymerization, this method suffers from several disadvantages, like the usage of a higher amount of surfactant and higher polydispersity (Plamper and Richtering 2017; Kehren et al. 2019; Tan et al. 2016).

Recently, particle replication in non-wetting templates (PRINT) method has been developed using photocurable perfluoropolyether-based molding material, which has low surface energy and thus prevents the formation of an interconnecting film. This approach resulted in monodisperse microgel particles with controlled size, shape, composition, and surface functionalities (Daly et al. 2020; Makvandi et al. 2021). Furthermore, microfluidic techniques have also been recently adopted for the design of microgel particles with dimensions of 1–30 µm and anisotropy (Headen, García, and García 2018). Here, emulsions of monomers or prepolymer solutions are prepared by using microfluidic devices by splitting the liquid stream into droplets, which in turn can be crosslinked either physically or chemically (Chen, Wang, and Doyle 2017).

Membrane emulsification is an attractive technique due to its simplicity, low energy demands, low surfactant requirements, and formation of uniform particles with controlled size (Lai et al. 2015). In this method, a polymer solution is passed through a Shirasu porous glass membrane having a defined pore size ranging from 0.1 to 18 µm and the resulting droplets lead to uniform- sized microgel particles. The distinguishing feature here is that the particle size is regulated by the chosen membrane instead of turbulent droplet breakup. Articles providing details of such methods, including membrane emulsification, can be referred to for further information regarding the synthesis of microgels with controlled properties (Agrawal and Agrawal 2018a; Ohta et al. 2018).

7.3 STIMULI-RESPONSIVE MICROGELS FOR DRUG DELIVERY

7.3.1 Microgels with Degradable Crosslinking Points

In recent years, booming interest has been shown in fabricating degradable microgels to ensure the body's clearance of the degraded byproducts. Various synthetic strategies have been developed in this direction based on different functional groups like hydrazone, acetal, ketal, disulfide, carbonate ester, and siloxane (Foster et al. 2017; Mackiewicz et al. 2015; Madrigal et al. 2018; Hou et al. 2018). These chemical crosslinking units can be further degraded by simply changing the conditions of the surrounding environment. It is to be noted that polymer networks prepared by the chemical crosslinking method exhibit higher stability, longer durability, and enhanced mechanical properties in comparison to physically crosslinked hydrogels. In this section, we discuss these approaches, and other articles reported in the literature can be consulted for detailed study.

Monodisperse, hydrazone crosslinked PNIPAM-based microgels ($\approx$400 nm in diameter) were synthesized by Mueller et al. (2018) by polymerization of hydrazide and aldehyde-functionalized PNIPAM. The experimental results of small-angle neutron scattering displayed homogeneously crosslinked internal morphology as compared to the core-shell morphology obtained in conventional precipitation polymerization. These hydrazine-crosslinked microgels could be degraded under acidic conditions. The gelation chemistry used here does not require additional cross-linkers, and thus the developed system holds great potential for cell encapsulation and drug release.

Wang et al. (2015) synthesized PVCL-co-*N*-(2-hydroxypropyl)methacrylamide (HPMA)-based nanogels via precipitation polymerization. These nanogels could be successfully used for controlled delivery of doxorubicin (DOX) due to the presence of an acid-labile ketal group containing 2,2-dimethacroyloxy-1-ethoxypropane (DMAEP) crosslinker (Wang et al. 2015). Here, the developed degradable nanogels exhibited higher DOX release under acidic conditions, while DOX leakage under neutral conditions was limited.

Furthermore, Bhuchar et al. (2012) reported cationic microgels synthesized, including 2,2-dimethacroyloxy-1-ethoxypropane as a crosslinker, which can be degraded under acidic conditions. These microgels were loaded with insulin based on ionic interaction, and the cargo could be effectively released under acidic conditions caused by the particles' disruption of the endosome.

Murthy et al. (2003) synthesized ovalbumin-loaded acrylamide-based acid-degradable microgels using an acetal crosslinker in an inverse microemulsion method. Here, *N,N*'-bisacryloyl-di-(2-aminoethoxy)-4-(1,4,7,10-tetraoxaundecyl) phenyl]methane was used as a crosslinker, which can degrade under acidic conditions. The use of this crosslinker provided stable microgels at pH 7.4, while half of the microgels degraded within 5 min in acidic medium. The presence of acid-labile acetal groups resulted in the phagosomal disruption of microgels, releasing protein antigens into the cytoplasm of target cells. Due to the capability of these microgels to activate ovalbumin-specific cytotoxic T lymphocytes, they showed great potential for vaccine delivery targeted against viruses and tumors (Murthy et al. 2003). Steinhilber et al. (2013) fabricated NIH 3T3 cell-laden acid-labile microgels based on the combination of azide–alkyne cycloaddition reactions and microfluidics techniques. Here, poly(ethylene glycol)-dicyclooctyne was used in combination with acid-labile benzacetal linkers containing poly(glycerol azide) as a precursor of microgels. It was found that at least 94% of the cells were viable inside the microgel particles and could be separated and cultured as per the requirement by decomposing the developed microgel-based scaffolds (Steinhilber et al. 2013) (Figure 7.3).

Lei et al. (2020) synthesized multifunctional nanogels able to respond to pH, redox, and ultrasound. Here, block copolymers of polymethacrylate and polyethyleneimine were self-assembled, followed by crosslinking with disulfide crosslinkers using Michael addition chemistry. The developed microgels could be successfully loaded with DOX and perfluorohexane drugs. The loaded drugs did not leak under physiological conditions and could be completely released once triggered by different stimuli (Lei et al. 2020). Mackiewicz et al. (2021) reported pH-responsive PAA-based microgels with a very high capacity for DOX loading. A *N,N*'-bis(acryloyl) cystamine (BAC) crosslinker was used to fabricate these microgels because BAC can degrade under the conditions exhibited by cancer cells. Furthermore, Cui et al.

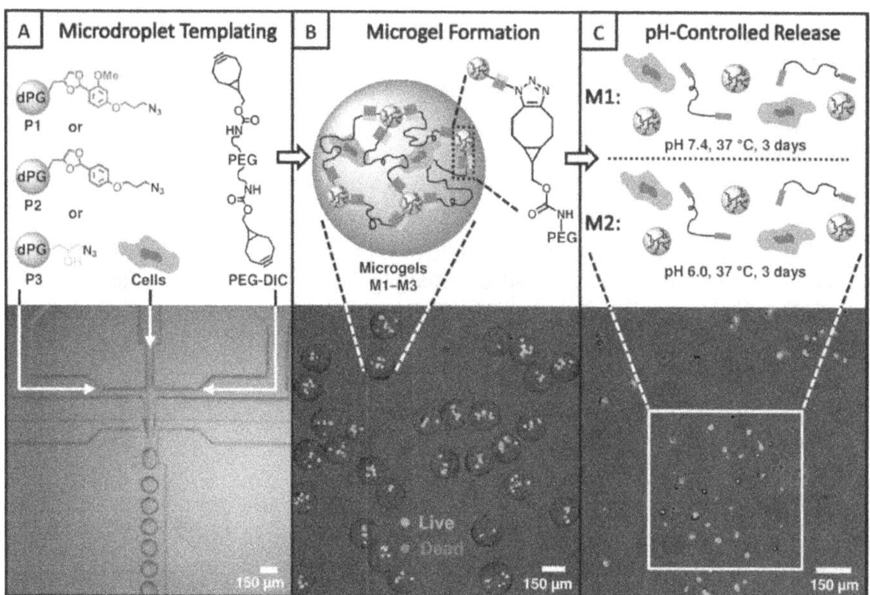

FIGURE 7.3 Acid-cleavable dPG-azide precursors P1–P3 used for microfluidic methods (a), formation of cell-loaded microgels M1-M3 and cell viability using fluorescence-based live (green)–dead (red) assays (b), pH change triggered release of cells encapsulated in microgels (c). Reproduced from Steinhilber et al. 2013, with permission.

(2017) designed PNIPAM-based temperature-responsive microgels, and it was possible to adjust their degradability by changing the ratio of BAC in the reaction mixture. These developed microgel particles successfully degraded under reducing conditions of glutathione (GSH), showing the possibility of being used as a drug carrier.

Van Thienen et al. (2007) explored the potential of carbonate ester-based crosslinking for developing dextran-based nanogels. Here, the developed system provided the opportunity to control the release of bovine serum albumin (BSA) and lysozyme by varying the amount of crosslinker used during the synthesis to crosslink the polymer network. Agrawal et al. (2013b) synthesized PVCL microgels with tunable size and thermoresponsive behavior by using modified polyalkoxysiloxane-based crosslinkers having different vinyl and PEG content. The presence of Si-O-Si bonds provided the possibility of degrading these microgels under basic conditions. However, owing to the very strong basic conditions required for microgel degradation here, the reported microgels could not be realized for pharmaceutical application.

7.3.2 Active and Passive Targeting for Drug Delivery

The enhanced permeation and retention (EPR) effect is an effective way of passively targeting cancer cells with drug-containing microgels. The EPR effect utilizes the higher porosity provided by the leaky vasculature of cancer cells, which results in enhanced permeation of macromolecular drug carriers (Yan et al. 2021). This is further supported by poor lymphatic drainage around these cells caused by rapid tumor growth (Villemin et al. 2019). Numerous microgel-based drug delivery systems have been investigated so far to target cancer sites based on the EPR effect. For example, Agrawal et al. (2017) created temperature- and pH-sensitive PVCL microgels functionalized with itaconic acid comonomers. Here, the size and VPTT of particles could be efficiently adjusted by varying the amount of comonomers during synthesis. It was observed that the drug-loaded microgels exhibited faster drug release in tumor environments than in normal physiological conditions.

Active targeting of cancer cells is another approach to ensuring drug delivery to the targeted biological area instead of affecting healthy cells. This is achieved by decorating the surface of microgels with various targeting ligands such as folic acid (FA), cRGD, galactose, glycyrrhizin, bisphosphonates, etc. (Agrawal and Agrawal 2018a; Clarke, and Lyon 2016; Campora et al. 2021; Soliman et al. 2021).

It has been reported that active targeting of malignant cells by ligand-decorated nanomaterials provides better efficiency than passively targeting nanomaterials (Mihalko et al. 2018). Soliman et al. (2021) developed folate-conjugated polyethylene oxide-/PAA-based nanogels for targeting cancer cells. These particles were tagged with the bioimaging radioisotope ^{99m}Tc. Experimental results exhibited higher biodistribution of developed particles conjugated to folic acid in tumor cells as compared to healthy cells. Transferrin-functionalized PNIPAM microgels designed by Zhang et al. (2017) for controlled release of DOX are another example of active targeting.

It is to be noted that passive targeting allows the accumulation of nanocarriers at the tumor site via the EPR effect, but it can't facilitate further internalization of the nanocarriers by cancer cells. In such a case, active targeting plays a very important role by allowing the targeted ligands to interact with the cell receptors or other overexpressed surface membrane proteins. The targeting ligands are uniquely identified by targeted cells, thus minimizing the undesired exposure of healthy cells to cytotoxic drugs and also minimizing multidrug resistance. Unique interactions between the ligands and receptors can further aid in the nanoparticle internalization by targeted cells. Active targeting-based drug delivery is also helpful in the case of drugs with short half-lives, as it allows the drug to be delivered directly to the targeted site.

7.3.3 Stimuli-Responsive Drug Release in Biological Environment

Numerous functional microgels have been developed in the last few years for achieving targeted drug delivery. Microgels exhibit stimulus sensitivity, causing changes in their swelling behavior and degradation, which can be used as an attractive tool for releasing drugs at the target site. In this regard, temperature-responsive microgels are an important class of colloids that shrink when the temperature is higher than volume phase transition temperature (VPTT), thus leading to drug release (Agrawal and Agrawal 2018a). This VPTT relies on the extent of solvent–polymer and polymer–polymer interactions, and it is significantly influenced by the chemical composition of the colloids (Agrawal, Agrawal, and Pich 2017). The elevated temperature in tumor cells and the additional possibility of inducing hyperthermia render these microgels a potential candidate for controlled drug delivery (Wiemer et al. 2017).

PNIPAM nanogels copolymerized with *N*-hydroxyethylacrylamide (HEAA) were fabricated by Bucatariu et al. (2014) using the precipitation polymerization method.

Nanogels were incorporated with propranolol drug, and its release was controlled by temperature. Propranolol was rapidly released below the VPTT (25°C), and the release rate was similar to the release of a free drug. On the other hand, experiments performed at 37°C and 42°C exhibited that some part of the loaded drug was immediately released in the first 5 minutes due to microgel collapse, followed by a prolonged release. Rejinold et al. (2014) fabricated fibrinogen-functionalized PNIPAM nanogels using coupling chemistry and coacervation methods. These nanogels were loaded with multiple drugs, namely 5-fluorouracil (5-FU) and megestrol acetate. Nanogels containing both drugs exhibited higher cell killing ability and internalization by breast cancer cells above their VPTT compared to separate dose of individual drug. This work was further extended to fabricate temperature-responsive PVCL microgels loaded with 5-FU and megestrol acetate for simultaneous delivery of more than one anticancer drug to the cancer site (Rejinold et al. 2015).

PVCL is not only temperature sensitive, nonionic and water-soluble but also biocompatible as it does not generate any toxic byproducts upon hydrolysis, as observed in the case of PNIPAM (Agrawal et al. 2013b). Hence, increasing attention is being paid to developing drug delivery systems based on PVCL. Lou et al. prepared temperature- and pH-sensitive PVCL-based microgels via precipitation polymerization by taking advantage of undecenoic acid functionality incorporated in the polymer network (2014). Cytotoxicity tests on 3T3 fibroblast cells showed that DOX could be successfully delivered by these microgels triggered by temperature and pH changes.

The variation of pH in different body parts has gained significant scientific interest for designing advanced drug delivery systems. The pH difference from pH 7.4 in the extracellular matrix to pH 4.0–4.5 in lysosomes and pH 5.0–5.5 in endosomes is a potential tool that can induce complete or partial degradation of the carrier and control drug release (Sauraj et al. 2020; Agrawal, Agrawal, and Pich 2017). Agrawal et al. (2017) prepared temperature and pH-sensitive PVCL-based microgels via hydrazine-based crosslinking, which can be broken under acidic conditions The microgels were prepared via precipitation polymerization employing diacetoneacrylamide (DAAM) and itaconic acid dimethyl ester (IADME) as functional units. Experimental results indicated that it was possible to adjust the size and VPTT of these microgels by tuning the concentration of protons in the surrounding environment, and these particles could be successfully loaded with the anticancer drug DOX. DOX-loaded microgels displayed low drug leaching in the blood due to strong electrostatic interaction at pH 7.4, while higher release was exhibited by biological conditions of tumor cells having lower pH (Figure 7.4).

Amphiphilic, pH-responsive AA and n-butyl acrylate (BuA)-based microgels were synthesized via microfluidic techniques by Lu et al. (2016). Hydrophobic droplets containing tetrahydropyranyl acrylate, BuA, ethylene glycol dimethacrylate as a crosslinker, and a photo-initiator were generated via a microfluidic platform. These hydrophobic droplets were photo-polymerized and subsequently hydrolyzed, producing anionic amphiphilic microgels. These microgels were capable of safeguarding and delivering both hydrophobic and hydrophilic model drugs owing to their amphiphilic nature. pH-responsive PNIPAM/PAA microgels were synthesized by Chen et al. (2021) and combined with thiolated polyethylene glycol and polyallyl amine-coated gold nanorods. These microgels were loaded with DOX, and their

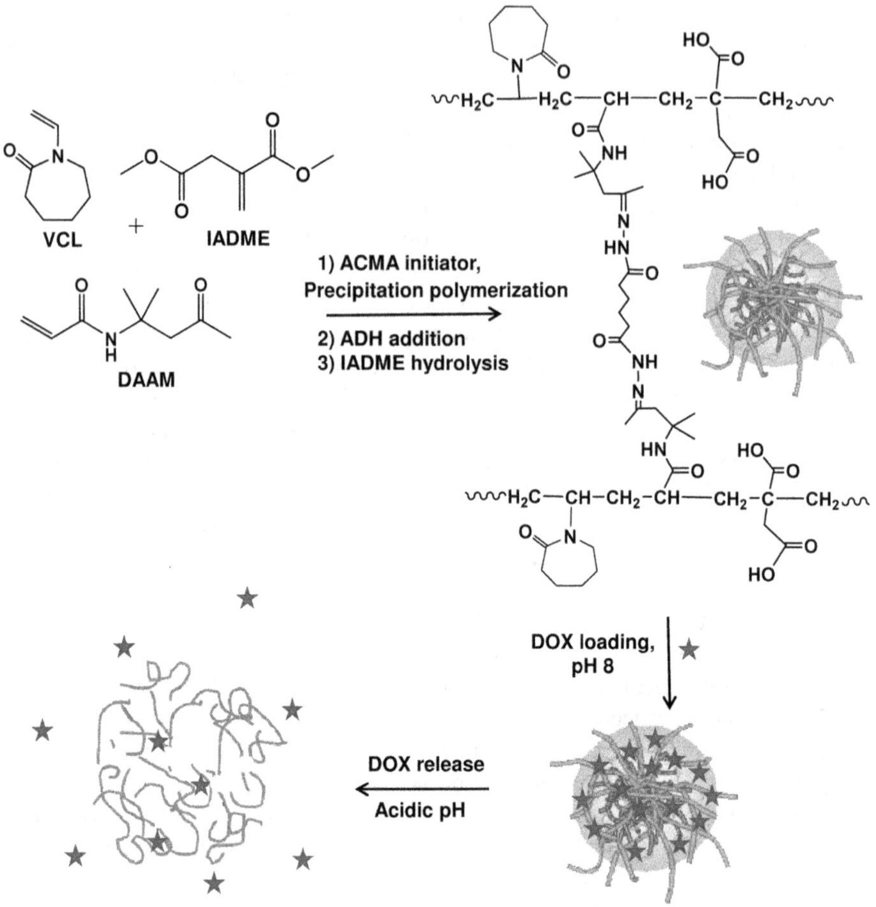

FIGURE 7.4 Synthesis of acid-labile hydrazone linkages based microgels that can degrade under acidic conditions, releasing the loaded drug. Reproduced from Agrawal, Agrawal, and Pich 2017, with permission.

electrostatic interaction varied as a function of pH. These microgels could effectively release DOX depending on the changes in temperature, pH and near-infrared light.

The difference in the amount of reducing GSH in the cytosol (2–10 mM) as compared to the extracellular fluids (2–20 μM) offers the opportunity to design redox-responsive drug carrier systems (Sauraj et al. 2020). Hence, numerous drug delivery carriers with disulfide bonds have been investigated as these bonds degrade under physiologically reducing conditions.

PVCL/MAA microgels that could respond to reducing conditions were reported by Wang et al. (2013b). These microgels were made degradable by using BAC crosslinkers. These microgels were efficiently charged with DOX as an anticancer drug based on the electrostatic interactions. Drugs could be successfully released by degradation of the particle induced by the reducing environment of GSH or dithiothreitol (DTT), which causes the breaking of disulfide linkages. Similarly,

Zhang et al. (2013) created phenylboronic acid-containing PNIPAM-based microgels using BAC crosslinkers in precipitation polymerization. These microgels were non-toxic and could effectively release loaded insulin upon treatment with temperature, pH, and glucose stimuli.

Ryu et al. (2010) used thiol–disulfide exchange chemistry to design nanogels using polymers consisting of an oligoethyleneglycol unit and pyridyl disulfide (PDS)-derived thioethylmethacrylate. Disulfide-crosslinked nanogels were prepared by treating a small percentage of PDS groups with a controlled amount of DTT, which resulted in free thiol groups that could in turn react with remaining PDS groups (Ryu et al. 2010). Lipophilic guest molecules were incorporated into the hydrophobic interior of nanogels. In the presence of a GSH-reducing environment, nanogels disintegrated, resulting in nile red release (Figure 7.5).

Jin et al. (2015) reported novel enzyme/redox/pH stimuli-sensitive MAA-based nanogels using BAC crosslinkers in a precipitation polymerization method. The surface of these nanogels was further decorated with polyethylene glycol (PEG) and folic acid, which enhanced blood circulation time and offered active targeting, respectively. Nanogels were able to encapsulate both hydrophilic DOX and hydrophobic paclitaxel (PTX) drugs. Drug release was expedited in an acidic environment

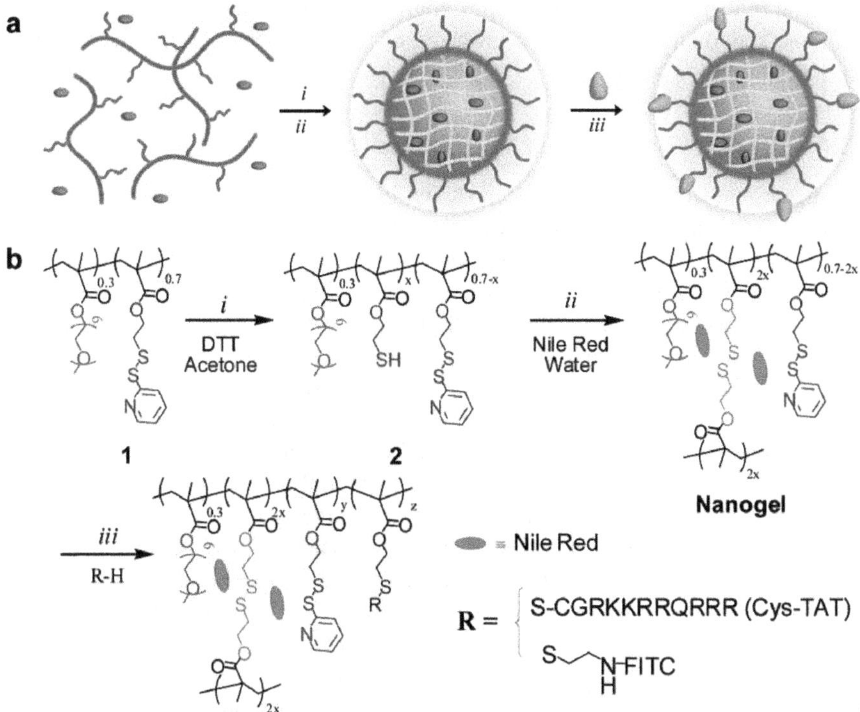

FIGURE 7.5 Schematic representation of biodegradable nanogel preparation. (a) Synthetic steps for the polymer and nanogel fabrication. (b) Breaking of the PDS group by DTT (i), crosslinked nanogel preparation (ii), and postmodification with Cys-TAT peptide or FITC (iii). Reproduced from Ryu et al. 2010, with permission.

supported by nanogel degradation. Nanogel degradation was triggered by protease via breaking amino bonds and by GSH via breaking disulfide bonds. Experimental results indicated that loading multiple drugs provided a synergistic effect for effective cancer therapy. Yang et al. (2016) developed disulfide-crosslinked PNIPAM/AA nanogels by precipitation polymerization using BAC as a crosslinker. These nanogels contained DOX as a payload, and further intracellular tracking experiments were performed to check their fate. Experimental results confirmed that DOX-containing nanogels could be transported to lysosomes, where they shrank due to the acidic environment and resulted in partial DOX release. Next, these nanogels entered the cytoplasm, where they degraded due to the high GSH concentration, and DOX was completely released, which in turn was finally translocated to the nucleus to exert cytotoxicity against cancer cells.

The major advantages of stimuli-responsive microgels are the ease of synthesis, postmodification, and possibility of using an aqueous medium, thus avoiding toxic organic solvents. However, to achieve efficient drug delivery, stimuli-responsive microgels must be biocompatible, biodegradable, and exhibit high drug loading efficiency and sustained drug release. Lower loading capacity results in low drug availability in the vicinity of cancer cells, which might lead to multidrug resistance. The other disadvantages associated with these systems include premature drug release into the bloodstream, high burst release, lower stability, lack of cytotoxic specificity, and gradual lowering of the pH of the system due to acidic degradation.

7.3.4 Remotely Controlled Drug Release

Significant research interest has been shown in developing microgels that offer the possibility of being utilized remotely by tuning the magnetic field or light (Wiemer et al. 2017). Magnetic microgels can be directed to the target area by changing an external magnetic field, leading to efficient drug delivery with reduced toxicity (Seyfoori et al. 2019). Hence, a variety of magnetic nanoparticles containing microgels have been reported in the literature (Yan et al. 2021; Cui et al. 2017).

Magnetite nanoparticles loaded with dual-responsive dextran microgels were synthesized by He et al. (2021). DOX, an anticancer drug, was loaded inside these dextran/magnetite hybrid microgels. Here, DOX-loaded magnetic microgels displayed controlled, noninvasive drug release due to substantial heating caused by the magnetic field. Hu et al. (2017) synthesized PNIPAM microgels with both temperature sensitivity and magnetic properties. Here, polyethyleneimine-functionalized magnetic nanoparticles and DOX were included inside the microgels. The developed system was further decorated with folic acid for the active, targeted delivery of drugs assisted by a magnetic field.

Matyjaszewski et al. fabricated poly(di(ethylene glycol) methyl ether methacrylate) (PM(EO)$_2$MA) magnetic microgels that can respond to changes in temperature. Microgels were synthesized using living radical polymerization and the inverse miniemulsion technique simultaneously. Here, bis(2-methacryloyloxyethyl) disulfide crosslinker was used for making the microgels degradable and thus suitable for drug release applications (2009). Oleic acid-coated Fe_3O_4 nanoparticles were incorporated in (PM(EO)$_2$MA) microgels based on their hydrophobic interaction with the microgel interior. Furthermore, it was possible to attract these microgels with the help of magnetic field stimuli, which also facilitated the sustained delivery of the model drug rhodamine B (Dong, Mantha, and Matyjaszewski 2009) (Figure 7.6).

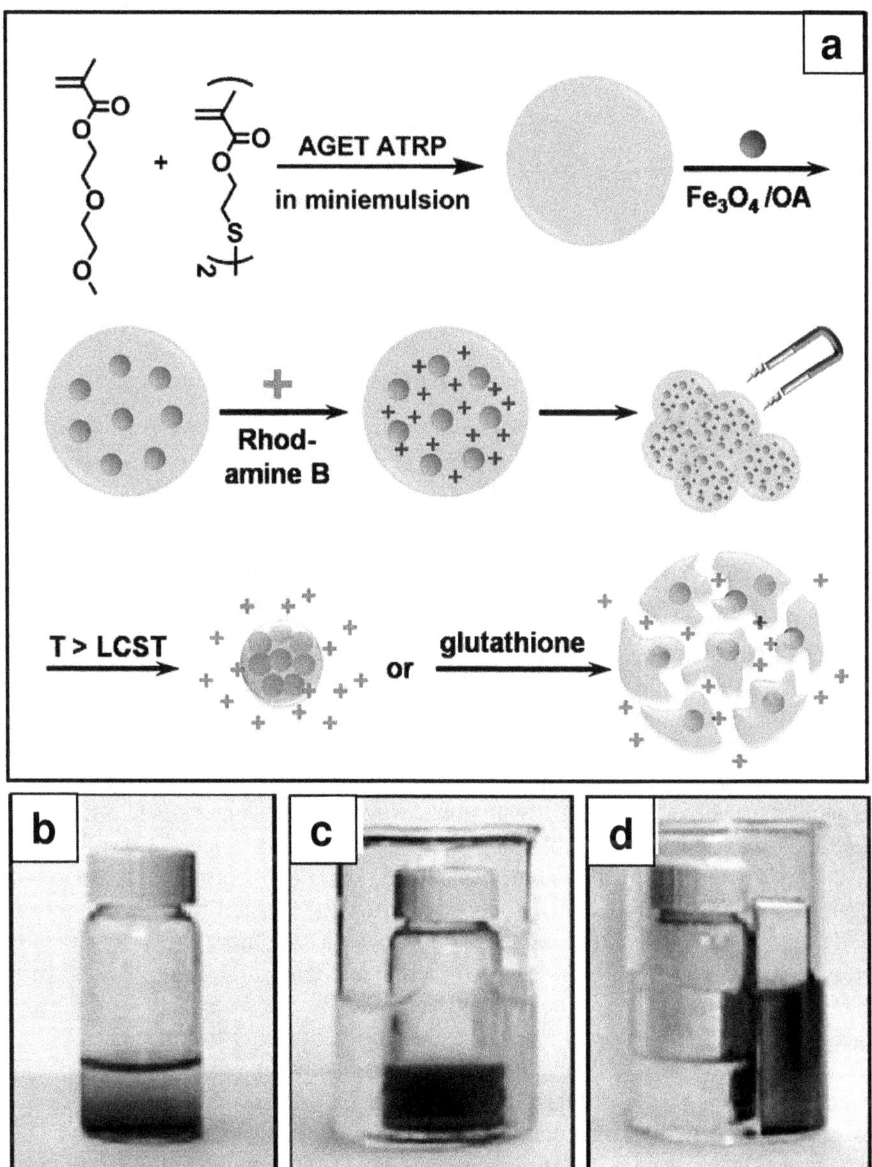

FIGURE 7.6 Fabrication of PM(EO)$_2$MA microgels, loading with Fe_3O_4 nanoparticles and rhodamine B, rhodamine B release triggered by change in temperature or reducing conditions (a). Digital photos of PM(EO)$_2$MA- Fe_3O_4 microgel dispersion at 40°C (b), in ice cold water without (c) and with a magnet (d). Reproduced from Dong, Mantha, and Matyjaszewski 2009, with permission.

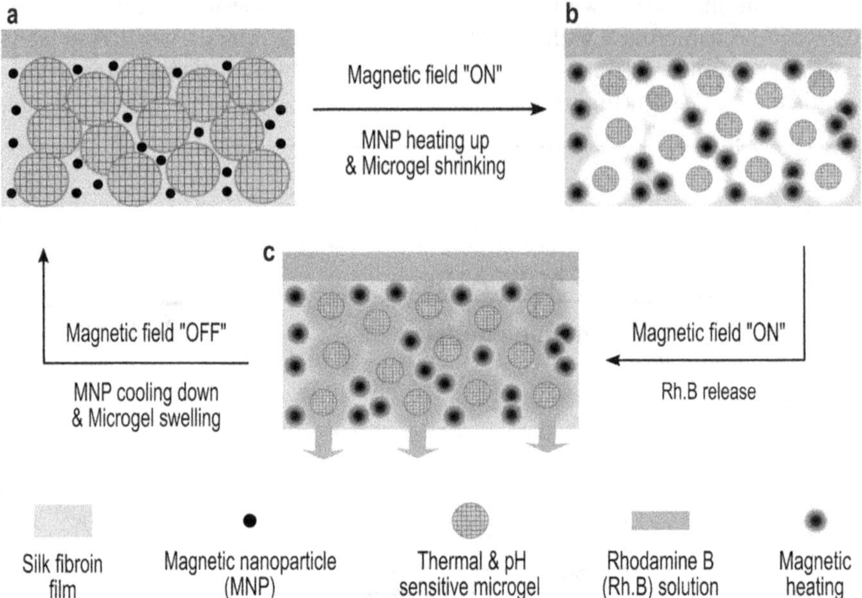

FIGURE 7.7 Silk film containing magnetic nanoparticles and microgels (a); shrinking of microgels and rhodamine B delivery when the magnetic field is on (b); swelling of microgels and no rhodamine B delivery when the magnetic field is off (c). Reproduced from Wang et al. 2020, with permission.

In another direction, Wang et al. (2020) explored the combination of magnetic nanoparticles and dual-responsive PNIPAM-based microgels embedded in silk fibroin film. Rhodamine B was loaded as a model drug in the developed film to check the controlled release on demand. Here, the application of an alternating magnetic field caused heat generation and the collapsing of microgel particles, resulting in drug release. Microgels swelled again upon switching the magnetic field off, and the release of loaded drugs could be stopped (Wang et al. 2020) (Figure 7.7).

In the last decade, light stimulus has gained booming interest from scientists for designing drug carriers, as this stimulus provides the possibility of having a drug delivery system with good spatiotemporal resolution. Additionally, various parameters such as wavelength, polarization direction and intensity can also be altered to achieve the desired effect without any direct touch. Hence, various light-responsive microgels have been reported for controlled drug release. For example, Wang et al. (2017b) created both light- and magnetic field-sensitive microgels with gold rods coated with magnetic ionic liquid and DNA. These DNA microgels were responsive to near-infrared light, which could be easily used for the controlled release of the model drug DOX. Lee et al. (2019) designed pheophorbide A-functionalized polyhydroxyethyl methacrylate core and chitosan shell-based microgels. The 5′-deoxy-5-fluorocytidine anticancer drug was also incorporated into the microgels. In the presence of near-infrared light, the microgel core generated reactive oxygen species, which also facilitated the drug release for effective colon cancer therapy. de Solorzano et al. (2020) investigated hollow gold NP-loaded PNIPAM microgels, which were biocompatible and collapsed upon exposure to light, offering the option of controlled drug release. Qi et al. (2017) made efforts to address the issue of controlling drug release remotely in a reproducible manner. In this regard, MAA-functionalized PNIPAM microgels in combination with Fe_3O_4 nanoparticles were developed. The VPTT of the microgels could be adjusted between 37°C and 46°C by changing the ratio of MAA and Fe_3O_4 during synthesis. The *in vivo* efficiency of this system was further investigated with an 808 nm laser, which displayed enhancement in drug release in a controlled way. In general, remotely operable nanocarriers provide the benefit of targeting the desired site and releasing the drug with a fast response time as a function of signal control from outside. However, the depth of penetration is a limitation here that should be addressed for the successful use of the developed materials.

7.4 STIMULI-RESPONSIVE MICROGELS AS THERANOSTICS

Magnevist, Omniscan, and Dotarem are some of the clinically used contrast agents. These are low molecular weight compounds facing the issue of lower r_1 relaxivity and short bioimaging times caused by short blood circulation intervals (Affram et al. 2020). In this regard, the smart combination of microgels and contrast agents offers tremendous scope for bioimaging applications by addressing the above-mentioned drawbacks. To improve the efficacy of cancer therapy, early diagnosis of cancer is crucial, along with monitoring its progression during treatment. Hence, it is required to prepare stimuli-responsive microgels that can be used not only for intracellular bioimaging with an increased signal-to-noise ratio but can also provide desired drug/gene delivery. This will lead to the development of bioimaging-guided therapy or theranostics, which holds immense promise for efficient and personalized medicine in the future.

In quest of exploring new theranostics, Theune et al. (2019) reported near-infrared and temperature-responsive nanogels (≈200 nm) based on polypyrrole, which were used for simultaneous photothermal and chemotherapy. The experimental results showed that the nanogel system could also be used as a photoacoustic bioimaging agent (Figure 7.8).

Zhang et al. (2019) synthesized CuS and DOX-loaded MAA-functionalized polyethylene glycol-based nanogels. The experimental results showed that the nanogels

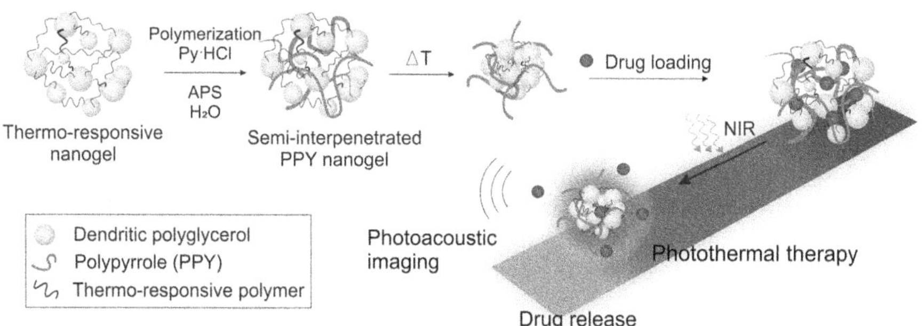

FIGURE 7.8 Scheme depicting polypyrrole-based temperature-sensitive, semi-interpenetrating nanogels for integrated photothermal therapy, drug delivery, and photoacoustic bioimaging. Reproduced from Theune et al. 2019, with permission.

enhanced (≈26 times) the photoacoustic bioimaging of interior regions, confirming the higher penetration power of the developed system. Furthermore, CuS-loaded nanogels disintegrated under near-infrared light, releasing the loaded anticancer drug (Zhang et al. 2019).

Wang et al. (2017a) incorporated carbon dots (QDs) in the interior of biocompatible, pH-sensitive chitosan-based nanogels. These hybrid nanogels could be loaded with DOX with high efficiency. DOX-loaded nanogels were further used on implanted tumors in a mouse model to inhibit their growth. The experimental results exhibited that both photothermal and chemotherapy options can be successfully integrated into these hybrid nanogels. Furthermore, Wu et al. (2020a) developed Ag–Au bimetallic NP cores and nonlinear poly(ethylene glycol) (PEG) shell-based hybrid nanogels. Nanogel particles were explored for B16F10 cell bioimaging by using strong visible fluorescence from the Ag–Au core. To investigate the potential for simultaneous drug delivery, nanogel particles were loaded with the model anticancer drug TMZ, which in turn could be successfully released by taking advantage of the higher temperature in the tumor environment and heat generated by external NIR irradiation.

Chiang et al. (2013) fabricated superparamagnetic iron oxide nanoparticles (SPIONs, 44 wt %) loaded hollow composite nanogels as a promising versatile theranostic system using poly(AA-co-2-methacryloylethyl acrylate (MEA))-g-PEG/PNIPAM-based pH/thermosensitive graft copolymer followed by in situ photopolymerization of MEA residues. Furthermore, the developed system was tested with HeLa cells and magnetically guided by applying a magnetic field only to one side. Experimental results confirmed that the use of a magnetic field enhanced the uptake of hybrid nanogels. This was further confirmed by ICP-AES measurements of intracellular iron concentrations with or without a magnetic field. Additionally, these hybrid nanogels exhibited remarkably enhanced transverse relaxivity (r_2) for magnetic resonance bioimaging, which could be further tuned by pH (Chiang et al. 2013) (Figure 7.9).

Wu et al. (2010b) synthesized CdSe quantum dots loaded on chitosan–poly(methacrylic acid) (chitosan–PMAA) nanogels, which could respond to pH stimuli. These nanogels could be used for photoluminescence bioimaging of mouse melanoma B16F10 cells. The anticancer drug TMZ was also released in response to a pH change in the pathological zone. Van Elk et al. (2015) designed alginate microgels, which in turn were combined with temperature-sensitive. Here, liposomes were loaded with fluorescein as a model drug and Prohance as a T_1 MRI contrast agent. Additionally, holmium ions were used as a crosslinker, which also acted as a T_2 MRI contrast agent. This system could be used for MR-guided cancer therapy *in vivo*.

Although significant efforts are being made to utilize microgels for drug delivery and theranostics, significant attention should be paid at various fronts to achieve the desired outcome. Taking advantage of the knowledge from various streams, scientists should join hands to synthesize microgels with tunable size and degradability and functionalize them with targeting ligands to obtain cytotoxic specificity. Furthermore, microgels should be designed in such a way that high loading efficiency of drugs/contrast agents could be achieved while avoiding their premature release in the bloodstream.

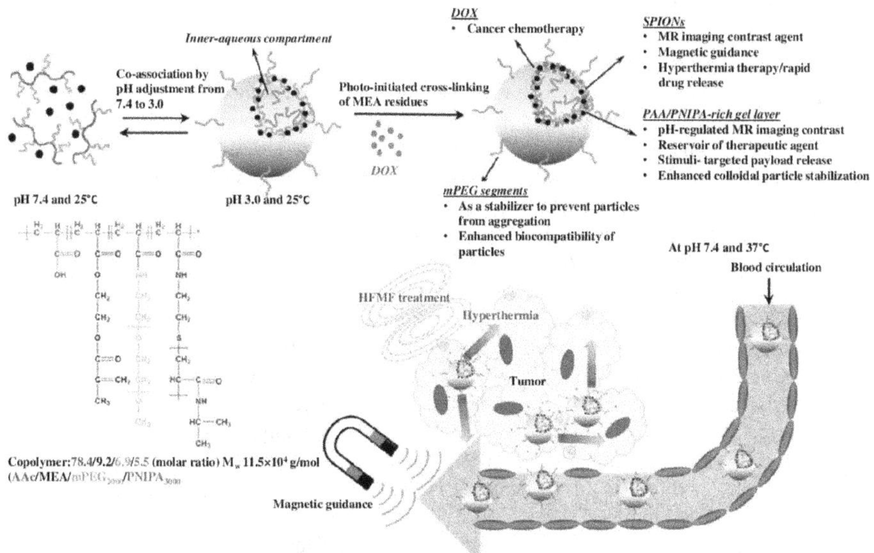

FIGURE 7.9 Preparation of DOX-loaded hollow hybrid nanogels having SPIONs as a theranostic system. Reproduced from Chiang et al. 2013, with permission.

7.5 CONCLUSIONS

In this contribution, we have discussed various developments in synthetic methods for designing multifunctional microgels with the required physicochemical properties and their use in drug delivery and theranostics.

Microgels and microgel-based advanced systems present immense promise for drug delivery owing to their stimuli-sensitive properties, facile synthesis, easy post-modification, compartments for different actions, and variety of chemical groups. Furthermore, their ability to quickly respond to changes in the surrounding environment due to particle flexibility and to overcome biological barriers due to network deformation may enhance in anticancer activity.

To achieve the widespread use of microgels in pharmaceutics, it is of prime importance to perform interdisciplinary research using cutting edge knowledge from various disciplines such as chemistry, material science, and biomedical engineering. Furthermore, microgels should be modified with required targeting ligands, high loading efficiency should be achieved, and leakage of loaded contrast agents should be addressed to use microgels as a versatile platform for drug delivery and theranostics.

ACKNOWLEDGMENTS

GA thanks Department of Science & Technology, India (No. INT/Korea/P-60) and Seed Grant by IIT Mandi (IITM/SG/GA/72).

Conflicts of Interest: The authors declare no conflicts of interest.

REFERENCES

Affram, Kevin, Taylor Smith, Shannon Helsper, Jens T. Rosenberg, Bo Han, Jose Trevino, and Edward Agyare. 2020. "Comparative study on contrast enhancement of magnevist and magnevist-loaded nanoparticles in pancreatic cancer PDX model monitored by MRI." *Cancer Nanotechnology* 11(1): 1–14. doi: 10.1186/s12645-020-00061-9.

Agarwal, Tarun, Sheri-Ann Tan, Valentina Onesto, Jia Xian Law, Garima Agrawal, Sampriti Pal, Wei Lee Lim, Esmaeel Sharif, Farnaz Dabbagh Moghaddam, and Tapas Kumar Maiti. 2021. "Engineered herbal scaffolds for tissue repair and regeneration: Recent trends and technologies." *Biomedical Engineering Advances* 2: 100015. doi: 10.1016/j.bea.2021.100015.

Agrawal, Garima, and Rahul Agrawal. 2018a. "Functional microgels: Recent advances in their biomedical applications." *Small* 14(39): 1801724. doi: 10.1002/smll.201801724.

Agrawal Garima, and Rahul Agrawal. 2018b. "Stimuli-responsive microgels and microgel-based systems: advances in the exploitation of microgel colloidal properties and their interfacial activity." *Polymers* 10 (4): 418. doi: 10.3390/polym10040418.

Agrawal, Garima, and Rahul Agrawal. 2019. "Janus nanoparticles: Recent advances in their interfacial and biomedical applications." *ACS Applied Nano Materials* 2 (4): 1738–57. doi: 10.1021/acsanm.9b00283.

Agrawal, Garima, Rahul Agrawal, and Andrij Pich. 2017. "Dual responsive poly(N-Vinylcaprolactam) based degradable microgels for drug delivery." *Particle & Particle Systems Characterization* 34 (11): 1700132. doi: 10.1002/ppsc.201700132.

Agrawal, Garima, Sangram K. Samal, Sushanta K. Sethi, Gaurav Manik, and Rahul Agrawal. 2019. "Microgel/Silica hybrid colloids: Bioinspired synthesis and controlled release application." *Polymer* 178: 121599. doi: 10.1016/j.polymer.2019.121599.

Agrawal, Garima, Marco Philipp Schürings, Patrick van Rijn, and Andrij Pich. 2013a. "Formation of catalytically active gold–polymer microgel hybrids via a controlled in situ reductive process." *Journal of Materials Chemistry A* 1 (42): 13244-51. doi: 10.1039/c3ta12370g.

Agrawal, Garima, Marco Schürings, Xiaomin Zhu, and Andrij Pich. 2012. "Microgel/SiO_2 hybrid colloids prepared using a water soluble silica precursor." *Polymer* 53 (6): 1189–97. doi: 10.1016/j.polymer.2012.01.051.

Agrawal, Garima, Andreas Ülpenich, Xiaomin Zhu, Martin Möller, and Andrij Pich. 2014. "Microgel-based adaptive hybrid capsules with tunable shell permeability." *Chemistry of Materials* 26 (20): 5882–91. doi: 10.1021/cm502358s.

Agrawal, Garima, Jingbo Wang, Berit Brüster, Xiaomin Zhu, Martin Möller, and Andrij Pich. 2013b. "Degradable microgels synthesized using reactive polyvinylalkoxysiloxanes as crosslinkers." *Soft Matter* 9 (22): 5380–90. doi: 10.1039/c3sm50248a.

Beningo, Karen A., and Yu-li Wang. 2002. "Fc-receptor-mediated phagocytosis is regulated by mechanical properties of the target." *Journal of Cell Science* 115 (4): 849–56. doi: 10.1242/jcs.115.4.849.

Bhuchar, Neha, Rajesh Sunasee, Kazuhiko Ishihara, Thomas Thundat, and Ravin Narain. 2012. "Degradable thermoresponsive nanogels for protein encapsulation and controlled release." *Bioconjugate Chemistry* 23 (1): 75–83. doi: 10.1021/bc2003814.

Birkholz, Mandy-Nicole, Garima Agrawal, Christian Bergmann, Ricarda Schröder, Sebastian J. Lechner, Andrij Pich, and Horst Fischer. 2016. "Calcium phosphate/microgel composites for 3D powderbed printing of ceramic materials." *Biomedical Engineering/Biomedizinische Technik* 61 (3): 267–79. doi: 10.1515/bmt-2014-0141.

Bucatariu, Sanda, Gheorghe Fundueanu, Irina Prisacaru, Mihaela Balan, Iuliana Stoica, Valeria Harabagiu, and Marieta Constantin. 2014. "Synthesis and characterization of thermosensitive poly (N-Isopropylacrylamide-Co-Hydroxyethylacrylamide) microgels as potential carriers for drug delivery." *Journal of Polymer Research* 21 (11): 1–12. doi: 10.1007/s10965-014-0580-7.

Campora, Simona, Reham Mohsen, Daniel Passaro, Howida Samir, Hesham Ashraf, Saif El-Din Al-Mofty, Ayman A. Diab, Ibrahim M. El-Sherbiny, Martin J. Snowden, and Giulio Ghersi. 2021. "Functionalized poly (N-Isopropylacrylamide)-based microgels in tumor targeting and drug delivery." *Gels* 7 (4): 203. doi: 10.3390/gels7040203.

Chen, Lynna, Kai Xi Wang, and Patrick S. Doyle. 2017. "Effect of internal architecture on microgel deformation in microfluidic constrictions." *Soft Matter* 13 (9): 1920–28. doi: 10.1039/C6SM02674E.

Chen, Ruixia, Jun Shi, Chongchong Liu, Jingguo Li, and Shaokui Cao. 2021. "In situ self-assembly of gold nanorods with thermal-responsive microgel for multi-synergistic remote drug delivery." *Advanced Composites and Hybrid Materials*. doi: 10.1007/s42114-021-00306-0.

Chiang, Wen-Hsuan, Viet Thang Ho, Hsin-Hung Chen, Wen-Chia Huang, Yi-Fong Huang, Sung-Chyr Lin, Chorng-Shyan Chern, and Hsin-Cheng Chiu. 2013. "Superparamagnetic hollow hybrid nanogels as a potential guidable vehicle system of stimuli-mediated MR imaging and multiple cancer therapeutics." *Langmuir* 29 (21): 6434–43. doi: 10.1021/la4001957.

Clarke, Kimberly C., and L. Andrew Lyon. 2016. "Microgel surface modification with self-assembling peptides." *Macromolecules* 49 (15): 5366–73.

Cui, Ruiguang, Zhijun Zhang, Jingjing Nie, and Binyang Du. 2017. "Tuning the morphology, network structure, and degradation of thermo-sensitive microgels by controlled addition of degradable cross-linker." *Colloid and Polymer Science* 295 (4): 665–78. doi: 10.1007/s00396-017-4056-2.

Daly, Andrew C., Lindsay Riley, Tatiana Segura, and Jason A. Burdick. 2020. "Hydrogel microparticles for biomedical applications." *Nature Reviews Materials* 5 (1): 20–43. doi: 10.1038/s41578-019-0148-6.

de Solorzano, Isabel Ortiz, Martin Prieto, Gracia Mendoza, Victor Sebastian, and Manuel Arruebo. 2020. "Triggered drug release from hybrid thermoresponsive nanoparticles using near infrared light." *Nanomedicine* 15 (3): 219–34. doi: 10.2217/nnm-2019-0270.

Doermbach, Karla, Garima Agrawal, Mark Servos, Susanne Schipmann, Sabrina Thies, Uwe Klemradt, and Andrij Pich. 2014. "Silica-coating of hematite nanoparticles using reactive water-soluble polyalkoxysiloxanes." *Particle & Particle Systems Characterization* 31 (3): 365–73. doi: 10.1002/ppsc.201300234.

Dong, Hongchen, Venkat Mantha, and Krzysztof Matyjaszewski. 2009. "Thermally responsive PM(EO)$_2$MA magnetic microgels via activators generated by electron transfer atom transfer radical polymerization in miniemulsion." *Chemistry of Materials* 21 (17): 3965–72. doi: 10.1021/cm901143e.

Fan, Xiaotong, Choon Peng Teng, Jayven Chee Chuan Yeo, Zibiao Li, Tingting Wang, Haiming Chen, Lu Jiang, Xunan Hou, Chaobin He, and Junqiu Liu. 2021. "Temperature and pH responsive light-harvesting system based on AIE-active microgel for cell imaging." *Macromolecular Rapid Communications* 42 (7): 2000716. doi: 10.1002/marc.202000716.

Farjami, Toktam, and Ashkan Madadlou. 2017. "Fabrication methods of biopolymeric microgels and microgel-based hydrogels." *Food Hydrocolloids* 62: 262–72. doi: 10.1016/j.foodhyd.2016.08.017.

Feng, Qi, Dingguo Li, Qingtao Li, Xiaodong Cao, and Hua Dong. 2022. "Microgel assembly: Fabrication, characteristics and application in tissue engineering and regenerative medicine." *Bioactive Materials* 9: 105–19. doi: 10.1016/j.bioactmat.2021.07.020.

Fettis, Margaret M., Yaohua Wei, Antonietta Restuccia, Justin J. Kurian, Shannon M. Wallet, and Gregory A. Hudalla. 2016. "Microgels with tunable affinity-controlled protein release via desolvation of self-assembled peptide nanofibers." *Journal of Materials Chemistry B* 4 (18): 3054–64. doi: 10.1039/C5TB02446C.

Foster, Greg A., Devon M. Headen, Cristina González-García, Manuel Salmerón-Sánchez, Haval Shirwan, and Andrés J. García. 2017. "Protease-degradable microgels for protein delivery for vascularization." *Biomaterials* 113: 170–75. doi: 10.1016/j.biomaterials.2016.10.044.

Giussi, Juan M., Marta Martínez Moro, Agustín Iborra, M. Lorena Cortez, Desiré Di Silvio, Irantzu Llarena Conde, Gabriel S. Longo, Omar Azzaroni, and Sergio Moya. 2020. "A study of the complex interaction between poly allylamine hydrochloride and negatively charged poly (N-Isopropylacrylamide-Co-Methacrylic Acid) microgels." *Soft Matter* 16 (4): 881–90. doi: 10.1039/C9SM02070E.

Gupta, Aastha, Ankur Sood, Ankita Dhiman, Nishith Shrimali, Ritu Singhmar, Prasenjit Guchhait, and Garima Agrawal. 2022a. "Redox responsive poly (allylamine)/Eudragit S-100 nanoparticles for dual drug delivery in colorectal cancer." *Biomaterials Advances* 143: 213184. doi: 10.1016/j.bioadv.2022.213184.

Gupta, Aastha, Ankur Sood, Erwin Fuhrer, Kristina Djanashvili, and Garima Agrawal. 2022b. "Polysaccharide-based theranostic systems for combined imaging and cancer therapy: Recent advances and challenges." *ACS Biomaterials Science & Engineering*. doi: 10.1021/acsbiomaterials.1c01631.

He, Lihua, Rong Zheng, Jie Min, Fulin Lu, Changqiang Wu, Yunfei Zhi, Shaoyun Shan, and Hongying Su. 2021. "Preparation of magnetic microgels based on dextran for stimuli-responsive release of doxorubicin." *Journal of Magnetism and Magnetic Materials* 517: 167394. doi: 10.1016/j.jmmm.2020.167394.

Headen, Devon M., José R. García, and Andrés J. García. 2018. "Parallel droplet microfluidics for high throughput cell encapsulation and synthetic microgel generation." *Microsystems & Nanoengineering* 4 (1): 1–9. doi: 10.1038/micronano.2017.76.

Hou, Yong, Wenyan Xie, Katharina Achazi, Jose Luis Cuellar-Camacho, Matthias F. Melzig, Wei Chen, and Rainer Haag. 2018. "Injectable degradable PVA microgels prepared by microfluidic technology for controlled osteogenic differentiation of mesenchymal stem cells." *Acta Biomaterialia* 77: 28–37. doi: 10.1016/j.actbio.2018.07.003.

Hu, Yunli, Weijun Liu, and Fanhong Wu. 2017. "Novel multi-responsive polymer magnetic microgels with folate or methyltetrahydrofolate ligand as anticancer drug carriers." *RSC Advances* 7 (17): 10333–44. doi: 10.1039/C6RA27114F.

Huang, Jing, Xi Geng, Brian M. Tissue, and S. Richard Turner. 2018. "Microgels from hydrophobic solid monomers via miniemulsion polymerization for aqueous lead and copper ion removal." *Reactive and Functional Polymers* 133: 136–42. doi: 10.1016/j.reactfunctpolym.2018.10.011.

Jin, Sha, Jiaxun Wan, Lizheng Meng, Xiaoxing Huang, Jia Guo, Li Liu, and Changchun Wang. 2015. "Biodegradation and toxicity of Protease/Redox/pH stimuli-responsive PEGlated PMAA nanohydrogels for targeting drug delivery." *ACS Applied Materials & Interfaces* 7 (35): 19843–52. doi: 10.1021/acsami.5b05984.

Kehren, Dominic, Catalina Molano Lopez, Stefan Theiler, Helmut Keul, Martin Möller, and Andrij Pich. 2019. "Multicompartment aqueous microgels with degradable hydrophobic domains." *Polymer* 172: 283–93. doi: 10.1016/j.polymer.2019.03.074.

Klinger, Daniel, and Katharina Landfester. 2012. "Stimuli-responsive microgels for the loading and release of functional compounds: Fundamental concepts and applications." *Polymer* 53 (23): 5209–31. doi: 10.1016/j.polymer.2012.08.053.

Kwok, Man-hin, Guanqing Sun, and To Ngai. 2019. "Microgel particles at interfaces: phenomena, principles, and opportunities in food sciences." *Langmuir* 35 (12): 4205–17. doi: 10.1021/acs.langmuir.8b04009.

Lai, Yao-Tong, Mayu Sato, Seiichi Ohta, Kazuki Akamatsu, Shin-ichi Nakao, Yasuyuki Sakai, and Taichi Ito. 2015. "preparation of uniform-sized hemoglobin–albumin microspheres as oxygen carriers by Shirasu porous glass membrane emulsification technique." *Colloids and Surfaces B: Biointerfaces* 127: 1–7. doi: 10.1016/j.colsurfb.2015.01.018.

Lee, Junghan, Ratchapol Jenjob, Enkhzaya Davaa, and Su-Geun Yang. 2019. "NIR-responsive ROS generating core and ROS-Triggered 5′-Deoxy-5-fluorocytidine releasing shell structured water-swelling microgel for locoregional combination cancer therapy." *Journal of Controlled Release* 305: 120–29. doi: 10.1016/j.jconrel.2019.05.016.

Lei, Bin, Miaoxin Chen, Yizhou Wang, Junqi Zhang, Shouhong Xu, and Honglai Liu. 2020. "Double security drug delivery system DDS constructed by multi-responsive (pH/redox/US) microgel." *Colloids and Surfaces B: Biointerfaces* 193: 111022. doi: 10.1016/j.colsurfb.2020.111022.

Lou, Shaofeng, Shan Gao, Weiwei Wang, Mingming Zhang, Qiqing Zhang, Chun Wang, Chen Li, and Deling Kong. 2014. "Temperature/pH dual responsive microgels of crosslinked poly (N-Vinylcaprolactam-co-Undecenoic Acid) as biocompatible materials for controlled release of doxorubicin." *Journal of Applied Polymer Science* 131 (23). doi: 10.1002/app.41146.

Lu, Bingyuan, Mark D. Tarn, Nicole Pamme, and Theoni K. Georgiou. 2016. "Microfluidically fabricated pH-responsive anionic amphiphilic microgels for drug release." *Journal of Materials Chemistry B* 4 (18): 3086–93. doi: 10.1039/C5TB02378E.

Mackiewicz, Marcin, Serife Dagdelen, Kamil Marcisz, Ewelina Waleka-Bargiel, Zbigniew Stojek, and Marcin Karbarz. 2021. "Redox-degradable microgel based on poly (acrylic acid) as drug-carrier with very high drug-loading capacity and decreased toxicity against healthy cells." *Polymer Degradation and Stability* 190: 109652. doi: 10.1016/j.polymdegradstab.2021.109652.

Mackiewicz, Marcin, Klaudia Kaniewska, Jan Romanski, Ewa Augustin, Zbigniew Stojek, and Marcin Karbarz. 2015. "Stable and degradable microgels linked with cystine for storing and environmentally triggered release of drugs." *Journal of Materials Chemistry B* 3 (36): 7262–70. doi: 10.1039/C5TB00907C.

Madrigal, Justin L., Shonit N. Sharma, Kevin T. Campbell, Roberta S. Stilhano, Rik Gijsbers, and Eduardo A. Silva. 2018. "Microgels produced using microfluidic on-chip polymer blending for controlled released of VEGF encoding lentivectors." *Acta Biomaterialia* 69: 265–76. doi: 10.1016/j.actbio.2018.01.013.

Maeda, Tomohiro, Yusuke Akasaki, Kazuya Yamamoto, and Takao Aoyagi. 2009. "Stimuli-responsive coacervate induced in binary functionalized poly (N-Isopropylacrylamide) aqueous system and novel method for preparing semi-IPN microgel using the coacervate." *Langmuir* 25(16): 9510–17. doi: 10.1021/la9007735.

Makvandi, Pooyan, Atefeh Zarepour, Xuanqi Zheng, Tarun Agarwal, Matineh Ghomi, Rossella Sartorius, Ehsan Nazarzadeh Zare, et al. 2021. "Non-spherical nanostructures in nanomedicine: From noble metal nanorods to transition metal dichalcogenide nanosheets." *Applied Materials Today* 24: 101107. doi: 10.1016/j.apmt.2021.101107.

Martin-Molina, Alberto, and Manuel Quesada-Pérez. 2019. "A review of coarse-grained simulations of nanogel and microgel particles." *Journal of Molecular Liquids* 280: 374–81. doi: 10.1016/j.molliq.2019.02.030.

Meyer-Kirschner, Julian, Michael Kather, Andrij Pich, Dirk Engel, Wolfgang Marquardt, Joern Viell, and Alexander Mitsos. 2016. "In-line monitoring of monomer and polymer content during microgel synthesis using precipitation polymerization via Raman spectroscopy and indirect hard modeling." *Applied Spectroscopy* 70 (3): 416–26. doi: 10.1177%2F0003702815626663.

Mihalko, Emily, Ke Huang, Erin Sproul, Ke Cheng, and Ashley C. Brown. 2018. "Targeted treatment of ischemic and fibrotic complications of myocardial infarction using a dual-delivery microgel therapeutic." *ACS Nano* 12 (8): 7826–37. doi: 10.1021/acsnano.8b01977.

Mueller, Eva, Richard J. Alsop, Andrea Scotti, Markus Bleuel, Maikel C. Rheinstädter, Walter Richtering, and Todd Hoare. 2018. "Dynamically cross-linked self-assembled thermoresponsive microgels with homogeneous internal structures." *Langmuir* 34 (4): 1601–12. doi: 10.1021/acs.langmuir.7b03664.

Murthy, Niren, Mingcheng Xu, Stephany Schuck, Jun Kunisawa, Nilabh Shastri, and Jean M.J. Fréchet. 2003. "A macromolecular delivery vehicle for protein-based vaccines: Acid-degradable protein-loaded microgels." *Proceedings of the National Academy of Sciences* 100 (9): 4995–5000.

Mutharani, Bhuvanenthiran, Palraj Ranganathan, and Shen-Ming Chen. 2020. "Stimuli-enabled reversible switched aclonifen electrochemical sensor based on smart PNIPAM/PANI-Cu hybrid conducting microgel." *Sensors and Actuators B: Chemical* 304: 127232. doi: 10.1016/j.snb.2019.127232.

Ohta, Seiichi, Kenichiro Hashimoto, Xiaoting Fu, Masamichi Kamihira, Yasuyuki Sakai, and Taichi Ito. 2018. "Development of human-derived hemoglobin–albumin microspheres as oxygen carriers using Shirasu porous glass membrane emulsification." *Journal of Bioscience and Bioengineering* 126 (4): 533–39. doi: 10.1016/j.jbiosc.2018.04.017.

Plamper, Felix A., and Walter Richtering. 2017. "Functional microgels and microgel systems." *Accounts of Chemical Research* 50 (2): 131–40. doi: 10.1021/acs.accounts.6b00544.

Qi, Xiaofang, Lu Xiong, Jing Peng, and Dongyan Tang. 2017. "Near infrared laser-controlled drug release of thermoresponsive microgel encapsulated with Fe_3O_4 nanoparticles." *RSC Advances* 7 (32): 19604–10. doi: 10.1039/C7RA01009E.

Rejinold, N. Sanoj, Thejus Baby, K.P. Chennazhi, and R. Jayakumar. 2014. "Dual drug encapsulated thermo-sensitive fibrinogen-graft-poly (N-Isopropyl Acrylamide) nanogels for breast cancer therapy." *Colloids and Surfaces B: Biointerfaces* 114: 209–17. doi: 10.1016/j.colsurfb.2013.10.015.

Rejinold, N. Sanoj, Thejus Baby, K.P. Chennazhi, and R. Jayakumar. 2015. "Multi drug loaded thermo-responsive fibrinogen-graft-poly (N-Vinyl Caprolactam) nanogels for breast cancer drug delivery." *Journal of Biomedical Nanotechnology* 11 (3): 392–402.

Richtering, Walter, and Brian R. Saunders. 2014. "Gel architectures and their complexity." *Soft Matter* 10 (21): 3695–702. doi: 10.1039/C4SM00208C.

Ryu, Ja-Hyoung, Siriporn Jiwpanich, Reuben Chacko, Sean Bickerton, and S. Thayumanavan. 2010. "Surface-functionalizable polymer nanogels with facile hydrophobic guest encapsulation capabilities." *Journal of the American Chemical Society* 132 (24): 8246–47. doi: 10.1021/ja102316a.

Sauraj, Kumar Vinay, Bijender Kumar, Ruchir Priyadarshi, Farha Deeba, Anurag Kulshreshtha, Anuj Kumar, Garima Agrawal, P. Gopinath, and Yuvraj Singh Negi. 2020. "Redox responsive Xylan-SS-curcumin prodrug nanoparticles for dual drug delivery in cancer therapy." *Materials Science and Engineering: C* 107: 110356. doi: 10.1016/j.msec.2019.110356.

Seyfoori, Amir, S.A. Seyyed Ebrahimi, Ehsan Samiei, and Mohsen Akbari. 2019. "Multifunctional hybrid magnetic microgel synthesis for immune-based isolation and post-isolation culture of tumor cells." *ACS Applied Materials & Interfaces* 11 (28): 24945–58. doi: 10.1021/acsami.9b02959.

Soliman, Moamen M., Tamer M. Sakr, Hassan M. Rashed, Ashraf A. Hamed, and Hassan A. Abd El-Rehim. 2021. "Polyethylene oxide–polyacrylic acid–folic acid (PEO-PAAc) nanogel as a^{99m}TC targeting receptor for cancer diagnostic imaging." *Journal of Labelled Compounds and Radiopharmaceuticals* 64 (14): 534–47. doi: 10.1002/jlcr.3952.

Sood, Ankur, Varun Arora, Sadhana Kumari, Ankita Sarkar, S. Senthil Kumaran, Shubhra Chaturvedi, Tapan K. Jain, and Garima Agrawal. 2021. "Imaging application and radiosensitivity enhancement of pectin decorated multifunctional magnetic nanoparticles in cancer therapy." *International Journal of Biological Macromolecules* 189: 443–54. doi: 10.1016/j.ijbiomac.2021.08.124.

Sood, Ankur, Aastha Gupta, and Garima Agrawal. 2021. "Recent advances in polysaccharides based biomaterials for drug delivery and tissue engineering applications." *Carbohydrate Polymer Technologies and Applications* 2: 100067. doi: 10.1016/j.carpta.2021.100067.

Sood, Ankur, Aastha Gupta, Ravi Bharadwaj, Pavana Ranganath, Neal Silverman, and Garima Agrawal. 2022. "Biodegradable disulfide crosslinked chitosan/stearic acid nanoparticles for dual drug delivery for colorectal cancer." *Carbohydrate Polymers* 294: 119833. doi: 10.1016/j.carbpol.2022.119833.

Steinhilber, Dirk, Torsten Rossow, Stefanie Wedepohl, Florian Paulus, Sebastian Seiffert, and Rainer Haag. 2013. "A microgel construction kit for bioorthogonal encapsulation and pH-controlled release of living cells." *Angewandte Chemie International Edition* 52 (51): 13538–43. doi: 10.1002/anie.201308005.

Tan, Shen, Zhengquan Lu, Jing Zhao, Jianan Zhang, Mingyuan Wu, Qingyun Wu, and Jianjun Yang. 2016. "Synthesis and multi-responsiveness of poly (N-Vinylcaprolactam-co-acrylic acid) core–shell microgels via miniemulsion polymerization." *Polymer Chemistry* 7 (24): 4106–11. doi: 10.1039/C6PY00544F.

Theune, Loryn E., Jens Buchmann, Stefanie Wedepohl, Maria Molina, Jan Laufer, and Marcelo Calderón. 2019. "NIR- and thermo-responsive semi-interpenetrated polypyrrole nanogels for imaging guided combinational photothermal and chemotherapy." *Journal of Controlled Release* 311–312: 147–61. doi: 10.1016/j.jconrel.2019.08.035.

Van Elk, Merel, Cyril Lorenzato, Burcin Ozbakir, Chris Oerlemans, Gert Storm, Frank Nijsen, Roel Deckers, Tina Vermonden, and Wim E. Hennink. 2015. "Alginate microgels loaded with temperature sensitive liposomes for magnetic resonance imageable drug release and microgel visualization." *European Polymer Journal* 72: 620–31. doi: 10.1016/j.eurpolymj.2015.03.013.

Van Thienen, T.G., Koen Raemdonck, Jo Demeester, and S.C. De Smedt. 2007. "Protein release from biodegradable dextran nanogels." *Langmuir* 23 (19): 9794–801. doi: 10.1021/la700736v.

Villemin, Elise, Yih Ching Ong, Christophe M. Thomas, and Gilles Gasser. 2019. "Polymer encapsulation of ruthenium complexes for biological and medicinal applications." *Nature Reviews Chemistry* 3 (4): 261–82. doi: 10.1038/s41570-019-0088-0.

Wang, Hailin, Garima Agrawal, Larisa Tsarkova, Xiaomin Zhu, and Martin Möller. 2013a. "Self-templating amphiphilic polymer precursors for fabricating mesostructured silica particles: A water-based facile and universal method." *Advanced Materials* 25 (7): 1017–21. doi: 10.1002/adma.201203840.

Wang, Hui, Sumit Mukherjee, Jinhui Yi, Probal Banerjee, Qianwang Chen, and Shuiqin Zhou. 2017a. "Biocompatible chitosan–carbon dot hybrid nanogels for NIR-imaging-guided synergistic photothermal–chemo therapy." *ACS Applied Materials & Interfaces* 9 (22): 18639–49. doi: 10.1021/acsami.7b06062.

Wang, Ya, Giovanni Boero, Xiaosheng Zhang, and Juergen Brugger. 2020. "Thermal and pH sensitive composite membrane for on-demand drug delivery by applying an alternating magnetic field." *Advanced Materials Interfaces* 7 (17): 2000733. doi: 10.1002/admi.202000733.

Wang, Yang, Jinshan Nie, Baisong Chang, Yangfei Sun, and Wuli Yang. 2013b. "Poly (Vinylcaprolactam)-based biodegradable multiresponsive microgels for drug delivery." *Biomacromolecules* 14 (9): 3034–46. doi: 10.1021/bm401131w.

Wang, Yang, Jin Zheng, Yefei Tian, and Wuli Yang. 2015. "Acid degradable poly (Vinylcaprolactam)-based nanogels with ketal linkages for drug delivery." *Journal of Materials Chemistry B* 3 (28): 5824–32. doi: 10.1039/C5TB00703H.

Wang, Yitong, Ling Wang, Miaomiao Yan, Shuli Dong, and Jingcheng Hao. 2017b. "Near-infrared-light-responsive magnetic DNA microgels for photon-and magneto-manipulated cancer therapy." *ACS Applied Materials & Interfaces* 9 (34): 28185–94. doi: 10.1021/acsami.7b05502.

Wei, Menglian, Xue Li, and Michael J. Serpe. 2019. "Stimuli-responsive microgel-based surface plasmon resonance transducer for glucose detection using a competitive assay with concanavalin A." *ACS Applied Polymer Materials* 1 (3): 519–25. doi: 10.1021/acsapm.8b00207.

Wiemer, Katharina, Karla Dörmbach, Ioana Slabu, Garima Agrawal, F. Schrader, T. Caumanns, S.D.M. Bourone, et al. 2017. "Hydrophobic superparamagnetic FePt nanoparticles in hydrophilic poly (N-Vinylcaprolactam) microgels: A new multifunctional hybrid system." *Journal of Materials Chemistry B* 5 (6): 1284–92. doi: 10.1039/C6TB02342H.

Wu, Bi-cheng, and David Julian McClements. 2015. "Microgels formed by electrostatic complexation of gelatin and OSA starch: Potential fat or starch mimetics." *Food Hydrocolloids* 47: 87–93. doi: 10.1016/j.foodhyd.2015.01.021.

Wu, Weitai, Jing Shen, Probal Banerjee, and Shuiqin Zhou. 2010a. "Core–shell hybrid nanogels for integration of optical temperature-sensing, targeted tumor cell imaging, and combined chemo-photothermal treatment." *Biomaterials* 31 (29): 7555–66. doi:10.1016/j.biomaterials.2010.06.030.

Wu, Weitai, Jing Shen, Probal Banerjee, and Shuiqin Zhou. 2010b. "Chitosan-based responsive hybrid nanogels for integration of optical pH-sensing, tumor cell imaging and controlled drug delivery." *Biomaterials* 31 (32): 8371–81. doi: 10.1016/j.biomaterials.2010.07.061.

Xu, Wenjing, Andrey Rudov, Alex Oppermann, Sarah Wypysek, Michael Kather, Ricarda Schroeder, Walter Richtering, et al. 2020. "Synthesis of polyampholyte janus-like microgels by coacervation of reactive precursors in precipitation polymerization." *Angewandte Chemie* 132 (3): 1264–71. doi: 10.1002/ange.201910450.

Yan, Jiaqi, Yichuan Wang, Meixin Ran, Rawand A. Mustafa, Huanhuan Luo, Jixiang Wang, Jan-Henrik Smått, et al. 2021. "Peritumoral microgel reservoir for long-term light-controlled triple-synergistic treatment of osteosarcoma with single ultra-low dose." *Small* 17 (31): 2100479. doi: 10.1002/smll.202100479.

Yang, Hao, Qin Wang, Shan Huang, Ai Xiao, Fuying Li, Lu Gan, and Xiangliang Yang. 2016. "Smart pH/Redox dual-responsive nanogels for on-demand intracellular anticancer drug release." *ACS Applied Materials & Interfaces* 8 (12): 7729–38. doi: 10.1021/acsami.6b01602.

Yin, Xiangchun, and Harald D.H. Stöver. 2003. "Hydrogel microspheres formed by complex coacervation of partially MPEG-grafted poly (Styrene-alt-Maleic Anhydride) with PDADMAC and cross-linking with polyamines." *Macromolecules* 36 (23): 8773–79. doi: 10.1021/ma034617n.

Zhang, Qiang, Juan Colazo, Darren Berg, Samuel M. Mugo, and Michael J. Serpe. 2017. "Multiresponsive nanogels for targeted anticancer drug delivery." *Molecular Pharmaceutics* 14 (8): 2624–28. doi: 10.1021/acs.molpharmaceut.7b00325.

Zhang, Xinjie, Shaoyu Lü, Chunmei Gao, Chen Chen, Xuan Zhang, and Mingzhu Liu. 2013. "Highly stable and degradable multifunctional microgel for self-regulated insulin delivery under physiological conditions." *Nanoscale* 5 (14): 6498–506. doi: 10.1039/C3NR00835E.

Zhang, Zihao, Xucheng Zhang, Yuxue Ding, Peihua Long, Jia Guo, and Changchun Wang. 2019. "NIR-induced disintegration of CuS-loaded nanogels for improved tumor penetration and enhanced anticancer therapy." *Macromolecular Bioscience* 19 (4): 1800416. doi: 10.1002/mabi.201800416.

8 Bioactive Glasses: Multifunctional Delivery Systems for Cancer Theranostic Applications

Saeid Kargozar, Sara Gorgani
Mashhad University of Medical Sciences

Sahar Mollazadeh
Ferdowsi University of Mashhad (FUM)

Farzad Kermani
Mashhad University of Medical Sciences

Francesco Baino
Politecnico di Torino

CONTENTS

8.1 Introduction ... 175
8.2 BGs: Structure, Types, and Properties ... 177
8.3 Synthesis Methods of BGs ... 179
8.4 BGs for Drug Delivery: From Ion Therapy to Drug Release ... 180
8.5 BGs in Cancer Theranostic Applications ... 183
8.6 Concluding Remarks and Future Outlook ... 186
References ... 187

8.1 INTRODUCTION

Cancer is considered the second leading cause of death worldwide and is one of the most burdensome diseases the healthcare system has to deal with because of its high prevalence levels in the population [1,2]. Therefore, numerous attempts have been made to develop and introduce effective therapies for managing diverse types of cancer. Understanding cancer biology is of utmost importance for researchers who aim to design and apply new medical tools and instruments for the treatment and diagnosis of malignancies. This can be seen as a way of defining six main characteristics of cancer, which were established by Hanahan and Weinberg in 2000 as

DOI: 10.1201/9781003251767-8

follows: (i) sustained cellular proliferative signaling; (ii) resistance to cellular apoptosis signals; (iii) physiological immortality of cells; (iv) stimulation of angiogenesis; and (v) metastasis and invasion of cancer cells into other tissues [3]. The list has been expanded by two further hallmarks, including reprogramming cellular energy metabolism and evading immune system attack. In addition to altering genomic stability, these biological phenomena have been recognized as contributing factors to the extraordinary diversity of neoplastic diseases.

Materials science and engineering have provided great opportunities for researchers and scientists who are trying to design and develop anticancer substances. With the help of chemical engineering possibilities, it is now possible to prepare smart materials capable of treating tumor cells while causing minimal damage to normal cells [4]. It has recently become apparent that bioactive glasses (BGs) are among the most promising anticancer materials [5,6]. BGs represent a special family of biocompatible materials with diverse applications in biomedical settings. The invention of these man-made substances belongs to the original work of Prof. Larry L. Hench at University of Florida in the early 1970s [7]. In fact, the first developed BG (45S5 Bioglass®) was a silicate-based glass with a formulation of $45SiO_2$–24.5CaO–$24.5Na_2O$–$6P_2O_5$ (wt. %). This chemical composition was later commercialized and is being sold in different forms by several pharmaceutical companies. In spite of the fact that BGs are typically used to treat hard tissue defects (e.g., bone lesions), a number of recent studies have identified their therapeutic capacity for treating soft tissue injuries as well [8–12]. Aside from their excellent biocompatibility and ability to bond with living tissues (i.e., bioactivity), BGs also have several other characteristics that make them ideal for bioengineering applications, including their ability to stimulate cell proliferation, differentiation, and growth [13]. Moreover, some experimental studies have also provided insight into the stimulatory effect of BGs on new blood vessel formation, which has also been confirmed in some experimental studies [14,15].

Specific formulations of BGs have been found to be suitable compositions for cancer therapy strategies. There is evidence that the addition of specific elements to the basic composition of BGs (e.g., copper (Cu) and iron (Fe)) leads to the generation of magnetic anticancer materials as a result of their magnetic properties [16,17]. On this matter, different mechanisms have been proposed for taking the most benefit of anticancer glasses; for example, they are being used for hyperthermia and photothermal therapy (PTT) of malignant cells. Additionally, BGs containing particular elements (e.g., iron (Fe)) produce a high level of reactive oxygen species (ROS), which promote tumor cell apoptosis [18]. In addition, a subclass of BGs, known as mesoporous BGs (MBGs), can be used to load and deliver a wide variety of natural and synthetic medicines and bioactive molecules with anticancer properties [19]. Since MBGs contain mesoporous structures (pore sizes between 2 and 50 nm), they can be used as platforms for the localized delivery of anticancer agents [20]. It is now possible to make MBGs as smart anticancer drug delivery vehicles by opening and closing their pores with chemical molecules.

In this chapter, we first introduce different types of BGs and their synthesis and characterization approaches. Then, the therapeutic possibilities of BGs will be discussed for anticancer drug delivery as well as hyperthermia and PTT cancer therapy.

8.2 BGS: STRUCTURE, TYPES, AND PROPERTIES

Through enormous efforts in the glass and glass-ceramics fields, several compositions of BGs with diverse physicochemical, mechanical, and biological properties have been developed. On the basis of their chemical structure, BGs can be grouped into three major categories: silicate-based, borate-based, and phosphate-based. The BGs are routinely synthesized via mixing different inorganic oxides that serve as (i) network formers (e.g., SiO_2, B_2O_3, and P_2O_5), (ii) network modifiers (e.g., Na_2O, CaO, MgO, and K_2O), and (iii) intermediate oxides (e.g., Al_2O_3, ZnO, ZrO_2, and TiO_2). Both soft and hard tissues can be bonded with BGs since they have surface-reactive properties. In fact, after BGs are exposed to physiological fluids (e.g., blood) for several hours or days, a layer of hydroxycarbonate apatite (HCA) forms on the BG surface. It is usually the chemical composition and the synthesis method of BGs that determine how the HCA layer forms. This property is termed "bioactivity," which is the "fingerprint" of BGs. In addition, a large processing window makes it possible to produce different types of BG-based constructs for potential use in tissue engineering. Both the features mentioned above (i.e., bioactivity and a large processing window) are determined by the glass network connectivity (NC). In line with this statement, the NC of BGs is responsible for maintaining a balance between the processing properties of the BG and its bioactivity [21]. In a glass network, the NC determines the number of bridging oxygens (n) per glass-forming unit (Q). The NC for most BGs is between 1.9 and 2.6. BGs with lower NC (1.9–2.0) have higher bioactivity and the subsequent capability of tissue bonding. According to Equation (8.1), it is theoretically possible to calculate the NC of simple silicate-based BGs (NC_{Si}):

$$NC_{Si} = \frac{4[SiO_2] - 2([M_2O] + [M'O])}{[SiO_2]} \tag{8.1}$$

where, $[SiO_2]$, $[M_2O]$, and $[M'O]$ correspond to silicon dioxide, alkali oxide, and alkaline earth oxide, respectively, based on their molar percentages (mol%).

The bioactivity and solubility of BGs may be evaluated by NC; a glass with a lower NC has a higher degradation rate. As mentioned earlier, the building units of BGs are presented as the Q^n symbol, in which Q represents the network-forming polyhedron and n denotes the number of bridging oxygen atoms. In this way, BG structures that have more bridging oxygens are more chemically resistant and have a higher melting point.

The SiO_4 tetrahedron is the structural unit in silicate glasses, and it can be connected to a maximum of four other silica tetrahedra through Si-O-Si bonds. It has been reported that Bioglass® 45S5 possesses an NC of 2.11, corresponding to a structure composed primarily of Q^2 silicate chains (89%) and Q^3 branching units (11%). The latter links the chains by bridging oxygen atoms [22]. Using Raman spectroscopy and nuclear magnetic resonance (NMR), it has been possible to determine the distribution of Q^n in a glass structure; for example, 29Si magic-angle-spinning (MAS) NMR spectroscopy can be used to estimate the relative amount of Q species in silicate-based BG structures compared to the actual NC [23–25]. It should be highlighted that this characterization technique may be useful in studying the effects of dopants on the BG structure; for example, determining the role of doped elements in the glass network as network modifiers or network formers is feasible by NMR spectroscopy [26,27].

Phosphate-based glasses are built with a tetrahedral unit of (PO_4^{3-}) building block; in order to form a 3D network, an orthophosphate tetrahedron can bond with a maximum of three neighboring units (Figure 8.1). Since oxygen atoms are not shared between phosphate tetrahedra, the terminal double bond in phosphate glasses is

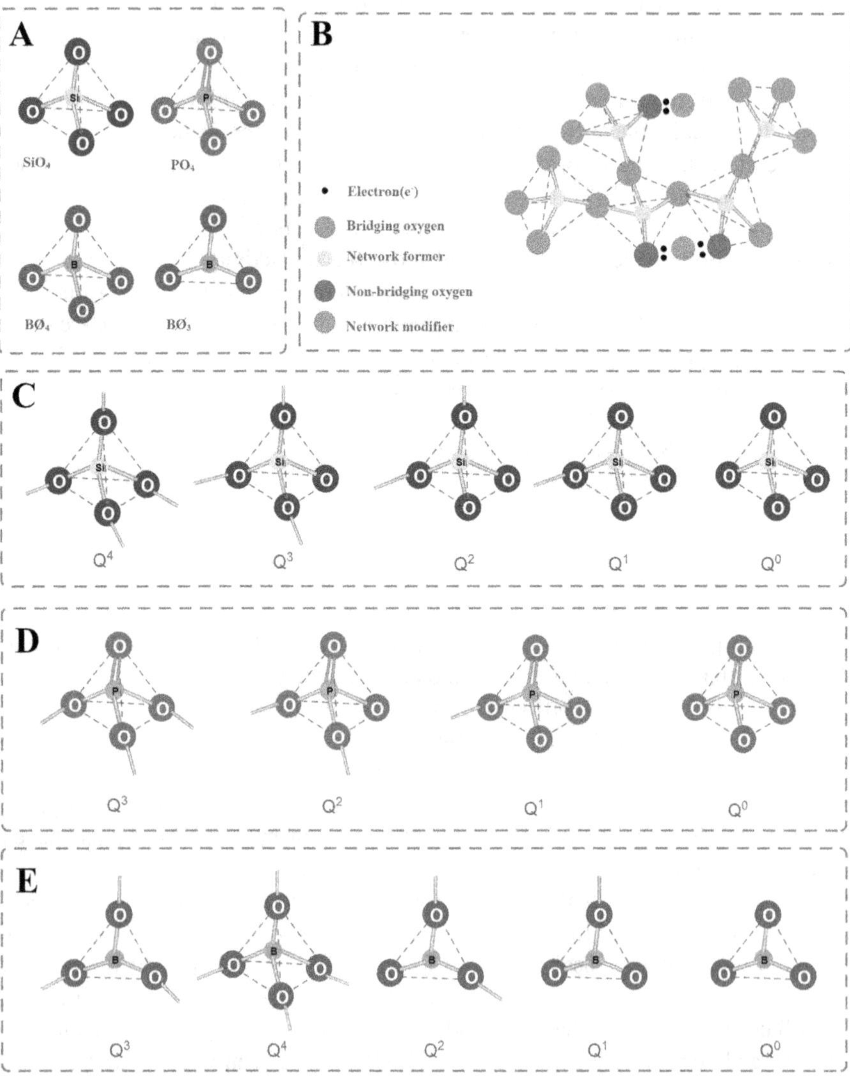

FIGURE 8.1 (a) Schematic representation of silicate-, phosphate-, and borate-based bioactive glass structural units. (b) Bridging/non-bridging oxygens in the silicate-based glass. (c–e) Illustrations of the possible Q^n species in silicate-, phosphate-, and borate-based BGs. (Reproduced from [29].)

limited to three (Q^3). Thus, phosphate glass has a lower NC value than silicate glass. The number of n can also be changed to form Q^2 by adding modifier cations in the same way as in silicate glasses. In phosphate-based BGs, 31P MAS NMR and Raman spectroscopy can be used to analyze the relative amounts and distributions of Q^n, respectively [24,28].

In the case of simple phosphate-based BGs, the following equation can be used to calculate NCp (Eq. 8.2):

$$NCp=\frac{3[P_2O_5]-2([M_2O]+[M'O])}{[P_2O_5]} \quad (8.2)$$

where $[P_2O_5]$, $[M_2O]$, and $[M'O]$ represent the molar percentage (mol%) of phosphorus pentoxide, alkali, and alkaline earth oxides, respectively.

Boron trioxide (B_2O_3) acts as the network former in borate-based glasses, and the planar BO3 trigonal group is the structural unit. This type of BG is well known for its high dissolution rates and reactivity (apatite-forming capability) in physiological environments, which are typically faster than boron-free silicate glasses. By replacing silica with boron (borosilicate glasses), borate-based glasses can be controlled in terms of degradation rate. For both hard and soft tissue healing, various bioactive borate glasses (e.g., 1393-B3) have been developed.

8.3 SYNTHESIS METHODS OF BGS

BGs can be synthesized in different ways, including by melt-quenching or sol-gel methods. Traditionally, glass compositions are produced by melting and quenching. In this method, raw materials (glass precursors of oxides and carbonates) were first mixed and homogenized and then treated at high temperatures (above 1200°C) to obtain a viscous liquid with casting ability. Finally, the molten glass is quenched into water or liquid nitrogen to obtain glass powders (frit) or cast into a pre-heated stainless-steel mold to have bulk glassy compounds [30,31]. The obtained glass powders could be easily used as such or ground for further applications, whereas the bulk glassy pieces obtained from the casting process should be annealed at about 500°C–600°C to eliminate any residual thermal stresses. It is also possible to produce BGs through the sol-gel process, which is a wet-chemical method that can be applied to a variety of conditions. Sol-gel processing starts with hydrolyzing glass former alkoxides (e.g., TEOS) or organometallic compounds (e.g., methoxide compounds) using deionized water and alcohol. In the next step, other water-soluble reagents (glass modifiers and/or intermediates) are added to the first sol at proper (30–45 minute) intervals. The formation of 3D networks occurred through simultaneous hydrolysis-condensation processes or delayed-condensation processes during the aging step (7–14 days). In the synthesis process of some BGs (e.g., 58S and 45S5 BGs), uniform gels could also be obtained very quickly by increasing the pH values [32]. Furthermore, the hydrothermal treatment could accelerate the gelation process [33,34]. The porosity and surface area of the glasses obtained are significantly influenced by the aging step (7–21 days). In order to remove the volatiles, the resulting gels should be dried in a two-step process, i.e., drying at a low temperature (about

70°C) for 24 hours and drying at a higher temperature (about 140°C–200°C). As the final step of the sol-gel process, the dried gels are heated to a temperature below the glass transition temperature (T_g) to densify the resulting network and eliminate volatile impurities. Sol-gel synthesis of glasses is possible in the presence of polymeric structure-directing agents (e.g., P123) to obtain mesoporous BGs (MBGs) with well-ordered nanopores (pore size = 2–50 nm) [17,27,28]. The melt-quenching and sol-gel methods usually required high temperatures (especially in the melting route), long duration (in the sol-gel approach), and expensive equipment and reagents. The discovery of a fast and low-cost method of synthesizing BGs would open up new research avenues in the future. SCS entails the rapid and self-propagating exothermic reaction between the fuel(s) (e.g., citric acid and urea) and the oxidizers (e.g., $Ca(NO_3)_2$ and $Fe(NO_3)_3$) in an aqueous or sol-gel medium [35–37]. The SCS method was recently proposed for the fabrication of bioceramics such as hydroxyapatite [38–40]. Several promising properties of SCS-synthesized nanoparticles have recently been observed, including high surface area and high surface charge. With proper tuning of various SCS parameters, including fuel type, fuel-to-oxidizer ratio (F/O), and the initial temperature of the synthesis process, the authors hope that this method can be applied to fabricating BGs containing aluminosilicate, silicate, phosphate, and borate glass compositions.

8.4 BGS FOR DRUG DELIVERY: FROM ION THERAPY TO DRUG RELEASE

In recent years, BGs have been the subject of a great deal of research regarding their potential for drug delivery. BGs exhibit significant properties for drug delivery, including excellent biocompatibility, compositional versatility, and exceptional stability in physiological fluids. By virtue of their structure, BGs can release therapeutic ions into surrounding biological environments. Accordingly, introducing doping elements into the BG network has become a routine method in the lab for providing targeted delivery of therapeutic dopants (e.g., copper and zinc) into desired locations. Apart from therapeutic applications, glasses doped with specific elements (e.g., europium and ytterbium) may be implemented for bioimaging strategies [41,42]. Despite all achievements, some practical points should be taken into consideration; for example, doped elements can change the dissolution rate, surface area, and pore size distributions in BGs [43–45]. For example, adding magnesium to sol-gel-based BG nanoparticles ($85SiO_2$–(15−x) CaO–xMgO, with x = 1, 3, 5, and 10 mol%) proved to enhance the specific surface area of the samples; the loading efficiency of the antibiotic Amoxicillin showed a decrease after increasing Mg content while its release kinetics increased [46]. Another important issue is that releasing ions from BG structures largely depends on the general type (silicate-, phosphate-, or borate-based glasses) and the specific chemical composition of BGs [47]. Under physiological conditions, borate and phosphate glasses degrade more quickly than silicate glasses; therefore, a burst release of therapeutic ions occurs during the incubation time [48].

It is important to note that there is a big difference between the release profile of ions from glass powders/particles and glass-based 3D constructs (scaffolds). In order to achieve the best in vitro and in vivo results, sustained release of ions is a crucial factor. The release profile of therapeutic ions can be greatly affected by the incorporation of BGs into polymeric substrates, and the release of dopants into the environment can be controlled more effectively with this method [49,50]. On the other hand, the addition of BGs to biopolymers may improve the hydrophilicity, bioactivity, and mechanical properties of the final construct. Furthermore, this can affect cell and tissue responses, degradation, and the drug release profile of polymers [51]. On this matter, using 3D printed layers of MBGs/sodium alginate-sodium alginate scaffolds (MBG/SA–SA), a dual-drug release system was generated [52]. A relatively fast release of bovine serum albumin (BSA) was observed in the SA layer, and a sustained release of ibuprofen (IBU) was observed in the MBG/SA layer after the two molecules were loaded into the SA layer and MBG layer, respectively. Human bone mesenchymal stem cells (hBMSCs) adhered more effectively to the layered MBG/SA–SA scaffolds, proliferated more, and differentiated osteogenically as compared to the SA scaffolds.

The BGs have been successfully loaded with substances that promote tissue repair and regeneration through antimicrobial, anti-inflammatory, immunomodulatory, and pro-angiogenic properties [53–55]. More importantly, anticancer drug-loaded BGs were also prepared for the battle against different types of malignancies. It is clear that sol-gel-based glasses (especially MBGs) are preferred to melt-quench BGs for drug delivery thanks to their inherently porous structure. Having well-ordered pores, MBGs provide the possibility of loading various therapeutic agents (synthetic or natural substances) into their channels and subsequent delivery to desired sites. There have been several reports that have clarified the potential of MBGs as stimulus-responsive delivery systems in tissue engineering and regenerative medicine; opening and closing the MBG channels are applicable using particular small molecules or chemical moieties for imparting a controlled release of the loaded drugs.

BG surfaces have been found to be suitable places for functionalization through diverse chemical compounds [56]. Due to their multifunctional properties, these biocompatible materials have been tested on a variety of natural and synthetic materials. For instance, Ferlenda et al. succeeded in grafting a natural antioxidant compound, *Rosa canina* bud extract, to a silica-based BG to prepare new multifunctional materials with a green approach [57]. They reported that the functionalizing process not only interferes with the bioactivity feature but also improves it. It should be mentioned that chemical linkers (e.g., EDC/NHS) can be utilized for the functionalization of BGs with different bioactive molecules. A cross-linking process involving EDC/NHS was employed to immobilize vancomycin onto amino-functionalized BG nanoparticles (BGNs) (see Figure 8.2) [58]. Surface coating of BGs with biopolymers was also proposed for providing sustained drug release platforms. At this point, foam-like BG scaffolds were coated with NHS-crosslinked gelatin and then loaded with the bioactive molecule icariin [59]. The reported data indicate that crosslinked gelatin coating is an appropriate method for surface modification of BGs to obtain a sustained release of drugs and improve mechanical strengths without any significant adverse effect on the sample bioactivity.

In some strategies, polymer-coated glasses have been used for biofunctionalizing bone implants to enhance their inherent properties, like low osteointegration, and eliminate adverse inflammatory and immunological reactions. In this regard, the anti-inflammatory and antioxidative molecule A-485 was loaded onto Mg-doped BG

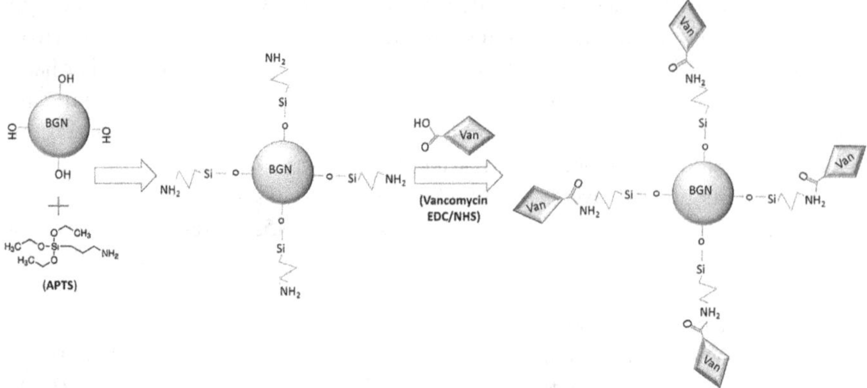

FIGURE 8.2 Schematic illustration of APTS molecules immobilizing on bioactive glass nanoparticles (BGN) and vancomycin molecules functionalizing them. (Reproduced with permission from [58].)

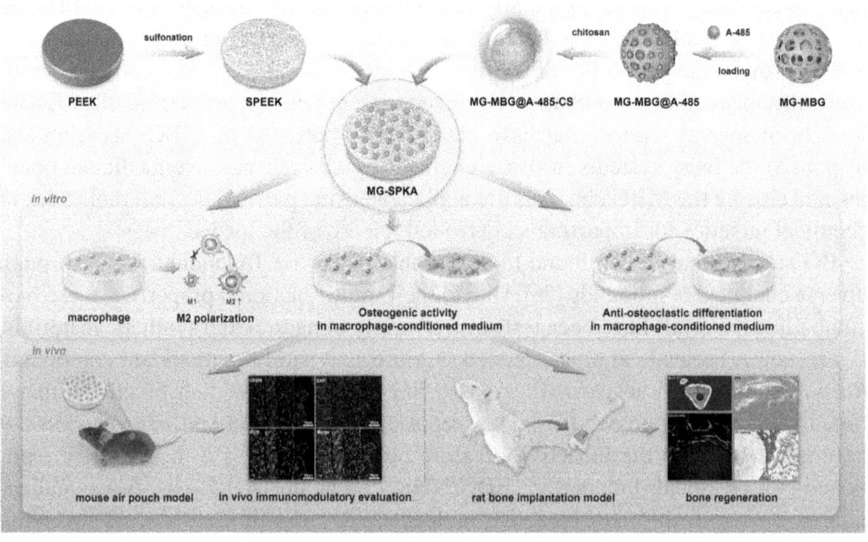

FIGURE 8.3 Schematic representation of the loading of A-485 (p300/CBP catalytic inhibitor with potent and selective activity) into the mesoporous bioactive glass (MBGs) and their immobilization on the surface of polyetheretherketone (PEEK). (Reproduced with permission from [60].)

nanoparticles and then dispersed in a chitosan solution to fabricate a composite, which was utilized for coating sulfonated polyetheretherketone (PEEK) by lyophilization (Figure 8.3) [60]. The obtained data showed a controlled release of A-485 from the prepared construct (named MG-SPKA) along with induced switching of macrophages to the M2 phenotype with enhanced expressions of IL-10, IL-4, and CD206. As well as inhibiting osteoclast differentiation, this BG-based drug delivery system also exhibited osteoimmunomodulatory properties and accelerated in vivo bone regeneration.

8.5 BGS IN CANCER THERANOSTIC APPLICATIONS

Globally, cancer remains one of the leading causes of death; therefore, numerous attempts have been made to find effective solutions for combating malignancies. Up to now, various types and formulations of BGs have been designed and examined for treating cancer (Table 8.1). As previously reported, BG particles can selectively enhance the toxicity of neoplastic stromal cells derived from bone and induce autophagy by activating MAPK signaling [61]. Apart from this issue, BGs can be doped with particular elements (e.g., Fe, Cu, Mn, etc.) for rendering and enhancing their anticancer activities [62]. It has been shown that Fe-doped mesoporous 45S5 BGs can produce reactive oxygen species (ROS) such as the OH free radicals, which are capable of destroying cancer cells in acidic environments (Figure 8.4a) [32].

TABLE 8.1
Different Additives Used in the Composition of BGs and BGs-Ceramics for Cancer Theranostic Applications

Additives/Dopants	Remarks
Iron oxides	Targeted drug delivery (Fe_3O_4 and γ-Fe_2O_3)
	Magnetite hyperthermia (Fe_3O_4 and γ-Fe_2O_3, FeO)
	Fenton reaction and potential for electrochemical reaction (Fe_2O_3)
	Enhanced bone formation and improve the crystallization of magnetite phase (Fe_2O_3)
	Photothermal therapy
	MRI contrast agent
Ferrites (MFe_2O_4)	Magnetite hyperthermia and targeted therapy (e.g., $MgFe_2O_4$, $LiFe_2O_4$, $MnFe_2O_4$, $SrFe_{12}O_{19}$)
	Enhance bioactivity (e.g., $SrFe_{12}O_{19}$)
	Photothermal therapy
Cobalt oxides	Ferrimagnetism and ferromagnetic property
	Enhancing the immunotherapy effects of cancer drugs
	Photothermal therapy
	Targeted therapy of cancer drugs
	Biosensor for cancer diagnose
Copper oxides	Cancer drug delivery
	Photothermal therapy
	Low toxicity with the ability of direct delivering to cancer cells
	Luminescence properties for cancer imaging
Zinc oxide	Management and chemoprevention of cancer cells
Gadolinium oxide	MRI contrast agent
	Cancer drug delivery
Samarium oxide	MRI contrast agent
	Bioimaging cancer theranostics
	Cancer drug delivery
Barium oxide	Computed tomography (CT)

Reproduced with some modifications from [64].

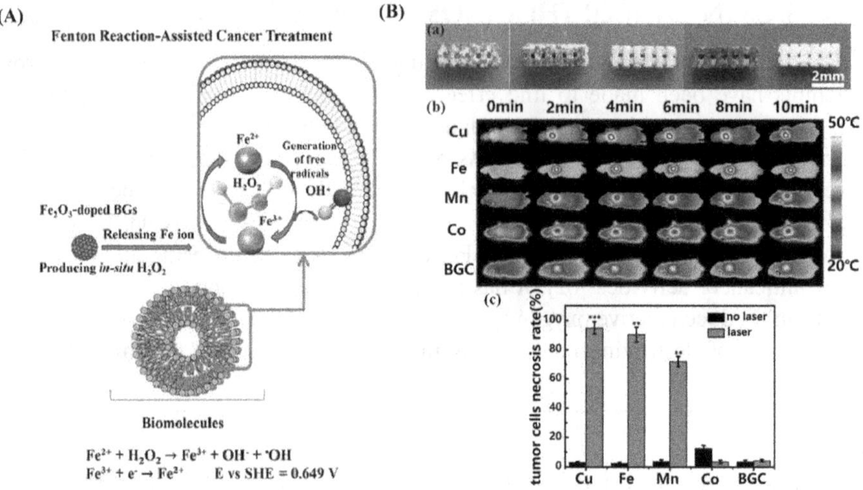

FIGURE 8.4 (a) The formation of reactive oxygen species (ROS) in the cancer cell environment through the mediated Fenton reaction ($Fe^{2+} + H_2O_2 \rightarrow Fe^{3+} + OH^- + OH$) with Fe-doped 45S5 BGs. Furthermore, the electrochemical potential changes through the ($Fe^{3+} + e^- \rightarrow$ E Fe^{2+}, E vs SHE = 0.649 V) may cause selective toxicity to cancer cells. (b) The photothermal effect of 3D printed Cu, Fe, Mn, and Co doped to bioactive glass-ceramic (BGC) and dopant-free BGC, the temperature of the scaffolds reached 53.4°C, 51.3°C, 46.7°C, and 43.3°C, and 39.9°C, respectively, under laser at 808 nm. (a), the fluorescence intensity of the BGC scaffolds under laser at 808 nm (b), the rate of tumor cell necrosis under laser at 808 nm. The suggested trend for photothermal therapy of the ions in this study is $Cu^{1/2+} > Fe^{2/3+} > Mn^{2/3+} > Co^{2/3\,+}$. (Reproduced with permission from [32,78].)

Furthermore, the electrochemical reaction of multivalent ions may be a critical factor in cancer cell apoptosis. It is well known that BGs can deliver drugs and molecules to fight cancer. In this regard, sol-gel synthesized silicate glass has been successfully used to deliver the anticancer drug DOX and the microRNA miR-7-FAM; the loaded BGs can significantly accelerate the apoptosis of tumor cells [63].

Loading and delivering anticancer drugs (e.g., doxorubicin) using MBGs has been recognized as a viable approach to cancer treatment [20]. In this regard, a variety of factors contribute to the outcome of the experiment [65]. These factors include the pH of the microenvironment, the dosage of the loaded drugs, and the degradation rate of the glasses. MBGs are commonly being surface-functionalized to enable targeted therapy for reducing the side effects of anticancer drugs as well as for enhancing the efficient killing of malignant cells. The surface modification of MBGs is being performed by using particular molecules (e.g., folate groups) that have specific receptors with high overexpression on the surface of tumor cells [66]. In some studies, drug-loaded MBGs were added to biopolymers to prevent the burst release of anticancer substances. For example, imatinib-loaded MBGs were mixed into a polyurethane matrix, and the obtained data indicated the sustained release of the drug in the first days of incubation in SBF (52%–84% release over 21 days) [67].

Hyperthermia treatment kills cancer cells by applying high temperatures for approximately one hour (typically 40°C–43°C). This approach can be combined with radiotherapy/chemotherapy to treat several types of malignancies, including those of the bones and soft tissues, such as those of the breast and skin [68]. However, if not properly localized, this method suffers from a critical restriction, i.e., non-targeted treatment of cancer cells and subsequent toxicity in normal cells and tissues [69]. Accordingly, magnetic biocompatible substances (e.g., inorganic nanoparticles) are being applied to elevate the temperature specifically on malignant cells locally. Upon administration of cancer-targeting magnetic nanoparticles (e.g., commercial superparamagnetic iron oxide nanoparticles (SPIONs)), an alternating magnetic field (AMF) is applied to raise the temperature of the nanoparticles inside the tumor. This approach results in the application of the generated heat to tumor cells, sparing the surrounding normal cells and tissues. While magnetic nanoparticles offer many advantages in the clinical setting, they also have some limitations, including a high nanoparticle concentration requirement and a sharp drop in heating efficiency within cells [70]. Recently, the use of magnetic bioactive glass-ceramics (e.g., F_3O_4-containing glasses) was suggested for hyperthermia treatment of cancer; they display unique features like excellent biocompatibility, reduced risk of material displacement in desired tissue, and regenerative potential of the damaged tissues (especially bone) [64,71]. Additionally, the successful fabrication of superparamagnetic and highly bioactive nanocomposites was reported through the incorporation of SPIONs into the 58S BG matrix ($58SiO_2$-33CaO-$9P_2O_5$, wt. %) [72]. As one of the newest cancer treatment methods, photothermal therapy eliminates cancer cells from the primary tumor and the lymph nodes at the earliest stage of metastasis. PTT can also be combined with other therapeutic modalities for treating metastatic cancer cells [73]. This method exhibits excellent merits for clinical settings due to its high specificity, minimal invasiveness, precise spatial-temporal selectivity, etc. Briefly, photoabsorbent inorganic nanoparticles (e.g., gold) convert the energy of the electromagnetic radiation (mostly infrared wavelengths) into heat, thus locally elevating temperature, which effectively facilitates tumor cell ablation [74]. Recently, BG nanoparticles have been proposed for use in the PTT of cancer; as an example, multifunctional Nd-Ca-Si silicate BGs and glass/alginate composite hydrogels were shown to emit fluorescence when exposed to an 808-nm laser in addition to their photothermal properties [75]. A linear correlation between fluorescence intensity and in situ temperature allows this system to select the optimal PTT temperature for effective tumor treatment with minimal damage to normal tissue. Another advantage of this composition for cancer therapy is related to its potential for repairing tissue damage caused by heat. In some studies, MBG particles have been proposed for simultaneous drug loading/release and PTT. Evidence suggests that Cu-doped MBGs have excellent drug loading and PTT properties, where drug release is well modulated by photothermal effects [76]. These kinds of strategies are suggested to address the inherent limitation of the PTT method, i.e., the inadequate penetration depth of near-infrared (NIR) light. On this point, there has been a great deal of attention paid to the development of manganese-doped MBGs loaded with chlorin e6 (Mn-MBG/Ce6) for the treatment of bone cancer and bone regeneration [77]. The addition of Mn to MBGs caused a controlled photothermal performance of the glasses without any adverse effect on the well-ordered mesoporous structure. Loading Ce6 into the Mn-MBG pores led to controlled NIR-triggered Ce6 release. Inducing mild hyperthermia and improving cellular uptake of Ce6 through a drug-loaded composition could enhance photodynamic therapy's efficacy without harming bone regeneration. It should also be mentioned that a 3D printed construct made of (Cu, Fe, Mn, Co)-doped BGs was developed for the treatment of photothermal tumors and regeneration of bone tissue [78]. The photothermal performance of the scaffolds showed a trend as Cu-BGC > Fe-BGC > Mn-BGC > Co-BG. Importantly, the final temperature of metal-doped BG scaffolds was dependent on the type of dopants, dopant contents, and laser power density (Figure 8.4).

It should finally be highlighted that the potential of BGs for simultaneous cancer therapy and bioimaging has also been well documented in some recent experimental studies. As an illustration, fetal bovine serum (FBS)-decorated europium-doped BG nanoparticles (EuBGN@FBS) were successfully developed and applied to enhance tumor targeting for cancer imaging and therapy [79]. EuBGN@FBS exhibits both controlled photoluminescence and pH-responsive drug release properties. The FBS coating of the glass samples resulted in their improved dispersibility in physiological environments, along with enhanced blood compatibility and cellular uptake.

8.6 CONCLUDING REMARKS AND FUTURE OUTLOOK

At present, biomedical glasses are marketed and routinely used in clinics for cancer treatment only in the form of radioisotope vectors (injectable insoluble Y_2O_3-Al_2O_3-SiO_2 microspheres) for the management of hepatocellular carcinoma [80]. However, BGs and, especially, MBGs are showing great promise for novel, multifunctional applications in the field of cancer treatment, especially bone cancer, following three major approaches: (i) hyperthermia, (ii) controlled release of drugs/ions, and (iii) photonic nanomedicine.

The magnetic hyperthermia technique is a powerful method of killing cancer cells that uses controlled heating and local temperature increases. SPIONs – namely, a non-glassy iron oxide material – are currently the only clinically-approved option to treat cancer via hyperthermia after being injected into the patient's body and driven to the diseased site [81]. The potential toxicity of SPIONs remains a concern despite some advantages, such as easy guidance and localization. There are several problems associated with the biodistribution, local accumulation, and long-term fate of iron oxide nanoparticles, which are non-degradable in vivo and can persist indefinitely in the body if not eliminated.

The use of magnetic BGs and glass-ceramics, incorporating magnetic phases like magnetite, can potentially overcome these drawbacks as the solubility of these materials in the biological environment can be modulated depending on their composition and texture, and the ionic dissolution products released from the glasses can be metabolized by living cells and tissues. A special class of glasses, i.e., MBGs, can slowly release anticancer drug molecules that were previously incorporated within the mesopores, thus allowing prolonged therapy [20]. Release kinetics can be tailored according to glass composition as well as the size, distribution, and shape of mesopores, which in turn depend on the MBG synthesis conditions. Furthermore, it has been recently reported that some metal-doped MBGs, such as Cu-containing

MBGs, can be used for multifaceted therapy of cancer by combining chemotherapy and PTT, where the thermal ablation of cancer cells upon NIR laser irradiation is performed concurrently with the local release of anticancer drugs modulated by the photothermal effect [76].

In vivo results in animal models showed that tumor shrinkage can be successfully achieved by using PTT and, in general, photonic nanomedicine, although targeting deep cancer is still a challenge to overcome [82]. In principle, reaching deep cancer might not be a problem by using micro-endoscopic approaches for delivering light to the cancer site; in this regard, miniaturized glass optical fibers could also be a valuable resource.

Combining diagnosis (cancer cell visualization) and therapy is also possible by properly designing BG composition; for example, Eu-doped BG nanoparticles can be uptaken in cells and visualized under fluorescent bioimaging [79].

In general, combining different BG-mediated treatments is a good strategy for obtaining synergistic effects and, thus, maximizing therapeutic efficacy; however, forecasting the extent and duration of the synergy, as well as the possible side effects, is a complex task that requires a tight alliance among biomaterials/glass scientists, oncologists, biologists and experts in processing large datasets.

REFERENCES

1. Siegel, R.L., et al.; Cancer statistics, 2022. *CA Cancer J Clin*, 2022. **72**(1): 7–33.
2. Kargozar, S., et al.; Hydroxyapatite nanoparticles for improved cancer theranostics. *J Funct Biomater*, 2022. **13**(3): 100.
3. Hanahan, D. and R.A. Weinberg; The hallmarks of cancer. *Cell*, 2000. **100**(1): 57–70.
4. Kargozar, S., S. Ramakrishna, and M. Mozafari; Chemistry of biomaterials: Future prospects. *Curr Opin Biomed Eng*, 2019. **10**: 181–190.
5. Westhauser, F., et al.; Selective and caspase-independent cytotoxicity of bioactive glasses towards giant cell tumor of bone derived neoplastic stromal cells but not to bone marrow derived stromal cells. *Biomaterials*, 2021. **275**: 120977.
6. Kargozar, S., et al.; Antioxidant effects of bioactive glasses (BGs) and their significance in tissue engineering strategies. *Molecules*, 2022. **27**(19): 6642.
7. Hench, L.L., et al.; Bonding mechanisms at the interface of ceramic prosthetic materials. *J Biomed Mater Res*, 1971. **5**(6): 117–141.
8. Jia, W., et al.; Glass-activated regeneration of volumetric muscle loss. *Acta Biomater*, 2020. **103**: 306–317.
9. Kargozar, S., et al.; Bioactive glasses and glass/polymer composites for neuroregeneration: Should we be hopeful? *Appl Sci*, 2020. **10**(10): 3421.
10. Wei, R., et al.; Preparation and in vitro evaluation of Lithium-doped bioactive glasses for wound healing with nerve repair potential. *Mater Lett*, 2021. **292**: 129629.
11. Kargozar, S., et al.; "Hard" ceramics for "Soft" tissue engineering: Paradox or opportunity? *Acta Biomater*, 2020. **115**: 1–28.
12. Kermani, F., et al.; Modified sol-gel synthesis of mesoporous borate bioactive glasses for potential use in wound healing. *Bioengineering (Basel)*, 2022. **9**(9): 442.
13. Kermani, F., et al.; Strontium- and cobalt-doped multicomponent mesoporous bioactive glasses (MBGs) for potential use in bone tissue engineering applications. *Materials*, 2020. **13**(6): 1348.
14. Kargozar, S., et al.; Bioactive glasses: Sprouting angiogenesis in tissue engineering. *Trends Biotechnol*, 2018. **36**(4): 430–444.

15. Kargozar, S., et al.; Synthesis, physico-chemical and biological characterization of strontium and cobalt substituted bioactive glasses for bone tissue engineering. *J Non-Cryst Solids*, 2016. **449**: 133–140.
16. Kargozar, S., et al.; Copper-containing bioactive glasses and glass-ceramics: From tissue regeneration to cancer therapeutic strategies. *Mater Sci Eng C Mater Biol Appl*, 2021. **121**: 111741.
17. Yazdanpanah, A., F. Moztarzadeh, and S. Arabyazdi, A heat-generating lithium-ferrite doped bioactive glass for cancer hyperthermia. *Phys B Condens Matter*, 2020. **593**: 412298.
18. El-Fiqi, A. and H.-W. Kim, Iron ions-releasing mesoporous bioactive glass ultrasmall nanoparticles designed as ferroptosis-based bone cancer nanotherapeutics: Ultrasonic-coupled sol–gel synthesis, properties and iron ions release. *Mater Lett*, 2021. **294**: 129759.
19. Salinas, A.J. and P. Esbrit, Mesoporous bioglasses enriched with bioactive agents for bone repair, with a special highlight of María Vallet-Regí's Contribution. *Pharmaceutics*, 2022. **14**(1): 202.
20. Kargozar, S., et al.; Mesoporous bioactive glasses (MBGs) in cancer therapy: Full of hope and promise. *Mater Lett*, 2019. **251**: 241–246.
21. Hmood, F., O. Goerke, and F. Schmidt, Chemical composition refining of bioactive glass for better processing features, part I. *Biomed Glas*, 2016. **4**(1): 82–94.
22. Brauer, D.S., Bioactive glasses-structure and properties. *Angew Chem Int Ed Engl*, 2015. **54**(14): 4160–81.
23. Lockyer, M.W.G., D. Holland, and R. Dupree, NMR investigation of the structure of some bioactive and related glasses. *J Non-Cryst Solids*, 1995. **188**(3): 207–219.
24. MacKenzie, K.J. and M.E. Smith, *Multinuclear Solid-State Nuclear Magnetic Resonance of Inorganic Materials*. 2002: Elsevier, Amsterdam.
25. Mollaei, Z., et al.; Elaboration of entropy with glass composition: A molecular dynamics study. *Mater Today Commun*, 2022. **33**: 104340.
26. Wajda, A., et al.; Influence of zinc ions on structure, bioactivity, biocompatibility and antibacterial potential of melt-derived and gel-derived glasses from CaO-SiO_2 system. *J Non-Cryst Solids*, 2019. **511**: 86–99.
27. Mollaei, Z., et al.; Configurational entropy as a simple input data for glass science and engineering. *Mater Today Commun*, 2022. **32**: 104153.
28. Fayon, F., et al.; Evidence of nanometric-sized phosphate clusters in bioactive glasses as revealed by solid-state 31P NMR. *J Phys Chem C*, 2013. **117**(5): 2283–2288.
29. Mehrabi, T., A.S. Mesgar, and Z. Mohammadi, Bioactive glasses: A promising therapeutic ion release strategy for enhancing wound healing. *ACS Biomater Sci Eng*, 2020. **6**(10): 5399–5430.
30. Jones, J.R., Reprint of: Review of bioactive glass: From Hench to hybrids. *Acta Biomater*, 2015. **23**: S53–82.
31. Vichery, C. and J.M. Nedelec, Bioactive glass nanoparticles: From synthesis to materials design for biomedical applications. *Materials (Basel)*, 2016. **9**(4): 288.
32. Kermani, F., et al.; Iron (Fe)-doped mesoporous 45S5 bioactive glasses: Implications for cancer therapy. *Transl Oncol*, 2022. **20**: 101397.
33. Anh Tuan, T., et al.; Simple and acid-free hydrothermal synthesis of bioactive glass $58SiO_2$–33CaO-$9P_2O_5$ (wt%). *Crystals*, 2021. **11**(3): 283.
34. Dang, T.H., et al.; Characterization of bioactive glass synthesized by sol-gel process in hot water. *Crystals*, 2020. **10**(6): 529.
35. Varma, A., et al.; Solution combustion synthesis of nanoscale materials. *Chem Rev*, 2016. **116**(23): 14493–14586.
36. Mollaei, Z., et al.; Crystallization behavior and density functional theory study of solution combustion synthesized silicon doped calcium phosphates. *Ceram Int*, 2022. **48**(10): 14349–14359.

37. Mollaei, Z., et al.; In silico study and experimental evaluation of the solution combustion synthesized manganese oxide (MnO_2) nanoparticles. *Ceram Int*, 2022. **48**(2): 1659–1672.
38. Kermani, F., et al.; Silicon-doped calcium phosphates; the critical effect of synthesis routes on the biological performance. *Mater Sci Eng C Mater Biol Appl*, 2020. **111**: 110828.
39. Kermani, F., et al.; Solution combustion synthesis (SCS) of theranostic ions doped biphasic calcium phosphates; kinetic of ions release in simulated body fluid (SBF) and reactive oxygen species (ROS) generation. *Mater Sci Eng C Mater Biol Appl*, 2021. **118**: 111533.
40. Kermani, F., et al.; Improved osteogenesis and angiogenesis of theranostic ions doped calcium phosphates (CaPs) by a simple surface treatment process: A state-of-the-art study. *Mater Sci Eng C Mater Biol Appl*, 2021. **124**: 112082.
41. Li, Q., et al.; Er3+/Yb3+ co-doped bioactive glasses with up-conversion luminescence prepared by containerless processing. *Ceram Int*, 2016. **42**(11): 13168–13175.
42. Fan, Y., et al.; Luminescent and mesoporous europium-doped bioactive glasses (MBG) as a drug carrier. *J Phys Chem C*, 2009. **113**(18): 7826–7830.
43. Chitra, S., et al.; Impact of copper on in-vitro biomineralization, drug release efficacy and antimicrobial properties of bioactive glasses. *Mater Sci Eng C Mater Biol Appl*, 2020. **109**: 110598.
44. Schuhladen, K., et al.; Dissolution of borate and borosilicate bioactive glasses and the influence of ion (Zn, Cu) doping in different solutions. *J Non-Cryst Solids*, 2018. **502**: 22–34.
45. Mutlu, N., et al.; Effect of Zn and Ga doping on bioactivity, degradation, and antibacterial properties of borate 1393-B3 bioactive glass. *Ceram Int*, 2022. **48**(11): 16404–16417.
46. Tabia, Z., et al.; Mesoporous bioactive glass nanoparticles doped with magnesium: Drug delivery and acellular in vitro bioactivity. *RSC Adv*, 2019. **9**(22): 12232–12246.
47. Schumacher, M., P. Habibovic, and S. van Rijt, Mesoporous bioactive glass composition effects on degradation and bioactivity. *Bioact Mater*, 2021. **6**(7): 1921–1931.
48. Mancuso, E., et al.; Sensitivity of novel silicate and borate-based glass structures on in vitro bioactivity and degradation behaviour. *Ceram Int*, 2017. **43**(15): 12651–12657.
49. Fathi, A., et al.; Three-dimensionally printed polycaprolactone/multicomponent bioactive glass scaffolds for potential application in bone tissue engineering. *Biomed Glas*, 2020. **6**(1): 57–69.
50. Terzopoulou, Z., et al.; Composite membranes of poly(epsilon-caprolactone) with bisphosphonate-loaded bioactive glasses for potential bone tissue engineering applications. *Molecules*, 2019. **24**(17): 3067.
51. Wu, C., et al.; The effect of mesoporous bioactive glass on the physiochemical, biological and drug-release properties of poly(DL-lactide-co-glycolide) films. *Biomaterials*, 2009. **30**(12): 2199–208.
52. Fu, S., et al.; 3D printing of layered mesoporous bioactive glass/sodium alginate-sodium alginate scaffolds with controllable dual-drug release behaviors. *Biomed Mater*, 2019. **14**(6): 065011.
53. Kermani, F., et al.; Calcium phosphate bioceramics for improved angiogenesis, in *Biomaterials for Vasculogenesis and Angiogenesis*. 2022, pp. 185–203. doi: 10.1016/B978-0-12-821867-9.00004-4.
54. Kargozar, S., et al.; Nanomaterials and scaffolds for tissue engineering and regenerative medicine, in *Nanomaterials and Nanotechnology in Medicine*. 2022, pp. 279–302. doi: 10.1002/9781119558026.ch11.
55. Kargozar, S., et al.; Nanotechnology for angiogenesis: Opportunities and challenges. *Chem Soc Rev*, 2020. **49**(14): 5008–5057.
56. Kargozar, S., et al.; Functionalization and surface modifications of bioactive glasses (BGs): Tailoring of the biological response working on the outermost surface layer. *Materials (Basel)*, 2019. **12**(22): p. 3696.

57. Ferlenda, G., et al.; Surface functionalization of a silica-based bioactive glass with compounds from rosa canina bud extracts. *ACS Biomater Sci Eng*, 2021. **7**(1): 96–104.
58. Zarghami, V., et al.; In vitro bactericidal and drug release properties of vancomycin-amino surface functionalized bioactive glass nanoparticles. *Mater Chem Phys*, 2020. **241**: 122423.
59. Reiter, T., et al.; Bioactive glass based scaffolds coated with gelatin for the sustained release of icariin. *Bioact Mater*, 2019. **4**(1): 1–7.
60. Huo, S., et al.; Dual-functional polyetheretherketone surface modification for regulating immunity and bone metabolism. *Chem Eng J*, 2021. **426**: 130806.
61. Fellenberg, J., et al.; Bioactive glass selectively promotes cytotoxicity towards giant cell tumor of bone derived neoplastic stromal cells and induces MAPK signalling dependent autophagy. *Bioact Mater*, 2022. **15**: 456–468.
62. Hooshmand, S., et al.; Mesoporous silica nanoparticles and mesoporous bioactive glasses for wound management: From skin regeneration to cancer therapy. *Materials (Basel)*, 2021. **14**(12): 3337.
63. Li, X., et al.; Bio-inspired bioactive glasses for efficient microRNA and drug delivery. *J Mater Chem B*, 2017. **5**(31): 6376–6384.
64. Miola, M., et al.; Glass-ceramics for cancer treatment: So close, or yet so far? *Acta Biomater*, 2019. **83**: 55–70.
65. Wu, C., W. Fan, and J. Chang, Functional mesoporous bioactive glass nanospheres: Synthesis, high loading efficiency, controllable delivery of doxorubicin and inhibitory effect on bone cancer cells. *J Mater Chem B*, 2013. **1**(21): 2710–2718.
66. Lin, H.M., H.Y. Lin, and M.H. Chan, Preparation, characterization, and in vitro evaluation of folate-modified mesoporous bioactive glass for targeted anticancer drug carriers. *J Mater Chem B*, 2013. **1**(44): 6147–6156.
67. Shoaib, M., et al.; Mesoporous bioactive glass-polyurethane nanocomposites as reservoirs for sustained drug delivery. *Colloids Surf B: Biointerfaces*, 2018. **172**: 806–811.
68. Crezee, J., N.A. Franken, and A.L. Oei, *Hyperthermia-Based Anti-cancer Treatments*. 2021, Multidisciplinary Digital Publishing Institute, Basel, p. 1240.
69. McWhinney, S.R., R.M. Goldberg, and H.L. McLeod, Platinum neurotoxicity pharmacogenetics. *Mol Cancer Ther*, 2009. **8**(1): 10–6.
70. Liu, X., et al.; Comprehensive understanding of magnetic hyperthermia for improving antitumor therapeutic efficacy. *Theranostics*, 2020. **10**(8): 3793–3815.
71. Borges, R., et al.; New sol-gel-derived magnetic bioactive glass-ceramics containing superparamagnetic hematite nanocrystals for hyperthermia application. *Mater Sci Eng C Mater Biol Appl*, 2021. **120**: 111692.
72. Borges, R., et al.; Superparamagnetic and highly bioactive SPIONS/bioactive glass nanocomposite and its potential application in magnetic hyperthermia. *Mater Sci Eng C Mater Biol Appl*, 2022. **135**: 112655.
73. Zou, L., et al.; Current approaches of photothermal therapy in treating cancer metastasis with nanotherapeutics. *Theranostics*, 2016. **6**(6): 762–72.
74. Shanmugam, V., S. Selvakumar, and C.S. Yeh, Near-infrared light-responsive nanomaterials in cancer therapeutics. *Chem Soc Rev*, 2014. **43**(17): 6254–87.
75. Ma, L., et al.; Multifunctional bioactive Nd-Ca-Si glasses for fluorescence thermometry, photothermal therapy, and burn tissue repair. *Sci Adv*, 2020. **6**(32): eabb1311.
76. Chang, L., Y. Liu, and C. Wu, Copper-doped mesoporous bioactive glass for photothermal enhanced chemotherapy. *J Biomed Nanotechnol*, 2018. **14**(4): 786–794.
77. Liu, Y., et al.; Mesoporous bioactive glass for synergistic therapy of tumor and regeneration of bone tissue. *Appl Mater Today*, 2020. **19**: 100578.
78. Liu, Y., et al.; 3D-printed scaffolds with bioactive elements-induced photothermal effect for bone tumor therapy. *Acta Biomater*, 2018. **73**: 531–546.

79. Chen, M., et al.; Multifunctional protein-decorated bioactive glass nanoparticles for tumor-specific therapy and bioimaging in vitro and in vivo. *ACS Appl Mater Interfaces*, 2021. **13**(13): 14985–14994.
80. Baino, F., et al.; Biomedical radioactive glasses for brachytherapy. *Materials (Basel)*, 2021. **14**(5): 1131.
81. Sedighi, O., et al.; A critical review of bioceramics for magnetic hyperthermia. *J Am Ceram Soc*, 2022. **105**(3): 1723–1747.
82. dos Santos, A.F., et al.; Photodynamic therapy in cancer treatment-an update review. *J Cancer Metastasis Treat*, 2019. **5**: 25.

9 Cryogels, Macroporous Hydrogels, as Promising Materials for Tissue Engineering and Drug Delivery

I. N. Savina
University of Brighton

CONTENTS

9.1 Introduction 193
9.2 Cryotropic Gelation as a Tool for the Preparation of Macroporous Scaffold 195
9.3 Functionalization of Cryogels to Increase Cell Response 196
9.4 Applications of Cryogels in Biomedical Field 197
9.4.1 Bone Regeneration 197
9.4.2 Nerve Regeneration 198
9.4.3 Wound Repair and Skin Regeneration 200
9.4.4 Pancreatic and Liver Tissue Engineering 201
9.4.5 Vascular Tissue Engineering 202
9.4.6 Drug and Cell Delivery 203
9.4.7 Biosensors 204
9.5 Conclusion 205
References 205

9.1 INTRODUCTION

The next generation of biomedical advances requires the development of new materials with unique properties to solve problems in medicine. Cryogels, hydrogels prepared by cryotropic gelation, have been proven to be a versatile and useful platform for the development of advanced materials for a range of applications ranging from bioseparation, drug and cell delivery, tissue scaffolds, and materials for screening processes [1–4]. Cryogels are hydrogels that, in addition to the properties of a hydrogel, such as hydrophilicity, the ability to hold large amounts of water without dissolving, and the ability to mimic a biological environment, also have a number of advantages

DOI: 10.1201/9781003251767-9

[5,6]. Cryogels have a porous structure with a high degree of interconnectedness of the pores, which ensures good mass transfer of solutes [7]. Their large pores are sufficient for cell migration, proliferation, and metabolic activity. In addition, the mechanical properties of cryogels are adjustable and can be adapted to different conditions depending on the tissue being modeled. All this makes cryogels an attractive material for the development of new advanced materials for biomedical applications.

Interest in the use of cryotropic gelation to obtain porous hydrogel has been growing over the past 20 years [2,8–10]. Cryotropic gelation uses solvent freezing as a tool to create a porous hydrogel material [11]. When the initial solution of the reagent is cooled at a temperature in the range of –12°C to –20°C, gelation occurs in the frozen sample as a result of physical or chemical crosslinking of the polymer and polymer precursors, resulting in the formation of a three-dimensional porous polymer matrix with a well-developed macro- and microstructure (Figure 9.1).

It is shown that the method of cryotropic gelation is more efficient than other methods based on the use of pore formers such as salt, sugar, silica, and others [2]. Pore formers must be removed after gelation, which includes an additional purification step and sometimes the use of organic solvents that can adversely affect cells. The washing step can lead to chemical contamination of the material, and using pore formers can result in the formation of a hydrogel with insufficient interconnectivity of the pores [2]. On the other hand, cryotropic gelation, which uses water crystals as pore-forming units, has been proven to be a robust and effective technique for the design of porous materials for biomedical applications [1,2,4,12,13]. The pore-forming units are removed simply by defrosting the cryogel.

This chapter discusses recent applications of cryogel-based materials in the biomedical field. The chapter begins with an introduction to cryotropic gelation to demonstrate the versatility of the method and how cryogel properties can be tailored to

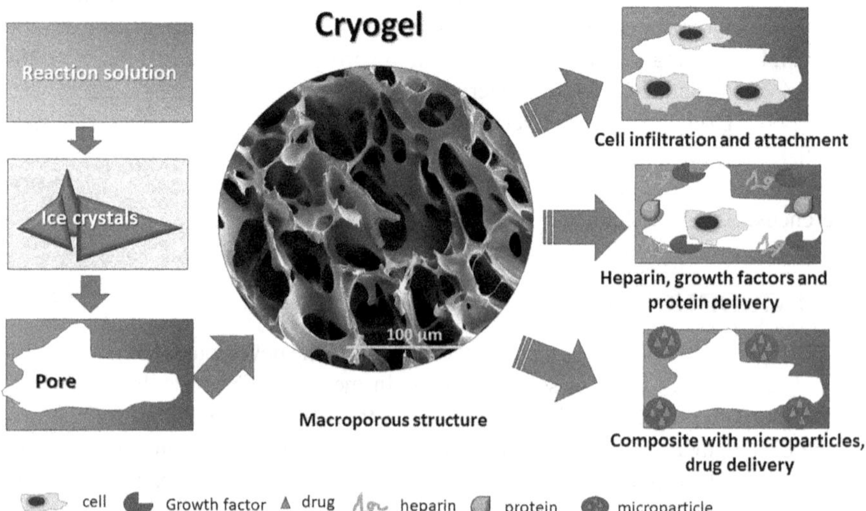

FIGURE 9.1 Schematic presentation of the cryogel preparation, cryogel macroporous structure, cell attachment and modification with heparin, growth factors, proteins and microparticles loaded with drugs.

any particular application. This is followed by a discussion of methods for adding additional functionality. Finally, recent research on the application of cryogel in the biomedical field, such as bone, nerve, skin, liver, and vascular regeneration, drug and cell delivery, and biosensor development, is discussed.

9.2 CRYOTROPIC GELATION AS A TOOL FOR THE PREPARATION OF MACROPOROUS SCAFFOLD

The term "cryotropic gelation" comes from the Greek words krios (frost) and tropos (cause) and explains the gel formation caused by cryogenic processing (freezing, storage in a frozen state, and thawing of the original gel precursor solution). It is known that temperature changes, especially cooling, can lead to the formation of hydrogels. For example, cooling a gelatin solution results in the formation of a gelatin hydrogel. However, we will not call such hydrogels "cryogels" unless they have gone through the freezing stage. The reason for this is that several processes occur during freezing: the solvent crystallizes, and all dissolved substances are pre-concentrated in a small volume of the unfrozen liquid phase. The concentration of the solute (polymer or monomer) increased in the liquid phase, supporting polymerization and crosslinking. As a result, the gel could be formed from solutions with a lower concentration of precursors, and freezing causes the formation of a gel with big pores. We can see this in the example of the formation of polyvinyl alcohol (PVA) and polysaccharide cryogels [14]. Solvent crystals are pure solvent crystals that create voids during polymer network formation. During thawing, these voids are filled with solvent and form

TABLE 9.1
Effect of Different Parameters on Cryogel Properties

Parameters	Effect	Reference
Cryogelation temperature	A lower cryogelation temperature results in smaller pores and thinner but denser pore walls.	[15,16]
Cooling rate	A lower cooling rate generally results in a larger pore size. For this to be effective, the crosslinking rate must be lower than the crystallization rate of the solvent. This also results in the preparation of aligned porous structures.	[15,17,18]
Monomer/ polymer concentration	Solutions with a higher monomer/polymer concentration result in cryogels with a smaller average pore size.	[16,19–21]
Polymer molecular weight	Using lower molecular weight polymers results in the formation of larger pores compared to gel formed using larger molecular weight polymers.	[17,22]
Crosslinking	Influence on the mechanical properties, swelling and stability of cryogels. Physical crosslinking results in gels that melt at higher temperatures and have smaller pores. Increasing the crosslinker concentration could lead to the formation of smaller pores.	[16,20,23,24]
Composite cryogels	By combining different polymers, adding particles, and adding fibers, the mechanical properties could be further tuned.	[25–27]

pores in the cryogel. The size of the solvent crystals and, therefore, the size of the pores will depend on many factors, such as freezing temperature, freezing rate, solute concentration, polymer precursor molecular weight, sample size, and others [1]. We summarize the effect of these parameters on the cryogel pore size and morphology in Table 9.1. Changing these parameters makes it possible to manipulate the cryogel porosity in terms of obtaining a cryogel of the desired morphology.

9.3 FUNCTIONALIZATION OF CRYOGELS TO INCREASE CELL RESPONSE

Additional modification of cryogels by introducing various peptides, proteins, growth factors (Figure 9.1), and nanoparticles may be used to stimulate tissue regeneration and induce a specific cell response. Cell adhesion to the engineered scaffold is a key process for successful regeneration. Materials that mimic the extracellular matrix (ECM) are more desirable because they provide cells with biological signals and regulate cell motility, growth, morphology, and differentiation. RGD is a tripeptide recognized by integrins and is the most common peptide used for scaffold modification. The introduction of RGD into the cryogel contributes to the maintenance of cell adhesion, proliferation, and regulation of cellular functions [28–32].

Other short peptides, such as laminin-derived IKVAV and YIGSR and fibronectin-derived LDV and REDV, have been used to modulate cellular responses in biomaterials. The use of short peptides is a good alternative to the use of natural proteins. They are more soluble, are stable, and can be incorporated into the scaffold at higher concentrations due to their small size. Peptides containing RGD and IKVAV motifs were grafted onto furan-modified HA-poly(ethylene glycol) (HA-PEG) cryogels [33]. RGD-modified cryogels promoted the spread and adherence of luminal epithelial breast cancer cells T47D. The replacement of RGD by IKVAV triggered the formation of 3D cellular spheroid structures similar to those observed in vivo [33]. Synergistic activity of RGD and GHK motifs on 3T3 and PC-12 cell proliferation has been observed [34]. Cryogel modification with RGD, GHK, and Cu^{2+} enhanced regenerative angiogenic responses in vitro by increasing human umbilical vein endothelial cell (HUVEC) proliferation, differentiation, and production of angiogenesis- and growth-factor-associated cytokines [35].

Immobilization of growth factors provides significant cell responses [36,37]. The immobilization of heparin (HEP) in the cryogel structure made it possible to load the cryogel with various biological factors that would be electrostatically coupled to the HEP (Figure 9.1). This creates a more suitable microenvironment for cell growth and tissue regeneration. Glial cell-derived neurotropic growth factor (GDNF) and nerve growth factor (NGF) were attached to star-PEG-HEP cryogel for neuroprotection application [36]. Vascular endothelial growth factor (VEGF) was attached to HEP-modified gelatin cryogel and supported neovascularization [37]. The formation of granulation tissue as well as functional neovascularization was facilitated by the sequential delivery of inflammation-modulating factors and wound healing factors (VEGF and FGF), which led to regenerative epithelization [38]. Similar results were observed after the incorporation of basic fibroblast growth factor (bFGF) into a chitosan-gluconic acid-PVA cryogel. Addition of bFGF accelerates wound healing [39].

Another strategy for improving cell response is embedding particles, which can not only improve the mechanical properties, create additional sites for the biological molecules binding, and increase specific surface area, but also induce different cellular responses. Examples of that were adding hydroxyapatite to the scaffold used in bone regeneration [40,41], coating with polydopamine nanoparticles to improve binding of ECM molecules [42,43], adding polypyrrole particles to add conductivity to the scaffold [43], and embedding particles with controlled drug release [44].

9.4 APPLICATIONS OF CRYOGELS IN BIOMEDICAL FIELD

The physicomechanical and structural properties of cryogel can be easily adapted to a wide range of biomedical applications. Mechanical properties, porosity, and biological response of cryogels can be adjusted to mimic particular tissue properties. In this part, we will give some examples of cryogels' applications in the biomedical field.

9.4.1 Bone Regeneration

Bone diseases and defects represent a key clinical problem, especially as they affect people over 50 years of age. Bone is able to regenerate and repair itself, but some critical size defects do not heal within a patient's lifetime and can only be repaired by a bone graft. Bone grafts, whether autografts or allografts, have several disadvantages, such as the risk of infection, immune rejection, cost, and donor site morbidity. Due to its mechanical strength and ability to prepare composite materials by combining different polymers and fillers, cryogel provides a suitable platform for the development of artificial bone grafts.

Strong cryogel matrices of silk fibroin were produced from silk fibroin solutions [13,45,46]. Cryogels had a Young's modulus of 50 to 126 MPa [46,47] and withstood a compression of about 90% at a pressure of 87–240 MPa, which makes them good candidates for fabrication of materials imitating bone [47]. The multiple networks and the increase in fibroin content significantly improved mechanical properties. Hickson *et al.* compared cryogels with traditional hydrogels in terms of finding the optimal material for designing a bone graft substitute [13]. *N*-Vinyl-2-pyrrolidone, chitosan-gelatin, and silk fibroin cryogels proved superior to hydrogels made from the same polymers in terms of porosity, swelling potential, and mechanical properties. To obtain a mechanically strong material, cryogels will be reinforced by adding fibers or nanoparticles. The introduction of bacterial cellulose fiber into poly(l-lactic) acid (PLLA) cryogels increased the compressive strength of the gel by a factor of four [48]. Their hydrophilic properties were better than those of the original PLLA. High-strength gelatin cryogels were prepared by adding poly(lactic-co-glycolic acid) (PLGA) microspheres [49]. Both PLGA and gelatin have been loaded with a high percentage of nanohyroxyapatite (HA). The preparation of the hybrid scaffold resulted in higher ultimate stress and a higher Young's modulus, which were 25 and 21 times higher than in the original cryogel scaffold, respectively. In in vitro studies, good cell proliferation and osteogenic differentiation of rabbit bone marrow-derived stem cells (rBMSCs) were observed, which was close to the natural environment, which, together with good mechanical strength, makes such hybrid cryogels good candidates for bone regeneration. To activate the cryogel scaffold's osteogenic ability, various bioactive factors and additives were added to the composition of cryogels. Hydroxyapatite nanoparticles are the most widely used in the preparation of bone regenerative materials as biocompatible inorganic materials. Thus, cryogel scaffolds prepared using type I collagen and nanocrystalline HA showed good results for 21 days, supporting the proliferation, differentiation, and individual functionality of human bone marrow stromal cells in a monoculture system [50]. Mature bone formation, including lacunae and mineralization, was observed after 12 weeks of subcutaneous and bone implantation in rats, demonstrating that the composite cryogel promotes tissue regeneration [50]. HA nanoparticles with zinc and cerium nanoparticles, which have biological and antibacterial activity, were incorporated into biodegradable poly(hydroxypropyl methacrylate) (HEMA) cryogels. Microbial activity was lower, and osteoblast cells (MG-63) showed strong adhesion and growth and attempted to create a continuous cell layer in nanocomposite cryogels in an in vitro test. Endochondral ossification was revealed in the in vivo test, which makes this material promising for clinical use [51]. It has been shown that an increase in VEGF in gelatin cryogels stimulates the healing of critical bone defects in the proximal tibia and the early phase of fracture healing [52].

Rayna and colleagues took a more sophisticated approach by preparing biocomposite cryogels composed of three different polymers: silk, chitosan, and agarose. HA and bioactive glass were additionally added to reinforce the cryogel [41]. Each component has been carefully selected as it adds individual properties to the final composite. Silk is mechanically strong; chitosan is biocompatible, is hemocompatible, and has antibacterial properties; and HA and bioglass have proosteogenic properties. Agarose was added as it can significantly improve the elastic properties of the matrix due to formation of interpenetrating networks and additional crosslinks. Agarose is also known to enhance chondrocyte proliferation. This scaffold was an optimal biodegradable carrier system for co-delivery of two active substances to bone in vivo, such as zoledronic acid and recombinant human bone morphogenic protein-2 (rhBMP-2). rhBMP-2 will bind to chitosan, silk fibroin, and HA, while zoledrone will bind to HA. Under the testing of this scaffold, sustained proliferation of both C2C12 cells and mesenchymal stem cells (MSCs) was observed for 6 weeks with upregulation of their phenotype toward osteogenic differentiation, and in vivo studies show the ability of the developed material to accelerate bone regeneration [41].

9.4.2 Nerve Regeneration

Damage to nerves, both in the peripheral nervous system and in the central nervous system, causes persistent cognitive, motor, or psychotic effects and dramatically reduces the quality of life of patients. There are limitations with using nerve grafts such as autologous grafts, which may cause loss of sensation, scarring, neuroma formation, and morbidity, while allogeneic grafts elicit a pro-inflammatory immune response, rapidly incapacitating transplanted cells. Cell transplantation by itself is not a viable option for regeneration, so the use of a scaffold can provide support and guidance to the cells to support regeneration. Cryogels in this case have a number of advantages since they are macroporous as well as soft and spongy but strong and reproducible, which makes them a useful material to address neuroscience challenges [53]. A comprehensive review on the application of the cryogel in neuroscience has recently been published [53,54]. Here we give several examples of the use of cryogels for solving problems in neurobiology.

Cryogels, made in the form of tubular structures, have been tested as nerve guidance conduits used to replace natural nerve autografts [18,55–57]. Gelatin cryogels prepared for peripheral nerve regeneration after neurorrhaphy have been shown to promote repair and prevent scar tissue invasion in a rat model [55]. An aligned chitosan-gelatin cryogel was made inside a polyurethane tube. Aligned, interconnected porous channels provide direction for directed axon growth and signals for Schwann cell adhesion and migration [18]. PC-12 cells were able to differentiate within the conduit and form long and parallel neurites along lamellar guide structures, which is important for nerve recovery. A conduit was prepared using methacrylated hyaluronic acid, methacrylic gelatin, and 4-arm poly(ethylene glycol)acrylate cryogel [58]. The cryogel-conduit provided a favorable microenvironment for rabbit Schwann cells and supported regeneration of axons and remyelination of the severed sciatic nerve. In the rat model, a partial recovery of sensory function was observed.

It has been demonstrated that electrical stimulation of neural cells enhances their growth and differentiation and can significantly improve the regeneration and sprouting of damaged axons in vitro and in vivo [59]. To increase the electrical conductivity of cryogels, scaffolds with electroconductive materials such as polypyrrole [60] or graphene [56] have been made. Amino-functionalized graphene-crosslinked collagen cryogel provided stable growth and proliferation of bone marrow mesenchymal stem cells and their stemness upon electrical stimulation. It also improved cell migration and proliferation when cryogel was transplanted into an injured spinal cord [56].

Cryogels have also been used for the delivery of cells to the injured site. Cryogels based on dextran or gelatin modified with laminin promoted the formation of artificial neural tissue in vitro by inducing the differentiation of stem cells derived from human umbilical cord blood [61]. Laminin is a main component of the brain's extracellular matrix and was used to mimic the environment of the brain. In a rat model, cryogel scaffolds could be transplanted into brain tissue or organotypic hippocampal slices. The cryogel did not cause inflammation or glial scarring when transplanted into the rat brain and promoted host neuroblast infiltration. An injectable laminin-coated carboxymethylcellulose alginate cryogel has been developed for non-invasive delivery using syringes [62]. The cryogel supported neuronal cell adhesion and spread. Cryogel mechanical properties protect cell viability and differentiated morphology, as well as scaffold integrity, during syringe injection. Star-PEG-HEP cryogel beads were prepared and functionalized with HEP-binding growth factors such as glial cell-derived neurotrophic growth factor (GDNF) and nerve growth factor (NGF) for neuroprotection [36]. The cryogels were compatible with PC-12 and MSC cells. The cryogel's high surface area-to-volume ratio offers a means of loading large amounts of drugs for delivery to the brain parenchyma. Cryogels allowed the proliferation and differentiation of neuron cells and maintained their viability after injection, which is important for the development of treatments for neurodegenerative diseases.

9.4.3 Wound Repair and Skin Regeneration

The skin is one of the most important organs of protection from the external environment. Extensive damage to the skin as a result of burns or chronic wounds can lead to significant complications and death. Current standard treatments include wound dressings, autografts, and allographs, but the effectiveness of these techniques is limited and requires research into new methods and materials that will stimulate skin repair. Many problems need to be addressed, such as poor adhesion to the wound, insufficient vascularization, infection, manufacturing costs, and a long shelf life. Cryogels, with their hydrophilic and elastic nature, adaptability to the wound bed, and macroporous, spongy morphology, which can prevent fluid accumulation in the wound as well as stimulate cell infiltration, appear to be a promising solution for creating advanced materials for wound healing.

Cryogels based on collagen and gelatin have been extensively studied as materials for wound healing [24,63–66]. It was shown that using gelatin based cryogels supports the formation of the neoepidermal layer by the seeded keratinocytes in vitro [63]. Infiltration of cells and biointegration in a porcine model demonstrate promotion of wound healing. It has been shown that the anisotropic morphology of cryogels obtained by unidirectional freezing can promote wound healing by creating a special environment for cells and controlling their migration. The smaller pores in the outer layer of the wound dressing restrict cell migration, while the placement of the larger pores of the material on the wound bed has the added benefit of increased flexibility to accommodate the roughness and curvature of the wound surface [63].

In the process of searching for the most biocompatible material for the manufacture of wound healing materials, platelet lysate (PL) was used. PL is an autologous blood product obtained by lysis of concentrated platelets. It contains a large number of growth factors and cytokines responsible for the regulation of angiogenesis and wound healing. Three-dimensional macroporous cryogels were produced from PL crosslinked by oxidized dextran with good potential for wound healing applications [67].

Adding transitional metals such as Zn, Cu, Co, and Ce improves wound healing [66,68,69]. Wound treatment with zinc-doped cryogel led to accelerated skin regeneration, accompanied by a decrease in leukocyte infiltration, a rapid passage of the inflammation and proliferation phases, and an increase in the formation of dermal components [66]. The addition of Cu and Zn to the gelatin cryogel did not disturb the organization of the intact skin but had a specific stimulating effect on various skin structures, including the vasculature. The addition of Co to the gelatin cryogel caused a significant reorganization of the skin layers and the appearance of multinucleated giant cells, along with intense angiogenesis in the dermis [69]. Cryogels of [2-(methacryloyloxy)ethyl]dimethyl-(3-sulfopropyl)ammonium hydroxide) or 3-[[2-(methacryloyloxy)ethyl]dimethylammonio]propionate and 2-hydroxyethyl methacrylate were loaded with miRNA146a-conjugated cerium oxide nanoparticles. Due to their radical scavenging properties, cerium oxide nanoparticles can reverse oxidative stress in diabetic wounds. Cerium oxide effectively delivers miRNA 146a, which promotes accelerated wound healing in diabetic mice [70].

Wounds are susceptible to bacterial infections, making it difficult to treat wounds in the clinic. To prevent bacterial contamination, different strategies have been used.

Antimicrobial cryogels have been prepared by the incorporation of silver [27,71,72]. Tannic acid and ferric ions (TA/Fe^{3+}) have been added to a chitosan and silk fibroin scaffold as a stimuli-responsive agent for photothermal therapy [73]. Increasing local temperature under near-infrared (NIR) illumination of Ta/Fe^{3+} cryogels kills both Gram-positive and Gram-negative bacteria, *Escherichia coli* and *Staphylococcus aureus,* providing antimicrobial activity. Animal studies have shown that this promotes wound healing without the use of antibiotics, making it a promising wound dressing [73]. Gelatin cryogels with polyvinylpyrrolidone and iodine were loaded with microparticles containing mannose-6-phosphate and human fibrinogen. These cryogels constantly release iodine, inhibiting microbial growth, and microparticles accelerate skin regeneration, preventing scarring [74]. Chitosan and silk fibroin cryogels embedded with NIR-responsive polydopamine (PDA) nanoparticles showed effective wound healing in skin defects in a rat model [75]. Cryogel effectively prevented bacterial infection of the wound due to photothermal therapy against *Staphylococcus aureus* and *Escherichia coli.* PDA nanoparticles have reactive catechol groups capable of retaining polypeptides and proteins, including growth factors, which creates favorable conditions for cell proliferation and tissue remodeling in the wound bed. Due to the ability of catechol groups to scavenge radicals, the amount of reactive oxygen species (ROS) produced in excess during inflammatory reactions was reduced [75].

Polyurethane-based cryogels with embedded exosomes with sustained oxygen-releasing properties were prepared [76]. In clinically complex, infected diabetic wounds, these cryogel dressings prevented infection and ulceration and improved wound healing with increased collagen deposition and re-epithelialization.

9.4.4 Pancreatic and Liver Tissue Engineering

Liver disease affects millions of people, and there are currently no effective treatments for the most severe cases. Liver transplantation is still the main treatment option. However, about 14% of patients die while waiting for a suitable transplant [77] and there is a need to develop effective treatments. In our work, we have developed a bioartificial liver device, an extracorporeal system, that can support or help restore liver function in patients with liver failure [30]. A HEMA-based cryogel cell scaffold with engineered surface properties and optimized fluid dynamics was prepared to support hepatocyte cells and the flow of blood through the bioreactor. The cryogel was modified with alginate, which inhibited nonspecific protein biofouling and augmented viable hepatocyte metabolic function. Modification with the RGD peptide significantly enhanced hepatocyte adhesion and metabolic activity.

Agarose–chitosan cryogels were prepared as a potential in vitro liver tissue model supporting primary hepatocytes for drug screening [78]. A cryogel with mechanical properties close to those of the liver was obtained. When cultivating hepatocyte cells in the cryogel, proliferation was observed with increased cellular metabolic activity, albumin secretion, and expression of the liver biomarker CYP450. This shows the potential of such materials for the development of an in vitro liver tissue model. Kumari *et al.* studied cryogels of PEG-gelatin-alginate in vitro as a model of liver tissue for preclinical therapeutic testing [79]. Using poly(*N*-isopropylacrylamide) temperature-sensing cryogels, which are able to change surface properties from hydrophilic to hydrophobic in response to temperature, liver cells were cultured in the form of spheroids, which enhanced functionality. The size of the spheroids was controlled by the pore size of the cryogel and was about 100 μm, which prevents the state of hypoxia in the spheroid culture. Boulais *et al* created a biochip containing three-dimensional alginate cryogel in which hepatocyte cells were cultured under dynamic conditions [20]. The cryogels were created with mechanical properties that could mimic those of a healthy or pathological liver. This device can be used to develop robust in vitro liver microtissues to study drug toxicity and efficacy. It may also help to better understand the biology of liver cells, as the mechanical properties of healthy or pathological liver tissues can be replicated. Antibacterial agarose cryogel was obtained by encapsulation of silver nanoparticles coated with chitosan. The cryogel has good compatibility with mammalian cells and has been shown to be useful for engineering soft tissues such as the heart, kidney, pancreas, and liver [80].

9.4.5 Vascular Tissue Engineering

Vascular transplants are often unavailable due to a lack of donors. Even when such treatment is available, these grafts can cause thrombosis, hyperplasia, calcification, and inflammatory reactions. Similarly, currently used heart valves degrade over time and can fail due to tearing or calcification. Thus, there is a need to develop new materials, and cryogel may offer some solutions.

It was shown that HEMA–gelatin cryogel provides a native environment for myocardial cell proliferation and differentiation with increased metabolic activity and the formation of tubular structures [81]. The mechanical strength, stiffness, and elasticity of cryogel make it possible to use these materials for engineered cardiac and skeletal tissue. The incorporation of conductive polymer polypyrrol into hybrid gelatin-methacrylate and poly(ethylene glycol)diacrylate cryogel significantly improves the cardiomyocytes behavior by increasing the expression of connexin-43 and α-actinin, both essential for the maturation of the myocardium and synchronous contraction [43]. Implantation of cardiomyocytes seeded in cryogel into infarcted myocardium in rats reduces the infarct size by 43% and improves cardiac function. It was shown that PVA-based cryogels are extremely well suited for developing cartilage and vascular materials due to their mechanical properties. PVA-gelatin cryogels were prepared by freeze-thawing a mixture of gelatin and PVA [82]. PVA provides suitable mechanical properties, while gelatin stimulates adhesion and proliferation of endothelial cells. PVA cryogels did not have large pores, which is good for this application since low porosity helps to retain endothelial cells on the gel surface and reduce their infiltration. Application of linear shear stress to PVA-gelatin cryogels dramatically increases endothelial cell proliferation and promotes neoendothelialization, making the cryogels a promising material for the development of artificial arterial grafts [82]. In another study, PVA cryogels were fabricated for use as leaflets in the tricuspid valve [83]. In a more recent work, Mohammadi *et al.* reinforced PVA cryogel with the addition of natural bacterial cellulose nanocomposite [84]. The cyclic flow demonstrated the ability of materials to open and close, and the strength of the cryogel allowed it to be temporarily compressed into a small ball for implantation without loss of mechanical integrity [83].

9.4.6 Drug and Cell Delivery

Besides providing 3D structure for the supporting cells growth and proliferation, cryogels have also been used for delivering drugs, therapeutics, vaccine and cells. Some examples of adding the drugs and growth factors to the cryogels have already been discussed in other parts of this book chapter. It should be noted that cryogels are not good candidates for loading small drug molecules for controlled release. Due to the large surface area and 3D structure of large interconnected pores, which provide good mass transfer with biological fluids, the small molecules are easily released from the polymer. Cryogels were characterized by a low loading capacity and an initial rapid burst release of the drug [85,86]. The properties of cryogels must be adjusted for controlled drug release. The polymer matrix of cryogel is very dense, which also makes it difficult to release large molecules such as proteins and requires controlled degradation of the cryogel [87]. The strategy is to use composites with nano- or microparticles [85,88] and molecularly imprinted polymers [89–91], which will control the release of drugs or proteins (Figure 9.1). For example, laponite nanoparticles have been used for the sustainable release of protein from alginate cryogel [85]. In another work, calcium carbonate microspheres were used for controlled delivery of ciprofloxacin for therapeutic intervention in osteoporosis and associated osteomyelitis [86]. Chang *et al.* used poly(D, L-lactide-co-glycolide) microspheres (PLGA) to encapsulate BMP-2 in a composite cryogel to facilitate supra-alveolar ridge augmentation [88]. A composite cryogel scaffold made of nanohydroxyapatite and collagen was used for local antibiotic delivery in the treatment of osteomyelitis. It has been observed that when loaded with BMP-2 and zoledronic acid, cryogel can completely eliminate infection in the rat femoral condyle and simultaneously accelerate bone healing in the dead space created during surgical procedures [92]. Controlled delivery of specific growth factors and chemokines has been achieved by incorporating HA into cryogels [36,37,93]. Injection of gelatin cryogels containing heparin loaded with VEGF into the ischemic hindlimbs of mice induced angiogenesis by controlling the release of VEGF [37].

Cell therapy is promising for the development of new treatments for the regeneration of damaged or diseased tissues. However, cells are easily damaged during injection and do not always remain localized in the affected tissue, making cell therapy less effective. Cryogels create a good protective environment for the cells; their elastic properties and mechanical strength allow the passage of cryogel microparticles loaded with the cells through the needle without damaging cells. Injection is a less invasive method for the delivery of the scaffold to the damaged tissue, and it is particularly beneficial for the cell delivery application. Considerable work has been done recently on the design of injectable cryogels [12].

Porous alginate cryogels were produced by cryotropic free radical polymerization of methacrylated alginate (MA-alginate) to create a porous alginate, which was then further crosslinked by calcium ions to enhance the cryogel toughness and injectability [94,95]. The obtained cryogels were used for cancer vaccination. The crosslinked

MA-alginate cryogel was seeded with irradiated breast cancer cells and preloaded with cytosine-phosphodiester-guanine oligonucleotide (CpG-ODN) and macrophage colony stimulating factor (GM-CSF). Irradiated breast cancer cells have been used as tumor antigens, and their transplantation into cryogels resulted in strong antigen-specific cellular and humoral responses in vivo. Efficient production of protective antitumor antibodies and activation of dendritic cells were noted, which provided an effective preventive effect against breast cancer in mice [95]. Combined chemo-immunotherapy was proposed by designing alginate cryogels containing GM-CSF, CpG-ODN and dextran nanoparticles loaded with Nutlin-3a (potent p53 activator). After peritumoral injection of cryogels in mice, the nanoparticles release over time and accumulate in tumor. The delivered Nutlin-3a was toxic to tumor cells and induced immunogenic cell death. In addition, GM-CSF and CpG-ODN released from the cryogel activate antigen-presenting cells, supporting the elimination of tumor cells [94].

Collagen-based cryogel scaffold coated with nanostructured PDA was used for developing mesenchymal stem cell therapy [36,42]. Growth factors were loaded into HEP-containing microcarriers and exhibit near-zero-order release kinetics. Cell-loaded microcarriers were injected through a thin cannula. The microcarriers protected the cells from damage during injection, and polydopamine was shown to increase cell viability and proliferation in the scaffold [36]. PEG-HEP cryogels were used for the transplantation of gene-modified MSCs, which were capable of sustained secretion of anti-CD33-antiCD3 antibody. The implanted cells release high levels of antibodies sufficient to trigger a T-cell-mediated antitumor response and regression of acute myeloid leukemia blast [31].

9.4.7 Biosensors

A biosensor is an analytical device that uses a biological component to detect the presence of chemicals. Compared to other detection methods, biosensors have a fast response, high sensitivity, low limits of detection (LOD), and a small size. A glucose biosensor based on a chitosan-bovine serum albumin cryogel with multi-walled carbon nanotubes (MWNTs), ferrocene, and glucose oxidase has been developed [96]. Glucose oxidase retains its enzymatic activity after inclusion in the composite cryogel. Sensitive electrochemical detection of glucose was observed as a result of the large surface area of the porous cryogel and the good electron transport supported by MWCNTs. The ferrocene trapped in the cryogel mediated electron transfer, which helped to avoid any interfering reactions. The biosensor has high stability of operation. It has been tested in more than 350 injections (RSD = 3.6%), with a concentration in a wide linear range from 0.010 to 30 mM and a low Michaelis-Menten constant (1.5 mM). Glucose determinations were not affected by dissolved oxygen or common blood sample interferences such as uric and ascorbic acids [96].

A highly sensitive and selective electrochemical immunosensor for measuring prostate-specific antigen (PSA) has been developed [97]. The cryogel consisted of chitosan, ionic liquid, graphene, and gold nanoparticles. It was biocompatible and porous, which provided more surface area available for gold nanoparticles (AuNPs) loading via amino groups, resulting in more anti-PSA being immobilized on AuNPs via chemisorption. Similarly, a cryogel composite of chitosan with MWCNTs decorated with AuNPs has been used for a highly sensitive non-enzymatic flow-based glucose sensor [98]. Nontipichet *et al.* synthesized a histamine biosensor based on a carbon electrode modified with multi-walled carbon nanotubes with electrodeposited Prussian blue and coated with a macroporous layer of a composite chitosan cryogel with AuNPs [99]. Cryogel, with its high specific surface area and conductivity, was an excellent material for diamine oxidase immobilization. The biosensor has demonstrated good reproducibility, high operational stability, excellent long-term stability, and good selectivity. The biosensor determined histamine levels in fish and shrimp with satisfactory recovery, and the results were consistent with those obtained using ELISA.

9.5 CONCLUSION

Recent studies reviewed here have shown that cryogels, due to their unique three-dimensional macroporous structure, adjustable physical and mechanical properties, and ability to mimic natural tissues, are a versatile platform for creating various biomaterials to solve emerging biomedical problems. A distinctive advantage of cryogels is the possibility of adding additional functionality by chemical modification or incorporation of particles and various polymers into the composition of the cryogel, which adds a new biological function and promotes regeneration. Cryogels are a promising material for solving a wide range of biomedical problems, from engineering scaffolds to support the development of bone, skin, vascular, and liver tissues to cells/drug carriers for transplantation and local delivery to appropriate sites. A deeper understanding of the mechanism of regeneration will stimulate the further development of new methods and therapeutic approaches to the regeneration and repair of biological tissues using cryogels. Further research is needed to understand the relationship between the physicochemical properties of cryogel and cell response, which will help develop materials with better response and regenerative capacity. In addition, cryogel scaling issues need to be addressed, especially in cases where cryogel production requires highly controlled and reproducible freezing conditions.

REFERENCES

1. I.N. Savina, M. Zoughaib, A.A. Yergeshov, Design and assessment of biodegradable macroporous cryogels as advanced tissue engineering and drug carrying materials, *Gels* 7(3) (2021) 79.
2. A. Memic, T. Colombani, L.J. Eggermont, M. Rezaeeyazdi, J. Steingold, Z.J. Rogers, K.J. Navare, H.S. Mohammed, S.A. Bencherif, Latest advances in cryogel technology for biomedical applications, *Advances in Therapy* 2(4) (2019) 45.
3. V.I. Lozinsky, I.Y. Galaev, F.M. Plieva, I.N. Savina, H. Jungvid, B. Mattiasson, Polymeric cryogels as promising materials of biotechnological interest, *Trends in Biotechnology* 21(10) (2003) 445–451.
4. I.N. Savina, R.V. Shevchenko, I.U. Allan, M. Illsley, S.V. Mikhalovsky, Chapter 6: Cryogels in regenerative medicine: Biomedical and biotechnological applications. In: *Supermacroporous Cryogels* (2016) 177. doi: 10.1201/b19676-9.

5. V.M. Gun'ko, I.N. Savina, S.V. Mikhalovsky, Cryogels: Morphological, structural and adsorption characterisation, *Advances in Colloid and Interface Science* 187 (2013) 1–46.
6. V.M. Gun'ko, I.N. Savina, S.V. Mikhalovsky, Properties of water bound in hydrogels, *Gels* 3(4) (2017) 30.
7. I. Savina, I. Galaev, Chapter 3: Production of synthetic cryogels and the study of porosity thereof: Biomedical and biotechnological applications. In: *Supermacroporous Cryogels* (2016) 91. doi: 10.1201/b19676-5.
8. V.I. Lozinsky, Cryostructuring of polymeric systems. 55. Retrospective view on the more than 40 years of studies performed in the ANNesmeyanov Institute of Organoelement compounds with respect of the cryostructuring processes in polymeric systems, *Gels* 6(3) (2020) 59.
9. P.A. Shiekh, S.M. Andrabi, A. Singh, S. Majumder, A. Kumar, Designing cryogels through cryostructuring of polymeric matrices for biomedical applications, *European Polymer Journal* 144 (2021) 110234.
10. M. Razavi, Y. Qiao, A.S. Thakor, Three-dimensional cryogels for biomedical applications, *Journal of Biomedical Materials Research Part A* 107(12) (2019) 2736–2755.
11. I.N. Savina, G.C. Ingavle, A.B. Cundy, S.V. Mikhalovsky, A simple method for the production of large volume 3D macroporous hydrogels for advanced biotechnological, medical and environmental applications, *Scientific Reports* 6 (2016) 21154.
12. L.J. Eggermont, Z.J. Rogers, T. Colombani, A. Memic, S.A. Bencherif, Injectable cryogels for biomedical applications, *Trends in Biotechnology* 38(4) (2020) 418–431.
13. K.R. Hixon, C.T. Eberlin, P.U. Kadakia, S.H. McBride-Gagyi, E. Jain, S.A. Sell, A comparison of cryogel scaffolds to identify an appropriate structure for promoting bone regeneration, *Biomedical Physics & Engineering Express* 2(3) (2016) 18.
14. V.I. Lozinsky, L.G. Damshkaln, R. Brown, I.T. Norton, Study of cryostructuration of polymer systems. XVIII. Freeze-thaw influence on water-solubilized artificial mixtures of amylopectin and amylose, *Journal of Applied Polymer Science* 78(2) (2000) 371–381.
15. D. Demir, N. Boelgen, Synthesis and characterization of injectable chitosan cryogel microsphere scaffolds, *International Journal of Polymeric Materials and Polymeric Biomaterials* 66(13) (2017) 686–696.
16. C. Oelschlaeger, F. Bossler, N. Willenbacher, Synthesis, structural and micromechanical properties of 3D hyaluronic acid-based cryogel scaffolds, *Biomacromolecules* 17(2) (2016) 580–589.
17. J. Wu, Q. Zhao, J. Sun, Q. Zhou, Preparation of poly(ethylene glycol) aligned porous cryogels using a unidirectional freezing technique, *Soft Matter* 8(13) (2012) 3620–3626.
18. A. Singh, P.A. Shiekh, M. Das, J. Seppälä, A. Kumar, Aligned chitosan-gelatin cryogel-filled polyurethane nerve guidance channel for neural tissue engineering: Fabrication, characterization, and in vitro evaluation, *Biomacromolecules* 20(2) (2019) 662–673.
19. K.H. Chang, H.T. Liao, J.P. Chen, Preparation and characterization of gelatin/hyaluronic acid cryogels for adipose tissue engineering: In vitro and in vivo studies, *Acta Biomaterialia* 9(11) (2013) 9012–9026.
20. L. Boulais, Cryogel-integrated hepatic cell culture microchips for liver tissue engineering, Bioengineering, Université de Technologie de Compiègne, 2020. https://tel.archives-ouvertes.fr/tel-03130501/document.
21. M. Madaghiele, L. Salvatore, C. Demitri, A. Sannino, Fast synthesis of poly(ethylene glycol) diacrylate cryogels via UV irradiation, *Materials Letters* 218 (2018) 305–308.
22. B. Ari, B. Yetiskin, O. Okay, N. Sahiner, Preparation of dextran cryogels for separation processes of binary dye and pesticide mixtures from aqueous solutions, *Polymer Engineering & Science* 60(8) (2020) 1890–1901.
23. Y.S. Hwang, C. Zhang, S. Varghese, Poly(ethylene glycol) cryogels as potential cell scaffolds: Effect of polymerization conditions on cryogel microstructure and properties, *Journal of Materials Chemistry* 20(2) (2010) 345–351.

24. I.U. Allan, B.A. Tolhurst, R.V. Shevchenko, M.B. Dainiak, M. Illsley, A. Ivanov, H. Jungvid, I.Y. Galaev, S.L. James, S.V. Mikhalovsky, S.E. James, An in vitro evaluation of fibrinogen and gelatin containing cryogels as dermal regeneration scaffolds, *Biomaterials Science* 4(6) (2016) 1007–1014.
25. C.-H. Chen, C.-Y. Kuo, Y.-J. Wang, J.-P. Chen, Dual function of glucosamine in gelatin/hyaluronic acid cryogel to modulate scaffold mechanical properties and to maintain chondrogenic phenotype for cartilage tissue engineering, *International Journal of Molecular Sciences* 17(11) (2016) 1957.
26. D.B. Raina, D. Larsson, F. Mrkonjic, H. Isaksson, A. Kumar, L. Lidgren, M. Tägil, Gelatin- hydroxyapatite-calcium sulphate based biomaterial for long term sustained delivery of bone morphogenic protein-2 and zoledronic acid for increased bone formation: In-vitro and in-vivo carrier properties, *Journal of Controlled Release* 272 (2018) 83–96.
27. L.P. Bagri, R.K. Saini, A.K. Bajpai, R. Choubey, Silver hydroxyapatite reinforced poly(vinyl alcohol)-starch cryogel nanocomposites and study of biodegradation, compressive strength and antibacterial activity, *Polymer Engineering & Science* 59(2) (2019) 254–263.
28. S.A. Bencherif, R.W. Sands, O.A. Ali, W.A. Li, S.A. Lewin, T.M. Braschler, T.Y. Shih, C.S. Verbeke, D. Bhatta, G. Dranoff, D.J. Mooney, Injectable cryogel-based whole-cell cancer vaccines, *Nature Communications* 6 (2015) 13.
29. P.B. Welzel, M. Grimmer, C. Renneberg, L. Naujox, S. Zschoche, U. Freudenberg, C. Werner, Macroporous StarPEG-heparin cryogels, *Biomacromolecules* 13(8) (2012) 2349–2358.
30. F. Bonalumi, C. Crua, I.N. Savina, N. Davies, A. Habstesion, M. Santini, S. Fest-Santini, S. Sandeman, Bioengineering a cryogel-derived bioartificial liver using particle image velocimetry defined fluid dynamics, *Materials Science and Engineering C: Materials for Biological Applications* 123 (2021) 14.
31. R. Aliperta, P.B. Welzel, R. Bergmann, U. Freudenberg, N. Berndt, A. Feldmann, C. Arndt, S. Koristka, M. Stanzione, M. Cartellieri, A. Ehninger, G. Ehninger, C. Werner, J. Pietzsch, J. Steinbach, M. Bornhauser, M.P Bachmann, Cryogel-supported stem cell factory for customized sustained release of bispecific antibodies for cancer immunotherapy, *Scientific Reports* 7 (2017) 42855.
32. J. Bruns, S. McBride-Gagyi, S.P. Zustiak, Injectable and cell-adhesive polyethylene glycol cryogel scaffolds: Independent control of cryogel microstructure and composition, *Macromolecular Materials and Engineering* 303(10) (2018) 1800298.
33. R.Y Tam, S.A. Fisher, A.E.G. Baker, M.S. Shoichet, Transparent porous polysaccharide cryogels provide biochemically defined, biomimetic matrices for tunable 3D cell culture, *Chemistry of Materials* 28(11) (2016) 3762–3770.
34. T.D. Luong, M. Zoughaib, R. Garifullin, S. Kuznetsova, M.O. Guler, T.I. Abdullin, In situ functionalization of Poly(hydroxyethyl methacrylate) cryogels with oligopeptides via β-cyclodextrin–adamantane complexation for studying cell-instructive peptide environment, *ACS Applied Bio Materials* 3(2) (2020) 1116–1128.
35. M. Zoughaib, D. Luong, R. Garifullin, D.Z. Gatina, S.V. Fedosimova, T.I. Abdullin, Enhanced angiogenic effects of RGD, GHK peptides and copper (II) compositions in synthetic cryogel ECM model, *Materials Science and Engineering C: Materials for Biological Applications* 120 (2021) 111660.
36. B. Newland, P.B. Welzel, H. Newland, C. Renneberg, P. Kolar, M. Tsurkan, A. Rosser, U. Freudenberg, C. Werner, Tackling cell transplantation anoikis: An injectable, shape memory cryogel microcarrier platform material for stem cell and neuronal cell growth, *Small* 11(38) (2015) 5047–5053.
37. I. Kim, S.S. Lee, S. Bae, H. Lee, N.S. Hwang, Heparin functionalized injectable cryogel with rapid shape-recovery property for neovascularization, *Biomacromolecules* 19(6) (2018) 2257–2269.

38. S. Jimi, A. Jaguparov, A. Nurkesh, B. Sultankulov, A. Saparov, Sequential delivery of cryogel released growth factors and cytokines accelerates wound healing and improves tissue regeneration, *Frontiers in Bioengineering and Biotechnology* 8 (2020) 345.
39. T. Takei, H. Nakahara, S. Tanaka, H. Nishimata, M. Yoshida, K. Kawakami, Effect of chitosan-gluconic acid conjugate/poly(vinyl alcohol) cryogels as wound dressing on partial-thickness wounds in diabetic rats, *Journal of Materials Science: Materials in Medicine* 24(10) (2013) 2479–2487.
40. C.L. Salgado, L. Grenho, M.H.V. Fernandes, B. Colaço, F.J. Monteiro, Biodegradation, biocompatibility, and osteoconduction evaluation of collagen-nanohydroxyapatite cryogels for bone tissue regeneration, *Journal of Biomedical Materials Research: Part A* 104(1) (2016) 57–70.
41. D.B. Raina, H. Isaksson, A.K. Teotia, L. Lidgren, M. Tagil, A. Kumar, Biocomposite macroporous cryogels as potential carrier scaffolds for bone active agents augmenting bone regeneration, *Journal of Controlled Release* 235 (2016) 365–378.
42. M. Razavi, S. Hu, A.S. Thakor, A collagen based cryogel bioscaffold coated with nanostructured polydopamine as a platform for mesenchymal stem cell therapy, *Journal of Biomedical Materials Research: Part A* 106(8) (2018) 2213–2228.
43. L. Wang, J. Jiang, W. Hua, A. Darabi, X. Song, C. Song, W. Zhong, M.M.Q. Xing, X. Qiu, Mussel-inspired conductive cryogel as cardiac tissue patch to repair myocardial infarction by migration of conductive nanoparticles, *Advanced Functional Materials* 26(24) (2016) 4293–4305.
44. P. Dwivedi, S. Bhat, V. Nayak, A. Kumar, Study of different delivery modes of chondroitin sulfate using microspheres and cryogel scaffold for application in cartilage tissue engineering, *International Journal of Polymeric Materials and Polymeric Biomaterials* 63(16) (2014) 859–872.
45. P.U. Kadakia, E. Jain, K.R. Hixon, C.T. Eberlin, S.A. Sell, Sonication induced silk fibroin cryogels for tissue engineering applications, *Materials Research Express* 3(5) (2016) 15.
46. F. Ak, Z. Oztoprak, I. Karakutuk, O. Okay, Macroporous silk fibroin cryogels, *Biomacromolecules* 14(3) (2013) 719–727.
47. B. Yetiskin, C. Akinci, O. Okay, Cryogelation within cryogels: Silk fibroin scaffolds with single-, double- and triple-network structures, *Polymer* 128 (2017) 47–56.
48. T. Kanno, H. Uyama, Unique ivy-like morphology composed of poly(lactic acid) and bacterial cellulose cryogel, *ACS Omega* 3(1) (2018) 631–635.
49. K.T. Shalumon, C.Y. Kuo, C.B. Wong, Y.M. Chien, H.A. Chen, J.P. Chen, Gelatin/nanohyroxyapatite cryogel embedded poly(lactic-co-glycolic Acid)/nanohydroxyapatite microsphere hybrid scaffolds for simultaneous bone regeneration and load-bearing, *Polymers* 10(6) (2018) 27.
50. C.L. Salgado, L. Grenho, M.H. Fernandes, B.J. Colaco, F.J. Monteiro, Biodegradation, biocompatibility, and osteoconduction evaluation of collagen-nanohydroxyapatite cryogels for bone tissue regeneration, *Journal of Biomedical Materials Research. Part A* 104(1) (2016) 57–70.
51. H. Zhou, H. Jiao, J. Xu, Y. Liu, S. Wei, Synthesis of poly hydroxypropyl methacrylate cryogel incorporated with Zn/Ce substituted hydroxyapatite nanoparticles for rejuvenation of femoral fracture treatment in a rat model, *Journal of Photochemistry and Photobiology. B, Biology* 201 (2019) 111651.
52. B.Y. Ozturk, I. Inci, S. Egri, A.M. Ozturk, H. Yetkin, G. Goktas, C. Elmas, E. Piskin, D. Erdogan, The treatment of segmental bone defects in rabbit tibiae with vascular endothelial growth factor (VEGF)-loaded gelatin/hydroxyapatite "cryogel" scaffold, *European Journal of Orthopaedic Surgery and Traumatology* 23(7) (2013) 767–774.
53. D. Eigel, C. Werner, B. Newland, Cryogel biomaterials for neuroscience applications, *Neurochemistry International* 147 (2021) 105012.

54. B. Newland, K.R. Long, Cryogel scaffolds: Soft and easy to use tools for neural tissue culture, *Neural Regeneration Research* 17(9) (2022) 1981–1983.
55. J. Tao, Y. Hu, S.J. Wang, J.M. Zhang, X. Liu, Z.Y. Gou, H. Cheng, Q.Q. Liu, Q.Q. Zhang, S.L. You, M.L. Gou, A 3D-engineered porous conduit for peripheral nerve repair, *Scientific Reports* 7 (2017) 13.
56. G. Agarwal, N. Kumar, A. Srivastava, Highly elastic, electroconductive, immunomodulatory graphene crosslinked collagen cryogel for spinal cord regeneration, *Materials Science and Engineering C: Materials for Biological Applications* 118 (2021) 19.
57. A. Singh, P.A. Shiekh, M. Das, J. Seppälä, A. Kumar, Aligned chitosan-gelatin cryogel-filled polyurethane nerve guidance channel for neural tissue engineering: Fabrication, characterization, and in vitro evaluation, *Biomacromolecules* 20(2) (2019) 662–673.
58. S. Wu, M. Kuss, D. Qi, J. Hong, H.-J. Wang, W. Zhang, S. Chen, S. Ni, B. Duan, Development of cryogel-based guidance conduit for peripheral nerve regeneration, *ACS Applied Bio Materials* 2(11) (2019) 4864–4871.
59. I. Goganau, B. Sandner, N. Weidner, K. Fouad, A. Blesch, Depolarization and electrical stimulation enhance in vitro and in vivo sensory axon growth after spinal cord injury, *Experimental Neurology* 300 (2018) 247–258.
60. T. Vishnoi, A. Singh, A.K. Teotia, A. Kumar, Chitosan-gelatin-polypyrrole cryogel matrix for stem cell differentiation into neural lineage and sciatic nerve regeneration in peripheral nerve injury model, *ACS Biomaterials Science & Engineering* 5(6) (2019) 3007–3021.
61. M. Jurga, M.B. Dainiak, A. Sarnowska, A. Jablonska, A. Tripathi, F.M. Plieva, I.N. Savina, L. Strojek, H. Jungvid, A. Kumar, The performance of laminin-containing cryogel scaffolds in neural tissue regeneration, *Biomaterials* 32(13) (2011) 3423–3434.
62. A. Beduer, T. Braschler, O. Peric, G.E. Fantner, S. Mosser, P.C. Fraering, S. Bencherif, D.J. Mooney, P. Renaud, A compressible scaffold for minimally invasive delivery of large intact neuronal networks, *Advanced Healthcare Materials* 4(2) (2015) 301–312.
63. R.V. Shevchenko, M. Eeman, B. Rowshanravan, L.U. Allan, I.N. Savina, M. Illsley, M. Salmon, S.L. James, S.V. Mikhalovsky, S.E. James, The in vitro characterization of a gelatin scaffold, prepared by cryogelation and assessed in vivo as a dermal replacement in wound repair, *Acta Biomaterialia* 10(7) (2014) 3156–3166.
64. R. Shevchenko, M. Eeman, I. Savina, I. Allan, S. James, M. Salmon, S. Mikhalovsky, S.E. James, A step towards an artificial skin: A novel supermacroporous anisotropic cryogel for wound healing applications, *International Journal of Artificial Organs* 33(7) (2010) 426–427.
65. M.B. Dainiak, I.U. Allan, I.N. Savina, L. Cornelio, E.S. James, S.L. James, S.V. Mikhalovsky, H. Jungvid, I.Y. Galaev, Gelatin–fibrinogen cryogel dermal matrices for wound repair: Preparation, optimisation and in vitro study, *Biomaterials* 31(1) (2010) 67–76.
66. D. Luong, A.A. Yergeshov, M. Zoughaib, F.R. Sadykova, B.I. Gareev, I.N. Savina, T.I. Abdullin, Transition metal-doped cryogels as bioactive materials for wound healing applications, *Materials Science & Engineering C-Materials for Biological Applications* 103 (2019) 13.
67. S. Seker, A.E. Elcin, Y.M. Elcin, Macroporous elastic cryogels based on platelet lysate and oxidized dextran as tissue engineering scaffold: In vitro and in vivo evaluations, *Materials Science & Engineering C-Materials for Biological Applications* 110 (2020) 11.
68. G. Sener, S.A. Hilton, M.J. Osmond, C. Zgheib, J.P. Newsom, L. Dewberry, S. Singh, T.S. Sakthivel, S. Seal, K.W. Liechty, M.D. Krebs, Injectable, self-healable zwitterionic cryogels with sustained microRNA - cerium oxide nanoparticle release promote accelerated wound healing, *Acta Biomaterialia* 101 (2020) 262–272.
69. A.A. Yergeshov, M. Zoughaib, R.A. Ishkaeva, I.N. Savina, T.I. Abdullin, Regenerative activities of ROS-modulating trace metals in subcutaneously implanted biodegradable cryogel, *Gels* 8(2) (2022) 118.

70. G. Sener, S.A. Hilton, M.J. Osmond, C. Zgheib, J.P. Newsom, L. Dewberry, S. Singh, T.S. Sakthivel, S. Seal, K.W. Liechty, M.D. Krebs, Injectable, self-healable zwitterionic cryogels with sustained microRNA - cerium oxide nanoparticle release promote accelerated wound healing, *Acta Biomaterialia* 101 (2020) 262–272.
71. Y. Huang, L. Bai, Y.T. Yang, Z.H. Yin, B.L. Guo, Biodegradable gelatin/silver nanoparticle composite cryogel with excellent antibacterial and antibiofilm activity and hemostasis for Pseudomonas aeruginosa-infected burn wound healing, *Journal of Colloid and Interface Science* 608 (2022) 2278–2289.
72. W.B. Wan, F. Cai, J.Y. Huang, S.X. Chen, Q. Liao, A skin-inspired 3D bilayer scaffold enhances granulation tissue formation and anti-infection for diabetic wound healing, *Journal of Materials Chemistry B* 7(18) (2019) 2954–2961.
73. Y.L. Yu, P.F. Li, C.L. Zhu, N. Ning, S.Y. Zhang, G.J. Vancso, Multifunctional and recyclable photothermally responsive cryogels as efficient platforms for wound healing, *Advanced Functional Materials* 29(35) (2019) 11.
74. S.G. Priya, A. Gupta, E. Jain, J. Sarkar, A. Damania, P.R. Jagdale, B.P. Chaudhari, K.C. Gupta, A. Kumar, Bilayer cryogel wound dressing and skin regeneration grafts for the treatment of acute skin wounds, *ACS Applied Materials & Interfaces* 8(24) (2016) 15145–15159.
75. L. Han, P.F. Li, P.F. Tang, X. Wang, T. Zhou, K.F. Wang, F.Z. Ren, T.L. Guo, X. Lu, Mussel-inspired cryogels for promoting wound regeneration through photobiostimulation, modulating inflammatory responses and suppressing bacterial invasion, *Nanoscale* 11(34) (2019) 15846–15861.
76. P.A. Shiekh, A. Singh, A. Kumar, Exosome laden oxygen releasing antioxidant and antibacterial cryogel wound dressing OxOBand alleviate diabetic and infectious wound healing, *Biomaterials* 249 (2020) 120020.
77. B. Carpentier, A. Gautier, C. Legallais, Artificial and bioartificial liver devices: Present and future, *Gut* 58(12) (2009) 1690–1702.
78. A. Tripathi, J.S. Melo, Preparation of a sponge-like biocomposite agarose-chitosan scaffold with primary hepatocytes for establishing an in vitro 3D liver tissue model, *RSC Advances* 5(39) (2015) 30701–30710.
79. J. Kumari, A.A. Karande, A. Kumar, Combined effect of cryogel matrix and temperature-reversible soluble-insoluble polymer for the development of in vitro human liver tissue, *ACS Applied Materials & Interfaces* 8(1) (2016) 264–277.
80. N. Kumar, D. Desagani, G. Chandran, N.N. Ghosh, G. Karthikeyan, S. Waigaonkar, A. Ganguly, Biocompatible agarose-chitosan coated silver nanoparticle composite for soft tissue engineering applications, *Artificial Cells, Nanomedicine, and Biotechnology* 46(3) (2018) 637–649.
81. D. Singh, V. Nayak, A. Kumar, Proliferation of myoblast skeletal cells on three-dimensional supermacroporous cryogels, *International Journal of Biological Sciences* 6(4) (2010) 371–381.
82. N.E. Vrana, P.A. Cahill, G.B. McGuinness, Endothelialization of PVA/gelatin cryogels for vascular tissue engineering: Effect of disturbed shear stress conditions, *Journal of Biomedical Materials Research: Part A* 94A(4) (2010) 1080–1090.
83. H. Jiang, G. Campbell, D. Boughner, W.-K. Wan, M. Quantz, Design and manufacture of a polyvinyl alcohol (PVA) cryogel tri-leaflet heart valve prosthesis, *Medical Engineering & Physics* 26(4) (2004) 269–277.
84. H. Mohammadi, D. Goode, G. Fradet, K. Mequanint, Proposed percutaneous aortic valve prosthesis made of cryogel, *Proceedings of the Institution of Mechanical Engineers, Part H: Journal of Engineering in Medicine* 233(5) (2019) 515–524.
85. S.T. Koshy, D.K.Y. Zhang, J.M. Grolman, A.G. Stafford, D.J. Mooney, Injectable nanocomposite cryogels for versatile protein drug delivery, *Acta Biomaterialia* 65 (2018) 36–43.

86. G. Pandey, N. Mittapelly, A. Pant, S. Sharma, P. Singh, V.T. Banala, R. Trivedi, P.K. Shukla, P.R. Mishra, Dual functioning microspheres embedded crosslinked gelatin cryogels for therapeutic intervention in osteomyelitis and associated bone loss, *European Journal of Pharmaceutical Sciences* 91 (2016) 105–113.
87. S.A. Bencherif, R.W. Sands, D. Bhatta, P. Arany, C.S. Verbeke, D.A. Edwards, D.J. Mooney, Injectable preformed scaffolds with shape-memory properties, *Proceedings of the National Academy of Sciences* 109(48) (2012) 19590–19595.
88. H.-C. Chang, C. Yang, F. Feng, F.-H. Lin, C.-H. Wang, P.-C. Chang, Bone morphogenetic protein-2 loaded poly(D, L-lactide-co-glycolide) microspheres enhance osteogenic potential of gelatin/hydroxyapatite/β-tricalcium phosphate cryogel composite for alveolar ridge augmentation, *Journal of the Formosan Medical Association* 116(12) (2017) 973–981.
89. K. Çetin, A. Denizli, 5-Fluorouracil delivery from metal-ion mediated molecularly imprinted cryogel discs, *Colloids and Surfaces B: Biointerfaces* 126 (2015) 401–406.
90. M. Bakhshpour, H. Yavuz, A. Denizli, Controlled release of mitomycin C from PHEMAH–Cu(II) cryogel membranes, *Artificial Cells, Nanomedicine, and Biotechnology* 46 (2018) 946–954.
91. K. Çetin, H. Alkan, N. Bereli, A. Denizli, Molecularly imprinted cryogel as a pH-responsive delivery system for doxorubicin, *Journal of Macromolecular Science, Part A* 54(8) (2017) 502–508.
92. I. Qayoom, E. Srivastava, A. Kumar, Anti-infective composite cryogel scaffold treats osteomyelitis and augments bone healing in rat femoral condyle, *Biomaterials Advances* 142 (2022) 213133.
93. B. Sultankulov, D. Berillo, S. Kauanova, S. Mikhalovsky, L. Mikhalovska, A. Saparov, Composite cryogel with polyelectrolyte complexes for growth factor delivery, *Pharmaceutics* 11(12) (2019) 15.
94. T. Bauleth-Ramos, T.Y. Shih, M.A. Shahbazi, A.J. Najibi, A.S. Mao, D.F. Liu, P. Granja, H.A. Santos, B. Sarmento, D.J. Mooney, Acetalated dextran nanoparticles loaded into an injectable alginate cryogel for combined chemotherapy and cancer vaccination, *Advanced Functional Materials* 29(35) (2019) 10.
95. T.Y. Shih, S.O. Blacklow, A.W. Li, B.R. Freedman, S. Bencherif, S.T. Koshy, M.C. Darnell, D.J. Mooney, Injectable, tough alginate cryogels as cancer vaccines, *Advanced Healthcare Materials* 7(10) (2018) 13.
96. A. Fatoni, A. Numnuam, P. Kanatharana, W. Limbut, C. Thammakhet, P. Thavarungkul, A highly stable oxygen-independent glucose biosensor based on a chitosan-albumin cryogel incorporated with carbon nanotubes and ferrocene, *Sensors & Actuators, B: Chemical* 185 (2013) 725–734.
97. J. Choosang, S. Khumngern, P. Thavarungkul, P. Kanatharana, A. Numnuam, An ultrasensitive label-free electrochemical immunosensor based on 3D porous chitosan-graphene-ionic liquid-ferrocene nanocomposite cryogel decorated with gold nanoparticles for prostate-specific antigen, *Talanta* 224 (2021) 9.
98. T. Kangkamano, A. Numnuam, W. Limbut, P. Kanatharana, P. Thavarungkul, Chitosan cryogel with embedded gold nanoparticles decorated multiwalled carbon nanotubes modified electrode for highly sensitive flow based non-enzymatic glucose sensor, *Sensors & Actuators, B: Chemical* 246 (2017) 854–863.
99. N. Nontipichet, S. Khumngern, J. Choosang, P. Thavarungkul, P. Kanatharana, A. Numnuam, An enzymatic histamine biosensor based on a screen-printed carbon electrode modified with a chitosan-gold nanoparticles composite cryogel on Prussian blue-coated multi-walled carbon nanotubes, *Food Chemistry* 364 (2021) 130396.

10 Constructing Three-Dimensional Microenvironments Using Engineered Biomaterials for Bone and Cartilage Tissue Regeneration

Ketki Holkar, Isha Behere, and Ganesh Ingavle
Symbiosis International (Deemed University)

CONTENTS

10.1 Introduction 214
10.2 Bone Microenvironment 215
10.3 Effect of 2D and 3D Microenvironment on MSCs and their Secretome 217
10.4 Properties of Scaffolds Required for BTE 217
10.5 Recent Approaches in Reconstructing Native Bone Microenvironment Using 3D Culture Models 218
10.5.1 Bone Organoids 219
10.5.2 Cell-Free Approach 220
10.6 Growth Factors in Bone Regeneration 221
10.7 3D Printing 222
10.8 Interpenetrating Network Hydrogels 223
10.9 Mineralized Microenvironment 224
10.10 Three-Dimensional Microenvironment for Cartilage Tissue 224
10.11 Prospects of the 3D Microenvironment 227
10.11.1 Biomaterial Types and Geometry 227
10.11.1.1 Hydrogels 227
10.11.1.2 Interpenetrating Network 227
10.11.1.3 Cryogels 228

DOI: 10.1201/9781003251767-10

10.11.2 Nanofibers 228
10.12 Incorporating Chondro-Inductive Molecules 228
10.13 Extracellular Vesicles/Secretome for Improved Chondrogenesis 229
10.14 Future Perspectives 229
10.15 Conclusion 230
References 230

10.1 INTRODUCTION

Bone is vascularized tissue known for its load-bearing potential and the fact that it can heal and remodel itself considerably. The bone can suffer from various injuries and diseases, whereas the self-regenerative potential of the bone is limited in elderly and immune-compromised people. The current treatments used to cure these problems are allograft, autograft, and natural filler material, which are costly and may elicit an immune response [1]. Hence, there is a need for a tissue-engineered approach to create operative replacements for damaged or diseased tissues. In bone tissue engineering (BTE), scaffolds are used as temporary replacements for native tissue that help the regeneration of lost tissue and support bone structurally. The ideal scaffold for any bone tissue application should possess biocompatibility, biodegradability, and three essential properties: osteoconduction, osteoinduction, and osteogenesis. The critical players for BTE highlight architectural properties such as surface topography, porosity, and mechanical strength. These favor cell attachment and proliferation, the exchange of gases and nutrients, and a biocompatible and biodegradable scaffold that should imitate the *in vivo* extracellular matrix (ECM) microenvironment.

The hyaline cartilage protects the subchondral bone, called articular cartilage (AC). It is a load-bearing soft tissue that covers the diarthrodial joints' surface. AC injuries are a peculiar and challenging medical condition due to the tissue's inability to regenerate. Cartilage regeneration is hampered by poor vascularity, a lower cell population, and a thick ECM. Swelling, joint pain, further tissue degradation, and inflammation can result from untreated cartilage defects caused by osteoarthritis or injury, eventually necessitating a total joint replacement [2]. Cartilage repair and regeneration aim to create fully integrated tissue at the articular surface and subchondral bone regeneration with mechanical and chemical qualities identical to the original cartilage. Current allograft implants and traditional therapies like autologous chondrocyte implantation and osteochondral transplantation do not produce fully integrated tissues, tissues with native matrix stiffness, or tissues with a similar biochemical composition as native articular cartilage. Developing improved alternative strategies for treating bone and cartilage-related disorders is a significant area requiring immediate intervention from the scientific community to overcome the abovementioned issues. Many researchers have indicated the progression of biomaterial-based 3D cell culture platforms to increase mesenchymal stem cell (MSC)-to-microenvironment exchanges, leading to improved bone and cartilage healing. *In vitro* bone and cartilage tissue regeneration has already been extensively studied using a variety of two-dimensional (2D) and 3D culture-based biomaterial experimental approaches. The essential criteria for such design systems include simple construction and the ability to recognize a combination of physical and biological cues from the native microenvironment. However, their success depends on identifying the most effective and therapeutically applicable methodologies for engineering biocompatible scaffolds and native microenvironments that allow cells to grow, proliferate, and differentiate into a specific lineage.

10.2 BONE MICROENVIRONMENT

The native microenvironment of bone is a highly dynamic structure consisting of different types of cells, ECM, growth factors, collagen, and non-collagen proteins and cytokines. Based on functions, the bone microenvironment can be divided into three parts: the bone synthesis unit, the bone dissolving unit, and the hemopoietic unit, which contribute to the mineralization or repair of bone, the removal of old/damaged bone, or the reservoir of minerals and production of the majority of blood cells, respectively. MSCs are multipotent cells that can differentiate into non-blood cell components, including osteoblasts, adipocytes, and chondrocytes. MSCs can differentiate into osteoblasts and are responsible for bone formation, whereas osteoclasts derived from hematopoietic stem cells play a role in bone resorption. As a dynamic and unique microenvironment, the stem cell niche in bone tissue regulates MSC self-renewal, the equilibrium between their quiescent and proliferative phases, as well as the destiny and differentiation of their progeny. Communication between stem cells and their immediate environment, which includes surrounding cells, extracellular matrix components, secretome exchanges, cytokine gradients, and physical elements like oxygen tension, topography, and mechanical cues, controls these functions (Figure 10.1) [3–6]. The ideal biomaterial for tissue regeneration *in vivo* should be non-immunogenic, osteoconductive, and biodegradable. Biomaterials used in BTE are classified as natural polymers (derived from biological tissue, for example, hyaluronic acid, alginate, collagen, etc.), synthetic polymers (produced artificially, for example, polylactic acid (PLA), polyglycolic acid (PGA), etc.), ceramics (inorganic compounds, for example, hydroxyapatite, bioglass, etc.), and metals (magnesium, titanium and their alloys) [7,8]. Natural biomaterials are more readily available and break down into simpler compounds with little cytotoxicity or immunogenicity [9]. On the other hand, natural biomaterials have lesser mechanical strength and compositional variability from batch to batch. Unlike natural biomaterials, synthetic biomaterials are more malleable, have a uniform composition between batches, are mechanically more robust, and are simple to produce on a large scale. Synthetic biomaterials, however, are less biocompatible and can trigger an inflammatory reaction after degradation. Ceramics are osteoconductive, biodegradable, and either bio-inert or bioactive, depending on how they interact with the host tissues. However, their mechanical strength is limited. Metals are frequently utilized in BTE because of their great mechanical strength. However, inflammatory reactions brought on by metal corrosion and degradation have raised questions. Tissue engineering employs composite scaffolds, which are made up of two different types of materials combined to maximize each benefit. A few examples of composite scaffolds are calcium phosphate coating on metals, interconnected networks of synthetic and natural polymers, and hydroxyapatite/chitosan gelation [10]. Extracellular matrix proteins are secreted by osteoblasts, which regulate the mineralization process using hydroxyapatite and type I collagen, which supports the bone skeleton. Growth factors like bone morphogenetic proteins (BMPs), insulin-like growth factors (IGFs), platelet-derived growth factors (PDGFs), fibroblast growth factor (FGF), transforming growth factor-beta (TGF-β), vascular endothelial growth factor (VEGF), etc., plays an essential part in the bone remodeling process [11]. Many molecules are involved in the osteogenesis process *in vivo*, but the most critical transcription factors are Runt-related transcription factor 2 (Runx2) and Osterix. Runx2 is a master regulator of osteoblastogenesis and is necessary for MSCs to differentiate into osteoblasts. It also prevents MSCs from converting into adipocytes and chondrocytes. As a result, Runx2 null mice indicate a total absence of intramembranous and endochondral ossification because osteoblast differentiation is absent [12,13]. Osterix is a second transcription factor necessary for osteoblast differentiation, as evidenced by the complete absence of osteoblasts and the ability of perichondrial mesenchymal cells to condense and differentiate into chondrocytes in osterix-null mice [14]. Runx2 is found in the MSCs of osterix-null mice, whereas osterix is not generated in Runx2 null mice, implying that osterix is triggered by Runx2 and is a downstream gene of Runx2 [15].

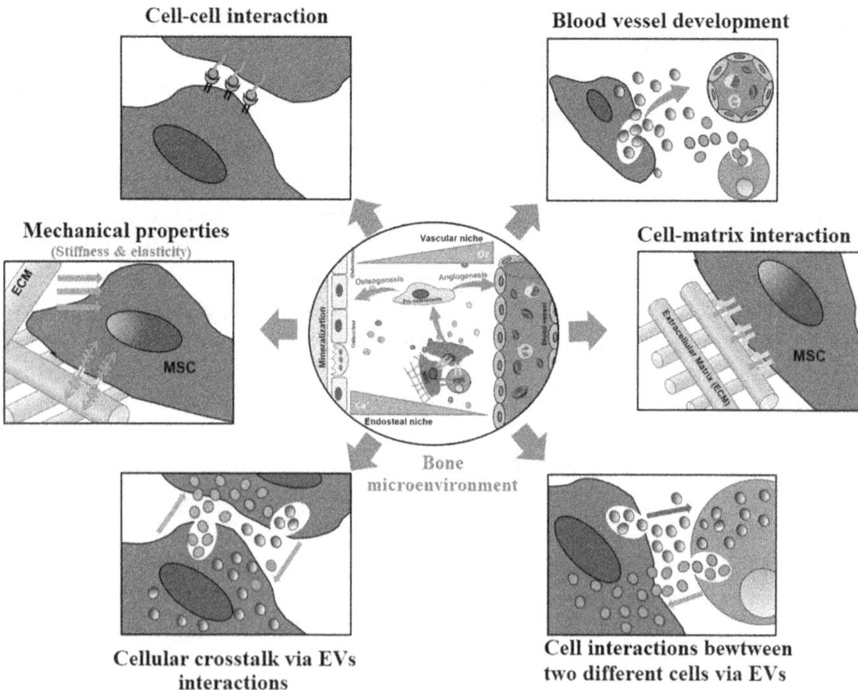

FIGURE 10.1 The cartoon illustrates the different components and cellular activities in the bone marrow environment. Microenvironmental cues such as mechanical forces (stiffness, elasticity, and compression), stem cell secretome (extracellular vesicles, growth factors and cytokines), cell-matrix interactions (collagen and fibronectin), and cell-cell interactions (notch signaling and cell adhesion molecules) converse in a complex fashion to impact various signaling pathways and ultimately determine stem cell fate.

In a healthy individual, osteoblasts and osteoclasts are maintained equally, irrespective of the fact that their functions are contrary to each other, thereby conserving the homeostasis of bone. As bone is a highly vascular tissue, BTE scaffolds are also considered to support osteogenesis and angiogenesis when bone regeneration is considered. Though bone has higher mechanical strength, it is susceptible to breakage or disease, making it fragile. Hence, understanding the molecular mechanism of bone remodeling is essential to designing a 3D scaffold for early osteogenesis and angiogenesis in damaged bone.

10.3 EFFECT OF 2D AND 3D MICROENVIRONMENT ON MSCS AND THEIR SECRETOME

Most basic stem cell research is done on 2D cell formats, primarily using flat plastic surfaces. However, culturing these stem cells in 2D formats affects their growth dynamics, differentiation potential, and loss of multipotency [16–18]. MSCs are thus being cultivated in 3D environments with (hydrogel culture) or without scaffolds (spheroid culture) to address these problems [19,20]. In 2D cell culture formats, cell-to-cell interactions are only available at the cells' edges, but 3D systems allow cell-cell, cell-matrix interactions, and physical and mechanical stimuli from all angles, similar to endogenous structures [21,22] (Figure 10.2). The 3D microenvironment encourages proliferation and signaling while increasing the release of angiogenic EVs and anti-inflammatory compounds [23]. Compared to 2D lab conditions, bioreactors are considered an inexpensive choice for large-scale EV manufacturing [24,25]. The release of therapeutically more efficient EVs can be modulated by several factors, including biophysical stimuli, cellular reprogramming, hypoxic conditions, and priming with active agents [23,26,27]. Genetic modification can be employed as an alternate strategy, and MSCs could be immortalized, lowering the expense involved with starting from primary cells every time. This might provide a consistent supply of EVs with minimal batch-to-batch variations [28–31]. Hence, providing stem cells with a 3D microenvironment during culture would increase their therapeutic potential and their secretome as it imitates native bone conditions.

10.4 PROPERTIES OF SCAFFOLDS REQUIRED FOR BTE

Bone has a 3D microenvironment that cannot be replicated using gold-standard 2D approaches; hence, 3D scaffolds can recreate the bone-mimetic structure. The scaffolds used for BTE should have some crucial properties or characteristics. The first factor is biocompatibility, which is vital as scaffolds integrate seamlessly with the host tissue without activating their immune response. The second factor is porosity, so the biomaterial should possess an open pore and interconnected pores, providing a larger surface area to volume ratio to allow cell migration growth and support neovascularization. It is also mandatory for the precise diffusion of nutrients and gases and for eliminating metabolic waste products.

The third factor is pore size; the smaller the pores, the more the cell occlusion and restriction of cellular penetration and ECM production, and the larger the pores, the lower the mechanical strength of scaffolds. The fourth factor is surface properties, which affect cellular adhesion and proliferation and support osteoconduction.

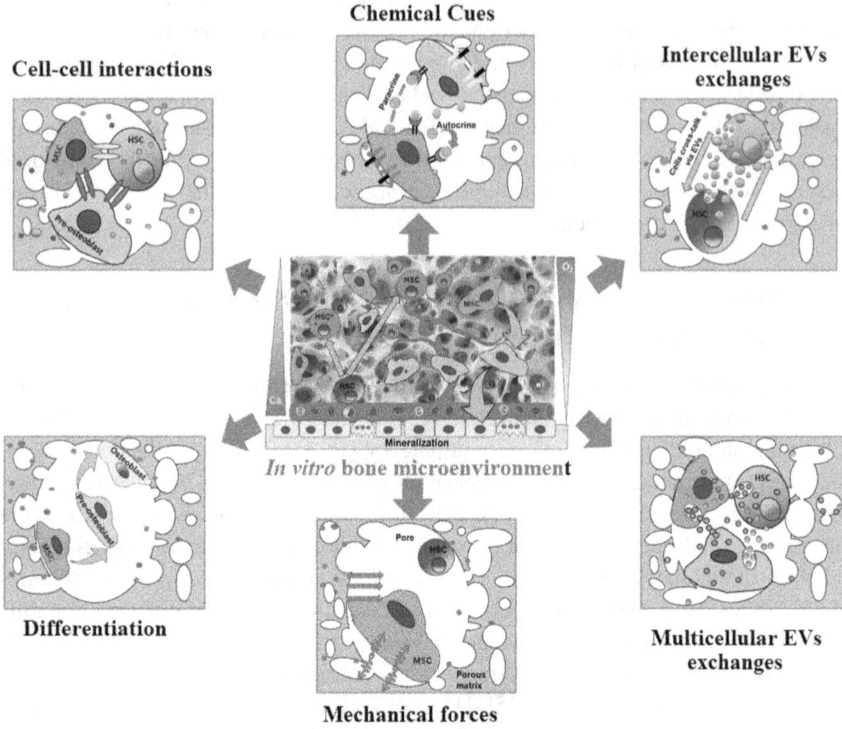

FIGURE 10.2 The *in vitro* bone microenvironment is depicted schematically with multiple interactions.

Literature suggests that a 'rougher' surface will facilitate cell migration and attachment more than a smooth surface. The fifth factor is osteoinduction, where stem cells are recruited at the bone defect site and differentiate into osteoblasts (Figure 10.2). However, the natural process of osteoinduction is not sufficient; hence, using osteoinductive scaffolds is the best alternative to initiate bone regeneration faster. The sixth factor is mechanical strength and biodegradability, as bone is a load-bearing tissue; the scaffold used for regeneration should have a similar mechanical strength to native bone (Figure 10.2). Also, as new tissue regenerates at the defect site, the scaffold should degrade simultaneously, for the same biodegradability of scaffolds must be considered [32]. Hence, all these critical parameters should be considered when constructing a 3D-engineered scaffold for BTE to regenerate bone in minimal time and efficiently.

10.5 RECENT APPROACHES IN RECONSTRUCTING NATIVE BONE MICROENVIRONMENT USING 3D CULTURE MODELS

Large bone defects, sometimes called critical-sized defects (CSDs), are challenging to treat since the patient's body does not naturally repair them. Due to the limitations of traditional bone transplants, bone organoids, extracellular vesicle (EV)-loaded

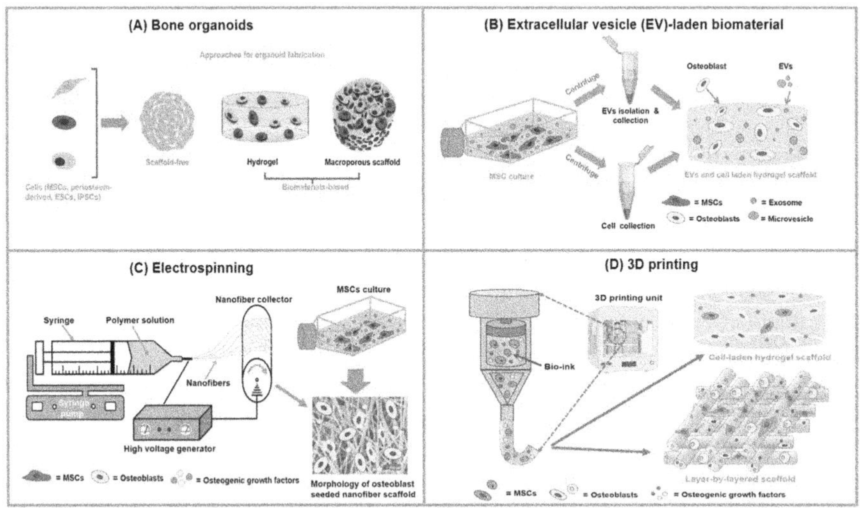

FIGURE 10.3 The schematic diagrams represent the scaffold-based 3D biomimetic scaffold fabrication process for bone tissue scaffold using (a) organoids, (b) EVs, (c) electrospinning, and (d) 3D printing techniques.

scaffolds (EVs), electrospun nanofiber-based and 3D printed-based scaffolds have become feasible choices for treating and reconstructing broken bones. Figure 10.3 depicts the whole approach of scaffold-based 3D biomimetic modeling, design, and fabrication for bone tissue scaffolds employing organoids, EVs, electrospinning, and 3D printing techniques. All of these cutting-edge technologies enable the incorporation of live cells and/or growth factors into scaffolds that attempt to mimic the biological and physicochemical composition of natural bone.

10.5.1 Bone Organoids

The native bone microenvironment is in 3D; however, current research in bone regeneration primarily focuses on the 2D study of cells. A 2D culture method homogeneously distributes drugs to all cells to study drug potential, resulting in incorrect results because the natural (*in vivo*) microenvironment is 3D and produces a drug gradient. Hence, animal models are being used to imitate the *in vivo* situation. However, their usage is limited due to the higher cost involved and their dissimilarity in physiology to humans. 3D culture systems can bridge the 2D culture system and the *in vivo* milieu to address the constraints. For example, bone organoids are 3D, self-organized bone tissue structures that create oxygen and metabolic factor gradients. The construction of bone organoids uses Matrigels and synthetic hydrogels to support their self-organization. The woven bone organoid model developed by Hofmann stimulates MSC development into a self-growing coculture of osteoblasts (immature bone cells) and osteocytes (mature bone cells) [33]. The constructed system demonstrated a self-renewing model that has the potential to recreate the woven bone, also called osteogenesis *in vitro* [33].

10.5.2 Cell-Free Approach

Extracellular vesicles (EVs) are cell-secreted nanosized bilayered vesicles involved in paracrine signaling. These can be categorized into three types based on biogenesis and size: apoptotic bodies, microvesicles (MVs), and exosomes (Exos) [34]. As apoptotic bodies play a role in apoptosis, most regenerative studies focus on MVs and Exos for their therapeutic potential. EVs carry growth factors, mRNAs, miRNAs, proteins, and DNA as their cargo [35]. They are better attractive cell-free applications for regenerative medicine. The osteoinductive potential of EVs has recently been explored in bone regeneration. EVs secreted from MSCs and pre-osteoblasts are essential regulators of bone function, critically involved in mineralization processes, and possess various osteoblast-specific factors as their cargo. Biomaterial-based sustained deliveries of EVs can reduce the dosage requirement of EVs for treatment and avoid frequent injections of EVs by providing their prolonged delivery; as a result, they have recently caught the attention of clinical researchers. Table 10.1 summarizes a few examples of biomaterial-assisted

TABLE 10.1
Summary of Biomaterial and EVs-Based Approaches Used in BTE

Source of EVs	Biomaterial Used	Type of EVs	Study Done	Findings	References
MC3T3 cells	Alginate hydrogel	MVs, Exos, Total EVs	3D, *In vitro* (MC3T3 cells)	Both the fractions of MC3T3-EVs are osteoinductive, but the cumulative effect of EVs shows maximum osteoinductive potential	[35]
Human BMSCs	HyStem-HP hydrogel	Exos	*In vitro* (Human osteoblasts) and *in vivo* (SD rats)	*In vitro* experiments were done in a 2D system. Critical-size bone regeneration was observed using BMSC-EVs through the action of miR-196a	[37]
Human BMSCs	3D collagen hydrogels	Exos	*In vitro* (HMSCs) and *in vivo* (athymic nude mice)	Pro-osteogenic exosomes from human BMSCs demonstrated osteoinductive potential in 2D and 3D *in vitro* studies, and subcutaneous implantation of scaffold showed good osteogenic and angiogenic potential in athymic nude mice	[38]
BMSCs	Alginate-polycaprolactone (PCL)	MVs	*In vitro* (HUVECs) and *in vivo* (nude mice)	Osteoinductive and angiogenic potential of BMSCs-derived MVs was observed	[39]

cell-free delivery of EVs. The ability to generate artificially designed EVs means that EV-loaded scaffolds may be the new era of medication delivery technologies. The 3D microenvironment of scaffolds is known to elicit the secretion of EVs with enhanced therapeutic potential compared to 2D culture. Hence, biomaterials can offer an exciting application in bone repair, either as a secretome-containing cell-free system or as the persistent delivery vehicle for EVs with modulated content for improved therapeutic potential [36].

10.6 GROWTH FACTORS IN BONE REGENERATION

Growth factors play a crucial role at the defect site *in vivo* to attract progenitors and inflammatory cells, differentiate stem cells into osteoblasts, and support neovascularization [40]. Several growth factors promote tissue growth and play a physiologic function in bone fracture repair. For regulating cell behavior in bone repair and osteogenesis, PDGFs, FGFs, BMPs, TGF-ß, IGFs, and VEGFs have shown promising applications [41]. The various stages of bone regeneration, which include the initial inflammatory phase, soft callus development, mineralization, and bone remodeling, necessitate the involvement of multiple GFs in precise spatiotemporal patterns. For example, recruitment of stem cells at the location of the defect, angiogenesis, and osteogenesis must occur sequentially in the bone-repair process; as a result, growth factors like PDGF, VEGF, and BMPs must have a synergistic impact for effective bone regeneration [42].

One of the vital growth factors involved in osteogenesis is BMP-2, which induces MSC differentiation into osteoblasts and the proliferation of osteoblasts [43]. Although the osteoinductive potential of BMP-2 is well known, its dosage, mode of delivery, etc., need to be standardized as coatings of BMP-2 to the scaffold might not produce consistent results, or a higher dosage can cause adverse effects like ectopic bone formation [44]. Hence, controlled, sustained, sequential, and stimuli-responsive release of growth factors is obligatory for efficient bone repair, similar to in vivo conditions. For example, fibronectin-based hydrogel scaffolds were used for the controlled delivery of BMP-2, and VEGF achieved osteogenesis and angiogenesis *in vivo* [45]. A few examples of biomaterial-assisted delivery of growth factors are summarized in Table 10.2. Recent research investigated the efficacy of synthetic peptides as a replacement for growth factors [46] for osteoinduction and immunity processes involved in bone regeneration [47]. The clinical studies showed growth factors used at higher doses resulted in adverse effects like bone formation at the abnormal site, an antibody-based immune response that can lead to cancer [48]. To avoid the adverse effects of the original growth factor, peptide sequences or small molecules (e.g., SVAK-12) having similar therapeutic effects are used [49–51]. However, because of the smaller size and rapid diffusion through the scaffold, the required dosage of this biomimetics is higher than the growth factor [50,52].

TABLE 10.2
Differential Release of Growth Factor Assisted Using Biomaterials for BTE

Growth Factor	Biomaterial Used	Loading Approach	Release Strategy	Findings	References
BMP-7	Nano-hydroxyapatite/Poly (2-hydroxyethyl methacrylate) hydrogel	Entrapment	Sustained delivery	Osteogenic differentiation of BMSCs	[53]
BMP-2	Nanocrystalline hydroxyapatite	Adsorption	Sustained	Osteogenic markers expressed significantly in *in vitro* study and ectopic bone formation in mice	[54]
rhBMP-2, VEGF	*O*-Carboxymethyl chitosan/hydroxyapatite collagen hydrogel	rhBMP-2 encapsulation in microspheres and VEGF encapsulation in chitosan/hydroxyapatite collagen hydrogel	Sustained and Sequential	The osteoinductive potential of dual growth factor encapsulated scaffold was observed *in vivo* and *in vitro* studies	[55]
BMP-2, FGF-2	Chitosan-collagen/poly(lactic acid)-poly(ethylene glycol)–poly(lactic acid) hydrogel	Entrapment/Microsphere encapsulation	Sequential	*In vivo* bone regeneration observed in rat skull defect model	[56]

10.7 3D PRINTING

It is also known as 'bioprinting', a standard method of placing cells in precise 3D arrangements. Unlike *in vitro* culture systems, the effect of single-cell interactions cannot be extrapolated to the tissue level as it is a much more complex system with different cell interactions. Hence, printing multiple cells will be more relevant for promising results in future bioprinting areas. To construct tissue architectures, a solution of biomaterials or a mixture of various biomaterials is commonly utilized as a hydrogel that encapsulates the required cell types throughout the bioprinting process. Acellular bioprinting and cellular bioprinting are the two types of 3D bioprinting [57]. Droplet-based, extrusion-based, and stereolithography are the three usual ways of cellular bioprinting, based on their processes of bioink deposition. Droplet-based bioprinting uses energy sources to pattern cell bioink micro-droplets with other active substances in an organized manner. It provides flexibility and precision in depositing biologicals such as cells, growth factors, and genes for tissue/

TABLE 10.3
Examples of 3D-Bioprinting Approaches Used in BTE

Biomaterial Used for 3D Printing	Type of Scaffold	Cells Used	Findings	References
Gelatin/alginate/ hydroxyapatite	Composite	Human BMSCs	Biocompatibility	[61]
Alginate, polydopamine nanoparticles, and tempo-oxidized cellulose nanofibrils	Hydrogels	MC3T3 cells	Osteoinductive, biocompatible, and mechanically more robust hydrogel was synthesized for BTE	[62]
Chitosan, glycerophosphate, hydroxyethyl cellulose, and cellulose nanocrystals	Hydrogels	MC3T3 cells	Osteogenesis observed in pre-osteoblasts with enhanced alkaline phosphatase secretion, mineralization, and ECM secretion	[63]

organ regeneration. Extrusion-based bioprinting employs mechanical or electromagnetic methods to deposit cells in a 'needle-syringe' fashion. Bioink injected by a deposition mechanism efficiently prints cell-laden filaments that create desired 3D structures during bioprinting. High-precision designs may be produced using stereolithography-based bioprinting, which employs laser energy to place cell-laden bioink in a reservoir through beam scanning. It has more advantages because of its exact control over biological deposition and high resolution [58]. 3D printing involves manufacturing implants based on specific shapes derived from computer-aided design (CAD) files. An FDA-approved 3D-printed porous device has been used as a cranial bone void filler [59]. Introducing shape-specific 3D-printed scaffolds for bone defects could be a landmark for BTE applications in the clinic. The 3D-bioprinting approach can also be used to create a bone disease model to avoid animal usage and investigate the mechanism of diseases or effects of drugs by mimicking osteoporosis or osteosarcoma conditions in the 3D microenvironment [60]. A summary of different 3D-bioprinting approaches used in BTE is discussed in Table 10.3.

10.8 INTERPENETRATING NETWORK HYDROGELS

Hydrogels mimic cell ECM with a porous structure and a higher swelling degree. Natural and synthetic polymers and their composites, have been used to synthesize hydrogels for a decade based on application. Natural polymers are preferred as they have higher biocompatibility and cell-binding sites but mostly lack mechanical strength. In contrast, synthetic polymers are explored primarily because of their holding ability as per the application and higher mechanical strength. The natural strength of cancellous bone is 10–50 MPa, which should be imitated to the maximum level in the scaffold to achieve efficient bone growth [64]. However, as the bone application requires scaffolds with higher mechanical strength, hydrogels do not have much mechanical strength as a single network. Therefore, to achieve up to fourfold increased mechanical strength compared to a single network, more than one network of polymers is used by the interpenetrating approach without affecting individual networks' physical or chemical properties [10]. Interpenetrating networks (IPNs) is one of the milestones in BTE.

10.9 MINERALIZED MICROENVIRONMENT

As discussed earlier, the mineral composition of bone is around 60%–70% calcium and phosphorus. Bone minerals, or hydroxyapatite, favor cell attachment, expansion, and osteoblastic differentiation of stem cells as they mimic natural bone conditions. Hence, it is widely used in most BTE scaffolds, and the biodegradation of hydroxyapatite causes the release of a phosphate group, which is utilized in the production of adenosine triphosphate (ATP). Increased levels of ATP activate osteoinductive genes, resulting in the osteogenic differentiation of stem cells [65]. The calcium to phosphorus ratio is the crucial factor that determines its acidity and solubility. In hydroxyapatite, this ratio is 1.67, causing lower acidity and solubility, whereas β-TCP has a Ca/P ratio close to 1.5, making it more degradable than hydroxyapatite [66]. Hence, the Ca/P ratio is a vital component in BTE scaffold fabrication, and scaffolds could be modified by creating nucleation sites for native stem cells. Scaffolds could be coated with hydroxyapatite, or a mineralized microenvironment can be made by encapsulating nano-hydroxyapatite crystal-coated microspheres into a scaffold for sustained delivery of minerals [67,68].

10.10 THREE-DIMENSIONAL MICROENVIRONMENT FOR CARTILAGE TISSUE

Indeed, the last 20 years have seen a considerable increase in biomaterial science, mechanobiology, and manufacturing techniques, all of which could potentially benefit cartilage regeneration. The development of biomaterials has led to the development of a broad range of formulations, from biocompatible and biodegradable polymers to the third-generation hydrogels now being used, which have cutting-edge chemistries to promote natural tissue regeneration [69–71]. Cell culture is one of the most fundamental processes in the biomaterials and tissue engineering fields. It includes removing cells from biological tissues, mimicking their *in vivo* survival environment to ensure advancement and reproduction, and keeping their primary structures and functions under sterile conditions with the appropriate temperatures, pH, and nutrition levels [72]. *In vitro* cell culture techniques available today include 2D adherent culture and 3D spherical culture, with the former being the more extensively utilized [73,74]. In this approach, a glass or polystyrene plate provides mechanical support for the cells, while external nutrition and metabolite elimination are maintained under the same conditions. The settings are well managed, and the cells are easy to inspect and collect. However, the 2D technique has limitations because it does not replicate complicated cell microenvironments. As cells develop in a limited environment in 2D culture, they are susceptible to contact inhibition, resulting in slower cell development and altered cell shape and function [75].

Cells in our bodies respond to stimuli from a very complex, 3D milieu by performing bioactivities. The composition and location of cell-ECM and cell-cell interactions alter fundamental cellular activities and are linked to organ function. When examining cell clusters in 3D culture systems, the aggregates create nutrient access and waste accumulation gradients. For example, the surfaces of aggregated spheroids have the highest amounts of proliferation; however, the cores of 3D cell bodies have the most significant quantity of dormant or necrotic cells [73]. As a result, it could be used in tissue engineering, regenerative medicine, drug discovery, toxicity testing, and organoid and assembly structure creation. Unfortunately, due to insufficient cultural contexts, 3D culture technology is still in its infancy, with high expenditures and a gap between culture and real-life happenings in the body. The current research priority is on how to continue to fortify technology to bring the 3D culture system closer to the native tissue microenvironment, how to achieve an efficient and automated culture system while lowering costs, and how to better exploit the benefits of diverse materials in the design due to cell viability and differentiation limitations.

As far as cartilage tissue is concerned, the 3D environment should be designed in a particular way that can give it enough mechanical strength and cell survivability. Using biomaterials as scaffolds to carry immunomodulatory cells, proteins, or medications could be an effective cartilage repair strategy. Creating an optimal cartilage model remains a difficult task in tissue engineering. Indeed, cartilage is a sophisticated structure that can endure high compressive stresses during daily activities. Capturing these mechanical properties by joining cells and scaffolds is one of the most challenging tasks in developing an *in vitro* cartilage model. This framework should enable cell proliferation, chondrogenic differentiation, and the retention of freshly created extracellular matrix within the scaffold, resulting in a tissue that accurately replicates cartilage architecture and properties [76]. Materials' physical qualities, such as stiffness, form, surface features, and pore size, can elicit various immunological responses [77]. To induce hyaline-like structures *in vitro*, mesenchymal stem cells must be seeded and grown in 3D configurations, which can take on a variety of shapes depending on the geometry and physicochemical qualities of the surrounding cells. The 3D structure of the cell determines its commitment to chondrogenic development. Because of loading transmission effects, dynamic loading, which is also a stimulus, can change the 3D configuration that determines differentiation, reversing the impact of adherent and non-adherent environments. Because the investigations look at how undifferentiated mesenchymal stem cells respond to diverse cell adhesion patterns in hydrogels and scaffolds, more research into the interaction of mechanical loading and 3D structure is required [78]. The scaffold can direct cartilage tissue growth by transporting seeded cells and growth nutrients to restore damaged cartilage. A biocompatible and biodegradable scaffold material with a flexible and porous 3D structure integrated with articular cartilage would be ideal [77]. Table 10.4 outlines recent achievements in constructing an optimal cartilage tissue engineering scaffold that mimics native microenvironment characteristics.

TABLE 10.4
Recent Developments in 3D Biomaterials-Based Models Explored Mimicking Cartilage-Related Microenvironment Factors to Study the Cartilage Tissue Regeneration

No.	Biomaterial	Polymer Used	Observation/Outcome	References
1.	Hydrogel	Tyrosine-crosslinked Alginate sulfate tyramine (ASTA)	Strong adherence to native cartilage with increased bond strength	[79]
2.	Hydrogel	Polyvinyl Alcohol/ Collagen II (PVA/ Col-II)	There are no adverse effects on cell viability or proliferation	[80]
3.	Injectable Hydrogels	Hyaluronate modified with β-cyclodextrin (β-CD) and adamantane (Ad)		
[HA-CD, HA-Ad]	*In vitro* and *in vivo*, chondrogenic differentiation, and ECM deposition. Significant evidence of cartilage tissue regeneration in defect model rats.			[81]
4.	Hydrogel	PCL-PEG-PCL diacrylate (IPN)	Low cytotoxicity, good biocompatibility	[82]
5.	Injectable IPN hydrogel	Alginate/cartilage ECM	Improved compression modulus, considerable capacity in mimicking the native cartilage tissue	[83]
6.	Cryogel	Hyaluronic acid	A favorable milieu for chondrocyte adhesion, proliferation, and matrix biosynthesis. Complete recovery of cryogels after injecting without disturbing the metabolism or viability of encapsulated cells	[84]
7.	Cryogel	Methacrylated Gelatin + Hyaluronic acid	GelMA has high mechanical stability due to cryogelation and chemical crosslinking. Appropriate pore size.	[85]
8.	Nanofibers	Polylactide (PLA)/ Gelatin + Chondroitin sulfate	Significant increase in Collagen II and Aggrecan markers *in vitro*. It inhibited inflammatory effects *in vivo*.	[86]

(*Continued*)

TABLE 10.4 (*Continued*)
Recent Developments in 3D Biomaterials-Based Models Explored Mimicking Cartilage-Related Microenvironment Factors to Study the Cartilage Tissue Regeneration

No.	Biomaterial	Polymer Used	Observation/Outcome	References
9.	Nanofibers	PLGA	Significantly increased chondrocyte adhesion and proliferation and aided in developing matured cartilage tissue.	[87]
10.	Nanofibers	PCL + dECM	Prominent chondrogenic differentiation	[88]

10.11 PROSPECTS OF THE 3D MICROENVIRONMENT

Constructing a concrete scaffold system mimicking the native tissue microenvironment to repair and rejuvenate avascular tissue is complex. However, it can be made possible with the help of existing biomaterial strategies with guided physical and biological microenvironment cues and material types.

10.11.1 Biomaterial Types and Geometry

10.11.1.1 Hydrogels

Hydrogels are gaining popularity due to their prospective applications, particularly in food, tissue engineering, cosmetics, and pharmaceutical administration. When exposed to an aqueous-based solvent, the hydrophilic nature of the 3D network members allows hydrogels to swell and absorb a massive amount of water [89]. With the correct combination of IPN polymers, a viable scaffolding system for cartilage tissue regeneration can be created.

10.11.1.2 Interpenetrating Network

A polymer composed of two or more networks partially integrated on a polymer scale but not covalently bound is referred to as an IPN. It is characterized as an IPN network because the two networks are physically connected but independent [67]. Compared with a single network, an IPN enhances mechanical properties and stability in tensile strength. Due to the complexity of its network, the most apparent advantage of this technology is that it provides a reinforced structure. IPN biomimetics also improve the final output loop structure. ECM-derived materials, on the other hand, can be non-crosslinked particles in the form of cartilage scaffolds or thermally crosslinked solutions at 37°C. The crosslinker should allow injectable hydrogels to gel reasonably while providing minimal cytotoxicity to the encapsulated cells [90]. The capacity to encapsulate live cells and the potential utility of IPN or semi-IPN scaffolds with superior mechanical integrity make the 3D structure more stable [10].

10.11.1.3 Cryogels

The scaffold should contain an interconnected open macroporous network for tissue engineering objectives to allow unimpeded cell penetration and transfer of nutrients, oxygen, and waste products. Cryogels are porous hydrogels with neutral, anionic, and cationic functionalities. They are 3D materials that are extensively crosslinked and have a dense network of interconnecting pores ranging in size from 1 to 100 μm. Such scaffolds are classified as selective adsorbents due to their outstanding structural characteristics and flow dynamics. Binding biomolecules in tissue engineering scaffolds promote cell proliferation and attachment [91]. The chemical interactions of a ligand with the polymeric backbone are at the heart of composite cryogels. The ligand is chosen and developed specifically for interaction with a biomolecule. To test the selective binding of biomolecules, supermacroporous composite cryogels are usually treated with a ligand. The absorptivity of a scaffold toward biomolecules is favorable for tissue regeneration and is dependent on factors such as scaffold structure, porosity, and mechanical integrity. It has been reported previously that 80%–90% porosity with a pore size of 50–135 μm is suitable for tissue regeneration [92]. Some synthetic polymers create resistance in adsorption capacity, but incorporating ECM components can tune the scaffold, making it feasible for a tissue to regenerate. For example, hyaluronic acid, the main ECM component of cartilage tissue, if added to the cryogels, can enable the adsorption capacity of water and other nutrients, thus creating a favorable microenvironment for cell adhesion, proliferation, and differentiation [93].

Imprinted cryogels are an ideal alternative to nonselective adsorbents because of their short diffusion path, short residence period, wide pores, and low pressure drop. However, large holes inside the cryogel have a low adsorption capability for specific molecules or ions. It is critical to improving the binding ability of extremely macroporous cryogels in actual adsorption phenomena. As a result, composite cryogels would be an excellent alternative for increasing surface area. This technique gives cryogels a more streamlined selection strategy and improved adsorption properties. Various methods for producing composite cryogels have been recorded, including embedding microbeads, polymer particles, nanoparticles, and the interlocking of IPN into cryogels [94].

10.11.2 Nanofibers

Nanofibers that are quickly drawn with the help of the electrospinning technique can also be used to regenerate cartilage tissue [95]. The mechanical properties of the scaffold will be improved by the layer-by-layer construction of a nanofiber sheet and an IPN hydrogel sheet. Incorporating relevant growth factors or stem cells into an IPN sheet will aid in depositing ECM and vascularizing newly formed tissue *in vivo*. *In vitro* and *in vivo*, adding/modifying the scaffold using peptides may help manage the scaffold's breakdown rates. The ideas, thoughts, and novel designs for this therapy technique are still in their infancy [96].

10.12 INCORPORATING CHONDRO-INDUCTIVE MOLECULES

The ability of a specific mix of growth factors and scaffolds to effectively induce cartilage regeneration has piqued the interest of modern researchers. A significant trend in cartilage tissue engineering is the development of a controlled delivery system that provides adequate structural support for the formation of neo-cartilage while enabling the spatiotemporal administration of growth factors to precisely and fully exercise their chondrogenic potential [97]. Growth factors are peptides that attach to transmembrane receptors on target cells, allowing them to increase, migrate, and differentiate. The signal transduction system may launch specific cellular processes when many receptors are engaged. MSC proliferation and chondrogenic differentiation were enhanced in the presence of TGF-ß, and ECM synthesis was improved, inhibiting ECM breakdown [98–100]. At the same time, IGF was responsible for maintaining cartilage homeostasis and repairing articular chondrocytes repairing. BMP was found to encourage the recruitment of ECM components such as collagen and proteoglycan and their production [101]. Similarly, IGF aided in the proliferation of chondrocytes and MSCs, enhanced ECM synthesis, and preserved the phenotype of cartilage [102].

10.13 EXTRACELLULAR VESICLES/SECRETOME FOR IMPROVED CHONDROGENESIS

Exosomes and microvesicles are EVs with bilayer lipids that store cargo or necessary information, such as nucleic acids and proteins. They regulate several biological processes, such as cell growth, mobility, and proliferation, and have a role in cell communication and signaling. EVs have recently received much attention in tissue engineering and regenerative medicine. Many *in vivo* and *in vitro* investigations have sought to assess these microstructures' chondrogenesis capability and involvement in cartilage regeneration [103]. The possibility of employing the MSC secretome as an alternative acellular form of cell treatment for various tissue injury reasons is being investigated. On the other hand, EVs supplied via bolus injections are swiftly sequestered and removed. Biomaterials provide delivery platforms to boost EV retention rates and healing efficacy. It is challenging to transfer EVs to disease sites in an efficient and controlled manner. However, restoring joint homeostasis and having a long-term positive influence on the healing process are crucial. Intra-articular EV injection, scaffold surface coating, intravenous EV injection, and embedding in a hydrogel matrix are all examples of EV delivery methods. Systemic EV injection can passively target inflammatory joints, as found in arthritic joints, because of increased synovial vascular permeability. Intra-articular EV injections can be combined with other treatments or regenerative cells and delivered directly to the diseased site.

10.14 FUTURE PERSPECTIVES

A complex interaction of physicochemical and biological parameters in the native stem cell niche influences stem cell fate. Engineering efforts to retain stemness and guide *ex vivo* differentiation have been inspired by native stem cell microenvironments. Controlling key determinants of stem cell fate, such as matrix topography (microscale structure), architecture, mechanics, biochemistry, and cell-cell and cell-matrix interactions, is possible with polymeric biomaterials. Developing a BTE scaffold that provides a microenvironment for stem cells is still in its early stages. Numerous issues like mechanical characteristics, degradation rate, architecture, topology, geometry, and biological activity must be addressed. The physiological activity of the cells in the presence of a biomaterial-based scaffold and the time necessary for MSC to differentiate into chondrocytes and osteoblasts as an essential clinical manifestation are critical elements to consider when constructing an ideal microenvironment with a bone and cartilage tissue engineering scaffold [104]. Furthermore, improving scaffold characteristics for successful bone and cartilage regeneration necessitates multi-length scale, multi-disciplinary approaches. 3D-printed shape-specific scaffolds can be alternatives to current traditional approaches for efficient bone and cartilage repair and the translation of tissue engineering-based therapies to the clinic. In addition, using bioreactors in tissue engineering to produce a microenvironment for bone and cartilage-related cells that can mimic the *in vivo* environment to aid the development of bone and cartilage tissue replacements is an essential strategy. However, because its bio-simulation of 3D structure and biochemical composition is not as excellent as scaffolds, combining these two technologies in stem cell culture, expansion, and guided differentiation will significantly advance bone and cartilage tissue engineering [105]. Increasing clinical popularity and industrial mass manufacturing are still a long way off for perfect bone and cartilage tissue engineering materials. However, advances in scaffold construction for bone and cartilage will be made with a more in-depth investigation into the bone and cartilage tissue microenvironment.

10.15 CONCLUSION

Bone and cartilage tissue engineering is an emerging field with economic benefits over traditional treatment strategies for bone damage or diseased conditions. The 3D microenvironment created in scaffolds mimics *in vivo* bone conditions, providing similar cell-cell and cell-matrix interactions. Recent advances in BTE, like the organoid model system, mineralized microenvironment, growth factors and their mimicry, 3D bioprinting, and IPN approach, could be the key to current limitations of BTE scaffold fabrication. Similarly, advances in 3D biomaterial scaffolding systems allow the articular cartilage to repair and rejuvenate. The 3D matrix is provided with an adequate framework that replicates the natural microenvironment of cartilage tissue by incorporating chondro-inducing growth factors and secretomes. Cartilage being an avascular and challenging tissue to regenerate, such 3D constructs/biomimetic systems enhance the therapeutic potential of chondrocytes and aesthetically repair the cartilage tissue.

REFERENCES

1. Oro F.B., Sikka R.S., Wolters B., Graver R., Boyd J.L., Nelson B., et al. Autograft versus allograft: An economic cost comparison of anterior cruciate ligament reconstruction. *Arthroscopy: The Journal of Arthroscopic & Related Surgery*. 2011;27:1219–25.
2. Sutherland A.J., Converse G.L., Hopkins R.A., Detamore M.S. The bioactivity of cartilage extracellular matrix in articular cartilage regeneration. *Advanced Healthcare Materials*. 2015;4:29–39.
3. Singh A., Yadav C., Tabassum N., Bajpeyee A., Verma V. Stem cell niche: Dynamic neighbor of stem cells. *European Journal of Cell Biology*. 2019;98:65–73.

4. Ceafalan L.C., Enciu A.-M., Fertig T.E., Popescu B.O., Gherghiceanu M., Hinescu M.E., et al. Heterocellular molecular contacts in the mammalian stem cell niche. *European Journal of Cell Biology*. 2018;97:442–61.
5. Wong V.W., Levi B., Rajadas J., Longaker M.T., Gurtner G.C. Stem cell niches for skin regeneration. *International Journal of Biomaterials*. 2012;2012:926059.
6. Schofield R. The relationship between the spleen colony-forming cell and the haemopoietic stem cell. *Blood Cells*. 1978;4:7–25.
7. Qi J., Yu T., Hu B., Wu H., Ouyang H. Current biomaterial-based bone tissue engineering and translational medicine. *International Journal of Molecular Sciences*. 2021;22:10233.
8. Qu H., Fu H., Han Z., Sun Y. Biomaterials for bone tissue engineering scaffolds: A review. *RSC Advances*. 2019;9:26252–62.
9. Aamodt J.M., Grainger D.W. Extracellular matrix-based biomaterial scaffolds and the host response. *Biomaterials*. 2016;86:68–82.
10. DeKosky B.J., Dormer N.H., Ingavle G.C., Roatch C.H., Lomakin J., Detamore M.S., et al. Hierarchically designed agarose and poly (ethylene glycol) interpenetrating network hydrogels for cartilage tissue engineering. *Tissue Engineering Part C: Methods*. 2010;16:1533–42.
11. Kowalczewski C.J., Saul J.M. Biomaterials for the delivery of growth factors and other therapeutic agents in tissue engineering approaches to bone regeneration. *Frontiers in Pharmacology*. 2018;9:513.
12. Komori T., Yagi H., Nomura S., Yamaguchi A., Sasaki K., Deguchi K., et al. Targeted disruption of Cbfa1 results in a complete lack of bone formation owing to maturational arrest of osteoblasts. *Cell*. 1997;89:755–64.
13. Otto F., Thornell A.P., Crompton T., Denzel A., Gilmour K.C., Rosewell I.R., et al. Cbfa1, a candidate gene for cleidocranial dysplasia syndrome, is essential for osteoblast differentiation and bone development. *Cell*. 1997;89:765–71.
14. Nakashima K., Zhou X., Kunkel G., Zhang Z., Deng J.M., Behringer R.R., et al. The novel zinc finger-containing transcription factor osterix is required for osteoblast differentiation and bone formation. *Cell*. 2002;108:17–29.
15. Komori T. Regulation of osteoblast differentiation by transcription factors. *Journal of Cellular Biochemistry*. 2006;99:1233–9.
16. Turinetto V., Vitale E., Giachino C. Senescence in human mesenchymal stem cells: Functional changes and implications in stem cell-based therapy. *International Journal of Molecular Sciences*. 2016;17:1164.
17. Ben-David U., Mayshar Y., Benvenisty N. Large-scale analysis reveals acquisition of lineage-specific chromosomal aberrations in human adult stem cells. *Cell Stem Cell*. 2011;9:97–102.
18. Bara J.J., Richards R.G., Alini M., Stoddart M.J. Concise review: Bone marrow-derived mesenchymal stem cells change phenotype following in vitro culture: Implications for basic research and the clinic. *Stem Cells*. 2014;32:1713–23.
19. Bartosh T.J., Ylöstalo J.H., Mohammadipoor A., Bazhanov N., Coble K., Claypool K., et al. Aggregation of human mesenchymal stromal cells (MSCs) into 3D spheroids enhances their antiinflammatory properties. *Proceedings of the National Academy of Sciences*. 2010;107:13724–9.
20. Bicer M., Cottrell G.S., Widera D. Impact of 3D cell culture on bone regeneration potential of mesenchymal stromal cells. *Stem Cell Research & Therapy*. 2021;12:31.
21. Cao J., Wang B., Tang T., Lv L., Ding Z., Li Z., et al. Three-dimensional culture of MSCs produces exosomes with improved yield and enhanced therapeutic efficacy for cisplatin-induced acute kidney injury. *Stem Cell Research & Therapy*. 2020;11:206.
22. Egger D., Tripisciano C., Weber V., Dominici M., Kasper C. Dynamic cultivation of mesenchymal stem cell aggregates. *Bioengineering*. 2018;5:48.

23. Almeria C., Weiss R., Roy M., Tripisciano C., Kasper C., Weber V., et al. Hypoxia Conditioned mesenchymal stem cell-derived extracellular vesicles induce increased vascular tube formation in vitro. *Frontiers in Bioengineering and Biotechnology.* 2019;7:292.
24. Watson D.C., Bayik D., Srivatsan A., Bergamaschi C., Valentin A., Niu G., et al. Efficient production and enhanced tumor delivery of engineered extracellular vesicles. *Biomaterials.* 2016;105:195–205.
25. Kwon S., Shin S., Do M., Oh B.H., Song Y., Bui V.D., et al. Engineering approaches for effective therapeutic applications based on extracellular vesicles. *Journal of Controlled Release.* 2021;330:15–30.
26. Noronha Nd.C., Mizukami A., Caliári-Oliveira C., Cominal J.G., Rocha J.L.M., Covas D.T., et al. Priming approaches to improve the efficacy of mesenchymal stromal cell-based therapies. *Stem Cell Research & Therapy.* 2019;10:131.
27. Katsuda T., Kosaka N., Takeshita F., Ochiya T. The therapeutic potential of mesenchymal stem cell-derived extracellular vesicles. *Proteomics.* 2013;13:1637–53.
28. Chen T.S., Arslan F., Yin Y., Tan S.S., Lai R.C., Choo A.B.H., et al. Enabling a robust scalable manufacturing process for therapeutic exosomes through oncogenic immortalization of human ESC-derived MSCs. *Journal of Translational Medicine.* 2011;9:1–10.
29. He J.-G., Li H.-R., Han J.-X., Li B.-B., Yan D., Li H.-Y., et al. GATA-4-expressing mouse bone marrow mesenchymal stem cells improve cardiac function after myocardial infarction via secreted exosomes. *Scientific Reports.* 2018;8:1–11.
30. Kang K., Ma R., Cai W., Huang W., Paul C., Liang J., et al. Exosomes secreted from CXCR4 overexpressing mesenchymal stem cells promote cardioprotection via akt signaling pathway following myocardial infarction. *Stem Cells International.* 2015;2015:659890.
31. Shi J., Zhao Y.-C., Niu Z.-F., Fan H.-J., Hou S.-K., Guo X.-Q., et al. Mesenchymal stem cell-derived small extracellular vesicles in the treatment of human diseases: Progress and prospect. *World Journal of Stem Cells.* 2021;13:49–63.
32. Salgado A.J., Coutinho O.P., Reis R.L. Bone tissue engineering: State of the art and future trends. *Macromolecular Bioscience.* 2004;4:743–65.
33. Chen S., Chen X., Geng Z., Su J. The horizon of bone organoid: A perspective on construction and application. *Bioactive Materials.* 2022;18:15–25.
34. Shao H., Im H., Castro C.M., Breakefield X., Weissleder R., Lee H. New technologies for analysis of extracellular vesicles. *Chemical Reviews.* 2018;118:1917–50.
35. Holkar K., Kale V., Ingavle G. Hydrogel-assisted 3D model to investigate the osteoinductive potential of MC3T3-derived extracellular vesicles. *ACS Biomaterials Science & Engineering.* 2021;7:2687–700.
36. Vermeulen S., Tahmasebi Birgani Z., Habibovic P. Biomaterial-induced pathway modulation for bone regeneration. *Biomaterials.* 2022;283:121431.
37. Qin Y., Wang L., Gao Z., Chen G., Zhang C. Bone marrow stromal/stem cell-derived extracellular vesicles regulate osteoblast activity and differentiation in vitro and promote bone regeneration in vivo. *Scientific Reports.* 2016;6: 21961.
38. Narayanan R., Huang C.-C., Ravindran S. Hijacking the cellular mail: Exosome mediated differentiation of mesenchymal stem cells. *Stem Cells International.* 2016;2016. doi: 10.1155/2016/3808674.
39. Xie H., Wang Z., Zhang L., Lei Q., Zhao A., Wang H., et al. Development of an angiogenesis-promoting microvesicle-alginate-polycaprolactone composite graft for bone tissue engineering applications. *Peer J.* 2016;4:e2040.
40. Kanczler J., Oreffo R. Osteogenesis and angiogenesis: The potential for engineering bone. *European Cells and Material* 2008;15:100–14.

41. Oliveira É.R., Nie L., Podstawczyk D., Allahbakhsh A., Ratnayake J., Brasil D.L., et al. Advances in growth factor delivery for bone tissue engineering. *International Journal of Molecular Sciences* 2021;22:903.
42. Shah N.J., Hyder M.N., Quadir M.A., Dorval Courchesne N.-M., Seeherman H.J., Nevins M., et al. Adaptive growth factor delivery from a polyelectrolyte coating promotes synergistic bone tissue repair and reconstruction. *Proceedings of the National Academy of Sciences.* 2014;111:12847–52.
43. Cho T.J., Gerstenfeld L.C., Einhorn T.A. Differential temporal expression of members of the transforming growth factor β superfamily during murine fracture healing. *Journal of Bone and Mineral Research.* 2002;17:513–20.
44. Groeneveld E., Burger E. Bone morphogenetic proteins in human bone regeneration. *European Journal of Endocrinology.* 2000;142:9–21.
45. Trujillo S., Gonzalez-Garcia C., Rico P., Reid A., Windmill J., Dalby M.J., et al. Engineered 3D hydrogels with full-length fibronectin that sequester and present growth factors. *Biomaterials.* 2020;252:120104.
46. Kesireddy V., Kasper F.K. Approaches for building bioactive elements into synthetic scaffolds for bone tissue engineering. *Journal of Materials Chemistry B.* 2016;4:6773–86.
47. Dang M., Saunders L., Niu X., Fan Y., Ma P.X. Biomimetic delivery of signals for bone tissue engineering. *Bone Research.* 2018;6:1–12.
48. Leijten J., Chai Y.C., Papantoniou I., Geris L., Schrooten J., Luyten F. Cell based advanced therapeutic medicinal products for bone repair: Keep it simple? *Advanced Drug Delivery Reviews.* 2015;84:30–44.
49. Saito A., Suzuki Y., Ogata S.I., Ohtsuki C., Tanihara M. Prolonged ectopic calcification induced by BMP-2–derived synthetic peptide. *Journal of Biomedical Materials Research Part A: An Official Journal of the Society for Biomaterials, The Japanese Society for Biomaterials, and The Australian Society for Biomaterials and the Korean Society for Biomaterials.* 2004;70:115–21.
50. Li J., Hong J., Zheng Q., Guo X., Lan S., Cui F., et al. Repair of rat cranial bone defects with nHAC/PLLA and BMP-2-related peptide or rhBMP-2. *Journal of Orthopaedic Research.* 2011;29:1745–52.
51. Kato S., Sangadala S., Tomita K., Titus L., Boden S.D. A synthetic compound that potentiates bone morphogenetic protein-2-induced transdifferentiation of myoblasts into the osteoblastic phenotype. *Molecular and Cellular Biochemistry.* 2011;349:97–106.
52. Wu B., Zheng Q., Guo X., Wu Y., Wang Y., Cui F. Preparation and ectopic osteogenesis in vivo of scaffold based on mineralized recombinant human-like collagen loaded with synthetic BMP-2-derived peptide. *Biomedical Materials.* 2008;3:044111.
53. Hou Y., Xu G., Guo Y., Shi J., Yuan W. In vitro evaluation of the nano-hydroxyapatite/hydrogel compound and its combination with BMP7 transfected bone marrow mesenchymal stem cells. *Journal of Biomaterials and Tissue Engineering.* 2017;7:1250–7.
54. Zhou M., Geng Y., Li S., Yang X., Che Y., Pathak J.L., et al. Nanocrystalline hydroxyapatite-based scaffold adsorbs and gives sustained release of osteoinductive growth factor and facilitates bone regeneration in mice ectopic model. *Journal of Nanomaterials.* 2019;2019. doi: 10.1155/2019/1202159.
55. Dou D., Zhou G., Liu H., Zhang J., Liu M., Xiao X., et al. Sequential releasing of VEGF and BMP-2 in hydroxyapatite collagen scaffolds for bone tissue engineering: Design and characterization. *International Journal of Biological Macromolecules.* 2019;123:622–8.
56. Min Q., Liu J., Yu X., Zhang Y., Wu J., Wan Y. Sequential delivery of dual growth factors from injectable chitosan-based composite hydrogels. *Marine Drugs.* 2019;17:365.

57. Bozkurt Y., Karayel E. 3D printing technology; methods, biomedical applications, future opportunities and trends. *Journal of Materials Research and Technology*. 2021;14:1430–50.
58. Cui H., Nowicki M., Fisher J.P., Zhang L.G. 3D bioprinting for organ regeneration. *Advanced Healthcare Materials*. 2017;6:1601118.
59. Probst F., Hutmacher D., Müller D., Machens H., Schantz J. Calvarial reconstruction by customized bioactive implant. *Handchirurgie, Mikrochirurgie, Plastische Chirurgie: Organ der Deutschsprachigen Arbeitsgemeinschaft fur Handchirurgie: Organ der Deutschsprachigen Arbeitsgemeinschaft fur Mikrochirurgie der Peripheren Nerven und Gefasse: Organ der V.* 2010;42:369–73.
60. Pavek A., Nartker C., Saleh M., Kirkham M., Khajeh Pour S., Aghazadeh-Habashi A., et al. Tissue engineering through 3D bioprinting to recreate and study bone disease. *Biomedicines*. 2021;9:551.
61. Luo Y., Lode A., Akkineni A.R., Gelinsky M. Concentrated gelatin/alginate composites for fabrication of predesigned scaffolds with a favorable cell response by 3D plotting. *RSC Advances*. 2015;5:43480–8.
62. Im S., Choe G., Seok J.M., Yeo S.J., Lee J.H., Kim W.D., et al. An osteogenic bioink composed of alginate, cellulose nanofibrils, and polydopamine nanoparticles for 3D bioprinting and bone tissue engineering. *International Journal of Biological Macromolecules*. 2022;205:520–9.
63. Maturavongsadit P., Narayanan L.K., Chansoria P., Shirwaiker R., Benhabbour S.R. Cell-laden nanocellulose/chitosan-based bioinks for 3D bioprinting and enhanced osteogenic cell differentiation. *ACS Applied Bio Materials*. 2021;4:2342–53.
64. Li Y., Liao C., Tjong S.C. Synthetic biodegradable aliphatic polyester nanocomposites reinforced with nanohydroxyapatite and/or graphene oxide for bone tissue engineering applications. *Nanomaterials*. 2019;9:590.
65. Shih Y.-R., Kang H., Rao V., Chiu Y.-J., Kwon S.K., Varghese S. In vivo engineering of bone tissues with hematopoietic functions and mixed chimerism. *Proceedings of the National Academy of Sciences*. 2017;114:5419–24.
66. Kim H.D., Amirthalingam S., Kim S.L., Lee S.S., Rangasamy J., Hwang N.S. Biomimetic materials and fabrication approaches for bone tissue engineering. *Advanced Healthcare Materials*. 2017;6:1700612.
67. Ingavle G., Avadhanam V., Zheng Y., Liu C., Sandeman S.J.B., Biomineralised interpenetrating network hydrogels for bone tissue engineering. *Bioinspired, Biomimetic and Nanobiomaterials*. 2016;5:12–23.
68. Hara E.S., Okada M., Nagaoka N., Nakano T., Matsumoto T. Re-evaluation of initial bone mineralization from an engineering perspective. *Tissue Engineering Part B: Reviews*. 2022;28:246–55.
69. Stampoultzis T., Karami P., Pioletti D.P. Thoughts on cartilage tissue engineering: A 21st century perspective. *Current Research in Translational Medicine*. 2021;69:103299.
70. Sancho-Tello M., Forriol F., de Llano J.J.M., Antolinos-Turpin C., Gómez-Tejedor J.A., Ribelles J.L.G., et al. Biostable scaffolds of polyacrylate polymers implanted in the articular cartilage induce hyaline-like cartilage regeneration in rabbits. *The International Journal of Artificial Organs*. 2017;40:350–7.
71. Fu T.-S., Wei Y.-H., Cheng P.-Y., Chu I., Chen W.-C. A novel biodegradable and thermosensitive poly (ester-amide) hydrogel for cartilage tissue engineering. *BioMed Research International*. 2018;2018:2710892.
72. Wu X., Su J., Wei J., Jiang N., Ge X. Recent advances in three-dimensional stem cell culture systems and applications. *Stem Cells International*. 2021;2021. doi: 10.1155/2021/9477332.
73. Duval K., Grover H., Han L.-H., Mou Y., Pegoraro A.F., Fredberg J., et al. Modeling physiological events in 2D vs. 3D cell culture. *Physiology*. 2017;32:266–77.

74. Seo J., Lee J.S., Lee K., Kim D., Yang K., Shin S., et al. Switchable water-adhesive, superhydrophobic palladium-layered silicon nanowires potentiate the angiogenic efficacy of human stem cell spheroids. *Advanced Materials.* 2014;26:7043–50.
75. Chaicharoenaudomrung N., Kunhorm P., Noisa P. Three-dimensional cell culture systems as an in vitro platform for cancer and stem cell modeling. *World Journal of Stem Cells.* 2019;11:1065.
76. Tortelli F., Cancedda R. Three-dimensional cultures of osteogenic and chondrogenic cells: A tissue engineering approach to mimic bone and cartilage in vitro. *European Cells and Materials.* 2009;17:1–14.
77. Yu W., Yin N., Yang Y., Xuan C., Liu X., Liu W., et al. Rescuing ischemic stroke by biomimetic nanovesicles through accelerated thrombolysis and sequential ischemia-reperfusion protection. *Acta Biomaterialia.* 2022;140:625–40.
78. Panadero J., Lanceros-Mendez S., Ribelles J.G. Differentiation of mesenchymal stem cells for cartilage tissue engineering: Individual and synergetic effects of three-dimensional environment and mechanical loading. *Acta Biomaterialia.* 2016;33:1–12.
79. Öztürk E., Stauber T., Levinson C., Cavalli E., Arlov Ø., Zenobi-Wong M. Tyrosinase-crosslinked, tissue adhesive and biomimetic alginate sulfate hydrogels for cartilage repair. *Biomedical Materials.* 2020;15:045019.
80. Lan W., Xu M., Zhang X., Zhao L., Huang D., Wei X., et al. Biomimetic polyvinyl alcohol/type II collagen hydrogels for cartilage tissue engineering. *Journal of Biomaterials Science, Polymer Edition.* 2020;31:1179–98.
81. Jeong S.H., Kim M., Kim T.Y., Kim H., Ju J.H., Hahn S.K. Supramolecular injectable hyaluronate hydrogels for cartilage tissue regeneration. *ACS Applied Bio Materials.* 2020;3:5040–7.
82. Su Z.C., Lin S.J., Chang Y.H., Yeh W.L., Chu I.M. Synthesis, characterization, and cytotoxicity of PCL–PEG–PCL diacrylate and agarose interpenetrating network hydrogels for cartilage tissue engineering. *Journal of Applied Polymer Science.* 2020;137:49409.
83. Shojarazavi N., Mashayekhan S., Pazooki H., Mohsenifard S., Baniasadi H. Alginate/cartilage extracellular matrix-based injectable interpenetrating polymer network hydrogel for cartilage tissue engineering. *Journal of Biomaterials Applications.* 2021;36:803–17.
84. He T., Li B., Colombani T., Joshi-Navare K., Mehta S., Kisiday J., et al. Hyaluronic acid-based shape-memory cryogel scaffolds for focal cartilage defect repair. *Tissue Engineering Part A.* 2021;27:748–60.
85. Jonidi Shariatzadeh F., Solouk A., Bagheri Khoulenjani S., Bonakdar S., Mirzadeh H. Injectable and reversible preformed cryogels based on chemically crosslinked gelatin methacrylate (GelMA) and physically crosslinked hyaluronic acid (HA) for soft tissue engineering. *Colloids Surf B Biointerfaces* 2021;203:111725.
86. Chen S., Chen W., Chen Y., Mo X., Fan C. Chondroitin sulfate modified 3D porous electrospun nanofiber scaffolds promote cartilage regeneration. *Materials Science and Engineering: C.* 2021;118:111312.
87. Shen Y., Xu Y., Yi B., Wang X., Tang H., Chen C., et al. Engineering a highly biomimetic chitosan-based cartilage scaffold by using short fibers and a cartilage-decellularized matrix. *Biomacromolecules.* 2021;22:2284–97.
88. Xu J., Fang Q., Liu Y., Zhou Y., Ye Z., Tan W.-S. In situ ornamenting poly (ε-caprolactone) electrospun fibers with different fiber diameters using chondrocyte-derived extracellular matrix for chondrogenesis of mesenchymal stem cells. *Colloids and Surfaces B: Biointerfaces.* 2021;197:111374.
89. Kadri R., Elkhoury K., Ben Messaoud G., Kahn C., Tamayol A., Mano J.F., et al. Physicochemical interactions in nanofunctionalized alginate/GelMA IPN hydrogels. *Nanomaterials.* 2021;11:2256.

90. Wang Y., Yu H., Yang H., Hao X., Tang Q., Zhang X. An injectable interpenetrating polymer network hydrogel with tunable mechanical properties and self-healing abilities. *Macromolecular Chemistry and Physics.* 2017;218:1700348.
91. Saylan Y., Denizli A. Supermacroporous composite cryogels in biomedical applications. *Gels.* 2019;5:20.
92. Zhou D., Shen S., Yun J., Yao K., Lin D.-Q. Cryo-copolymerization preparation of dextran-hyaluronate based supermacroporous cryogel scaffolds for tissue engineering applications. *Frontiers of Chemical Science and Engineering.* 2012;6:339–47.
93. Savina I.N., Zoughaib M., Yergeshov A.A. Design and assessment of biodegradable macroporous cryogels as advanced tissue engineering and drug carrying materials. *Gels.* 2021;7:79.
94. Shah S., Shaikh H., Memon N., Bhanger M.I., Qureshi T., Khan H., et al. Preparation, characterization, and binding profile of imprinted semi-IPN cryogel composite for aluminum. *Turkish Journal of Chemistry.* 2020;44:901–22.
95. Behere I., Pardawala Z., Vaidya A., Kale V., Ingavle G. Osteogenic differentiation of an osteoblast precursor cell line using composite PCL-gelatin-nHAp electrospun nanofiber mesh. *International Journal of Polymeric Materials and Polymeric Biomaterials.* 2021;70:1281–95.
96. Behere I., Ingavle G. In vitro and in vivo advancement of multifunctional electrospun nanofiber scaffolds in wound healing applications: Innovative nanofiber designs, stem cell approaches, and future perspectives. *Journal of Biomedical Materials Research Part A.* 2022;110:443–61.
97. Chen L., Liu J., Guan M., Zhou T., Duan X., Xiang Z. Growth factor and its polymer scaffold-based delivery system for cartilage tissue engineering. *International Journal of Nanomedicine.* 2020;15:6097.
98. Coricor G., Serra R. TGF-β regulates phosphorylation and stabilization of Sox9 protein in chondrocytes through p38 and Smad dependent mechanisms. *Scientific Reports.* 2016;6:1–11.
99. Derynck R., Zhang Y.E. Smad-dependent and Smad-independent pathways in TGF-β family signalling. *Nature.* 2003;425:577–84.
100. Ying J., Wang P., Zhang S., Xu T., Zhang L., Dong R., et al. Transforming growth factor-beta1 promotes articular cartilage repair through canonical Smad and Hippo pathways in bone mesenchymal stem cells. *Life Sciences.* 2018;192:84–90.
101. Whitty C., Pernstich C., Marris C., McCaskie A., Jones M., Henson F. Sustained delivery of the bone morphogenetic proteins BMP-2 and BMP-7 for cartilage repair and regeneration in osteoarthritis. *Osteoarthritis and Cartilage Open.* 2022;4:100240.
102. Liebesny P.H., Mroszczyk K., Zlotnick H., Hung H.-H., Frank E., Kurz B., et al. Enzyme pretreatment plus locally delivered HB-IGF-1 stimulate integrative cartilage repair in vitro. *Tissue Engineering Part A.* 2019;25:1191–201.
103. Song H., Zhao J., Cheng J., Feng Z., Wang J., Momtazi-Borojeni A.A., et al. Extracellular vesicles in chondrogenesis and cartilage regeneration. *Journal of Cellular and Molecular Medicine.* 2021;25:4883–92.
104. Birmingham E., Niebur G., McHugh P.E. Osteogenic differentiation of mesenchymal stem cells is regulated by osteocyte and osteoblast cells in a simplified bone niche. *European Cells and Materials.* 2012;23:13–27.
105. Hansmann J., Groeber F., Kahlig A., Kleinhans C., Walles H. Bioreactors in tissue engineering—principles, applications and commercial constraints. *Biotechnology Journal.* 2013;8:298–307.

11 Collagen-Based Functionalized Nanocomposite for Bone Tissue Regeneration

Sougata Ghosh
Kasetsart University
RK University

Sirikanjana Thongmee
Kasetsart University

Hisao Haniu
Shinshu University

Ebrahim Mostafavi
Stanford University School of Medicine

CONTENTS

11.1 Introduction 237
11.2 Collagen-Based Composites 239
  11.2.1 Hydroxyapatite 240
  11.2.2 Bioglass 240
  11.2.3 Chemical Polymers 242
  11.2.4 Natural Polymers 244
  11.2.5 Metal Nanoparticles 247
11.3 Conclusions and Future Perspectives 250
Acknowledgements 250
References 251

11.1 INTRODUCTION

Collagen constitutes almost one-third of the total proteins in the tissues and hence is predominantly found in both soft and hard tissues of mammals. Among the 28 different types of collagens, type I collagen is more abundant and widely distributed in the extracellular matrix (ECM) of different tissues, like bones, teeth, tendons, and

DOI: 10.1201/9781003251767-11

skin. The three interwoven chains (a-polypeptide chains) involving homotrimers or heterotrimers are the basic building blocks of collagen [1]. Thus, this natural protein is widely explored to develop biomaterial composites. Another significant advantage of collagen is its low immunogenicity, making it more popular for fabricating scaffolds with immense tissue engineering potential [2].

Collagen-based functionalized biomaterials can be fabricated essentially by rational crosslinking. Hence, collagen can be supplemented with other biomolecules such as alginate, glycosaminoglycans (GAG), elastin, hyaluronic acid, or chitosan. Physical crosslinking employing UV light and/or heat efficiently polymerizes the scaffolds, while chemical techniques involve treatment with formaldehyde or glutaraldehyde. However, enzymatic crosslinking agents such as transglutaminase are advantageous as they are more biocompatible and have more robust mechanical properties and resistance to enzymatic degradation [3].

Among various tissue engineering approaches, bone tissue engineering has gained much attention due to the complications during the treatment that often include non-unions, enormous tissue loss in traumatic injuries, postsurgical infections, or tumor-related bone resections [4]. Approximately two million bone graft-associated surgeries take place every year globally to address impairments in spontaneous healing. Hence, autografts, allografts, and xenografts are considered significant alternatives. Enormous challenges are often associated with these surgical procedures, including breaking of the donor site, loss of large segmental bones, mismatch due to morphologic alterations, and discomfort due to postsurgical pain. However, several limitations in grafting, like incompatibility, non-union, rapid erosion, and co-morbidities, have led to the exploration of novel scaffolds that can promote bone tissue regeneration and rapid healing [5]. There has been tremendous growth in the area of the grafting potential of collagen since the 19th century, as depicted in Figure 11.1 [5].

Collagen-based materials can be substituted with hydroxyapatite (HA), calcium phosphates, and bioactive glasses (BGs) for selective enhancement of the calcification capacity of bone. Since individually polymeric materials lack this property, fabrication of such composite materials helps cell adhesion and facilitates osseointegration. Furthermore, these materials can form an intermediate layer of HA, eventually forming a firm bond with bone at the implantation site [6]. Figure 11.2 illustrates the advancement in the field of nanomedicine that has led to the fabrication of effective

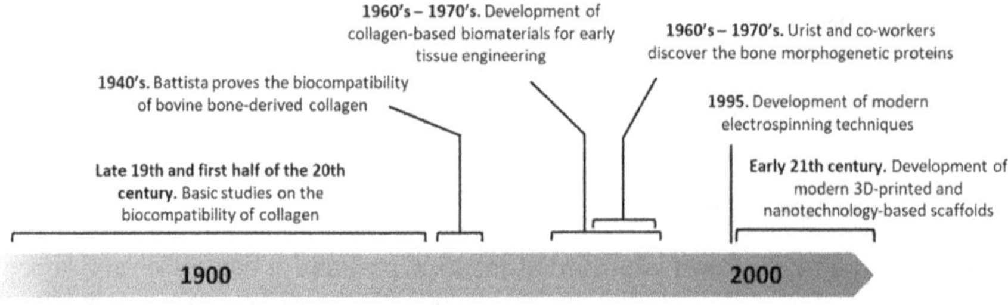

FIGURE 11.1 The timeline shows some of the major milestones in the development of collagen-based scaffolds for bone tissue engineering (BTE). Reprinted from [5].

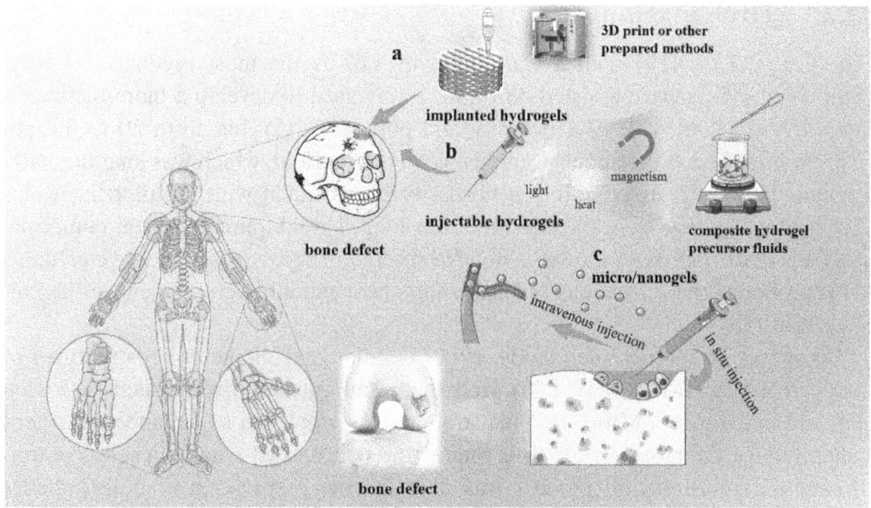

FIGURE 11.2 Different hydrogel systems based on biocompatible materials have been designed for obtaining ideal treatment in bone tissue engineering: (a) using 3D print technology, multi-crosslinking strategy, or nanoparticle composite design, various hydrogel scaffolds were implanted in bone defects through surgical intervention; (b) owing to the sol-gel property, rapid formation, and total filling of the defect site, injectable hydrogel can be easily injected into the bone injury site and formed a bionic scaffold under the external conditions of UV light, temperature change, or magnetic field effect. (c) In the field of nanotechnology applications, micro/nanogels have also gained wide application in bone tissue engineering because they possess two action pathways. One way is that micro/nanogels reach the lesion by intravenous injection; the other way is that an injectable hydrogel scaffold is formed by interconnected micro/nanogels in a bone defect. Reprinted with permission from [7]. Copyright © 2021 Wiley-VCH GmbH.

biomaterials for bone tissue engineering and drug delivery. Collagen-based three-dimensional (3D) bioprinted scaffolds, inorganic bone cement, and biocompatible hydrogels have provided potential therapeutic strategies for addressing bone injury [7]. Several techniques, like molecular self-assembly, electrospinning, and phase separation, are applied for generating biomimetic scaffolds comprised of collagen supplemented with other synthetic or natural polymers and nanomaterials [8,9].

In view of the background, this chapter elaborates on various collagen-based functionalized biomaterials with bone tissue engineering potential. Furthermore, the mechanisms behind the promotion of osteogenic induction, mineralization, and osseointegration are also discussed in detail.

11.2 COLLAGEN-BASED COMPOSITES

The major limitation of native collagen hydrogel is its low mechanical strength and high degradation rate. Hence, this section discusses several natural biopolymers, chemical polymers, BG, and even nanoparticles incorporated into collagen scaffolds to obtain multiple functionalities and superior mechanical properties.

11.2.1 Hydroxyapatite

HA ($Ca_{10}(PO_4)_6(OH)_2$) with a Ca/P ratio of 1.67 is the most predominant bone component. Microwave-assisted co-titration was used to develop a biomimetic collagen/HA scaffold with 72% porosity and pore sizes varying from 20 to 300 µm [10]. Prominent microchannels were visible in the scaffold, which was longitudinally aligned. The mineralized collagen fibrils were associated with intrafibrillar nano-HA crystallites that were mostly 10–30 nm long. Unlike pure collagen, composite scaffolds (with 75% HA) showed a notable six-fold increase in compressive modulus (3 MPa). Furthermore, increased tensile and shear moduli were evident in the collagen scaffold.

Likewise, in another such study, either cellular or lamellar microstructures of collagen-HA scaffolds were fabricated that were further incorporated with iron (Fe) and manganese (Mn) [11]. This strategy was employed to enhance the osteoinductivity of the biomaterials. It is interesting to note that a homogeneous or unidirectional freeze-drying process was used for the preparation of both lamellar and cellular structures, denoted by Col–HA-lamellar and Col–HA-cellular structures, respectively, from the intrafibrillar mineralized collagen hydrogels. Superior Young's modulus and high tensile strength were evident in the lamellar scaffolds, which favored adhesion of the osteoblast. The structure was dense with multiple collagen fibers that were both mineralized as well as interwoven, as evident from the scanning electron microscope (SEM) and transmission electron microscope (TEM) images in Figure 11.3. The lamellar scaffolds promoted osteogenic differentiation of the bone marrow mesenchymal stem cells (BMSCs). Significant gene expression was observed for collagen type I (Col1), osteoprotegerin (OPG), transcription factor Sp7 (Osterix), and Phex on day 14 while γ-carboxyglutamic acid-containing protein 1 (Bglapl) and DMP1 reached their peak on day 21. Incorporation of Fe/Mn in the collagen-based scaffolds was speculated to be a key determinant in promoting osteogenic gene expression.

11.2.2 Bioglass

Reinforcement of collagen-based scaffolds with BGs can lead to the enhancement of mechanical competence. The foam replica technique was used for the fabrication of collagen-coated highly porous 45S5 BG-based scaffolds [12]. Initially, the surface of the BG was cleaned so that the reactive –OH groups could be exposed, which were then functionalized with (3-aminopropyl)triethoxysilane (APTS) followed by immersion in a solution containing collagen. Gel formation occurred at 37°C, after which the scaffolds were dried at ambient temperature and treated with 1-ethyl-3-(3-dimethylaminopropyl)carbodiimide (EDC) and *N*-hydroxysuccinimide (NHS) for stabilization of the collagen layer due to crosslinking. Compressive strength of the composite scaffold was 0.18 ± 0.03 MPa. Sintering resulted in burning out of the sacrificial polyurethane (PU) foam, eventually exhibiting a hollow nature with highly interconnected pores ranging between 250 and 500 µm, identical to cancellous bone. Contraction of the collagen fibers during drying was accompanied

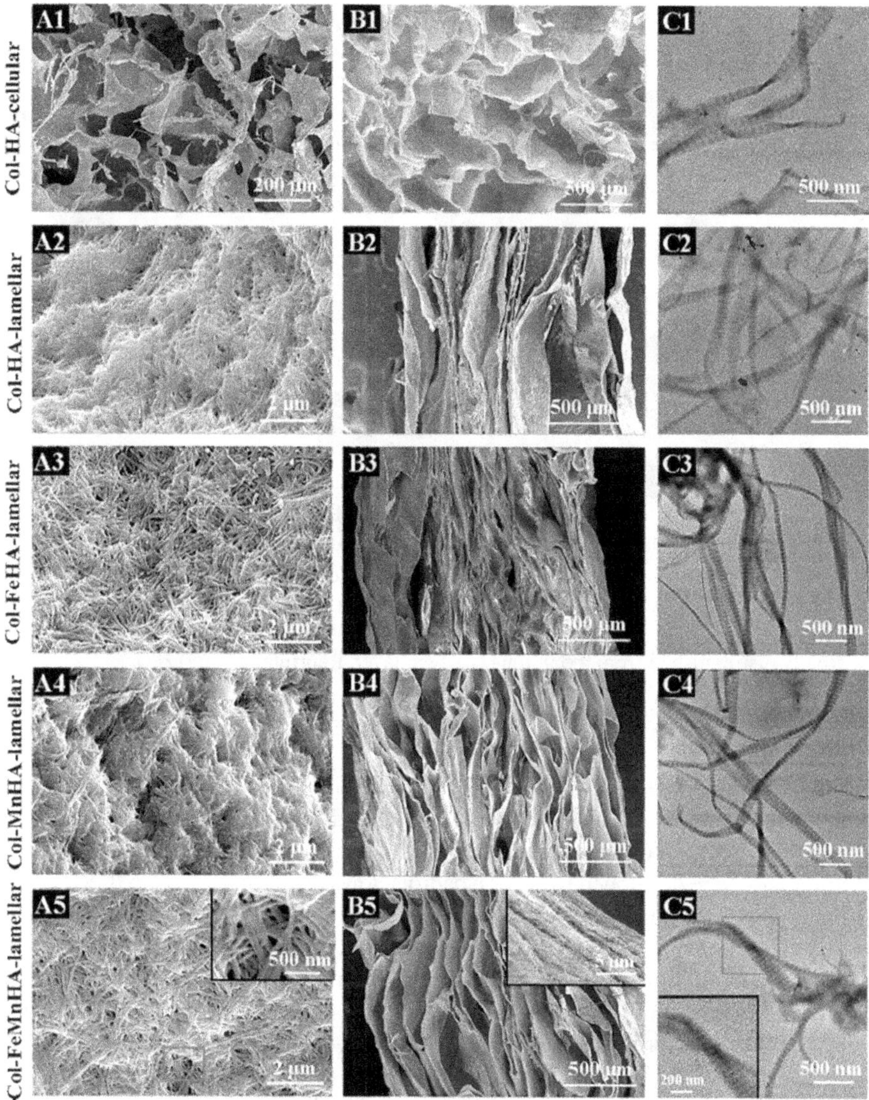

FIGURE 11.3 Surface (A1–A5) and cross-sectional (B1–B5) SEM morphologies and TEM (C1–C5) images of various scaffolds after freeze-drying. The insets in A5, B5, and C5 show the corresponding high-magnification images of the area of interest marked with red boxes. Reprinted with permission from [11]. Copyright © 2020 American Chemical Society.

by their orientation along the scaffold structure, finally covering the struts with a dense and homogenous layer, as evident from Figure 11.4. Scaffolds dipped in simulated body fluid (SBF) exhibited cauliflower shaped structures of HA deposited on the surface that completely covered the scaffolds after a period of 7 days. Osteoblast-like cells (MG-63) exhibited superior adherence and proliferation on the scaffold surface.

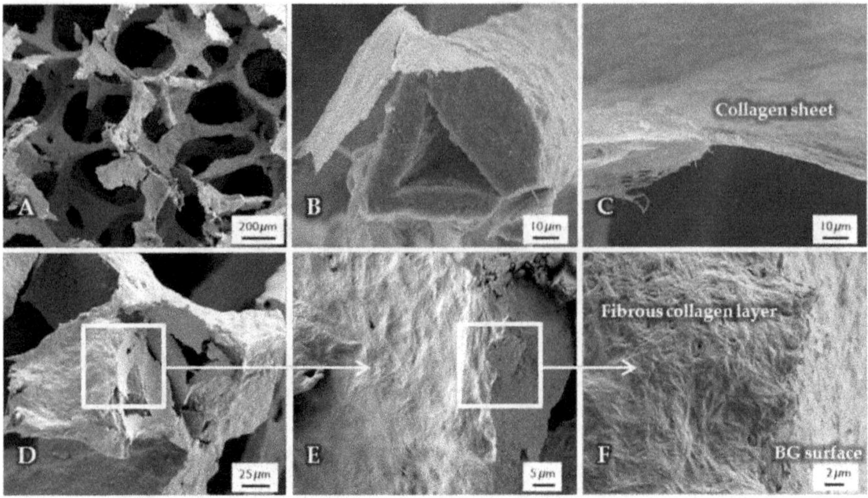

FIGURE 11.4 SEM images of uncrosslinked, collagen-coated BG-based scaffolds. The fibrous collagen layer can be clearly seen (b). After the coating process, the overall macroporosity of the scaffold is not affected (a). The collagen layer exhibits a thickness of a few micrometers (c). At the interface ((d–f), different magnifications), the rough BG surface can be clearly distinguished from the fibrous collagen layer. Reprinted from [12].

11.2.3 Chemical Polymers

Several chemically derived polymers are used for fiber matrix biofunctionalization, employing techniques like co-blending, physical adsorption, and covalent conjugation. Because of their close resemblance to the native tissue ECM, electrospun nanofiber matrices were developed using polycaprolactone (PCL) and chitosan (CS) blends [13]. Furthermore, the blend nanofibers were functionalized with type I collagen, which was accomplished by carbodiimide (EDC) coupling. The smooth nanofibers were 700–850 nm in diameter. The final collagen immobilization was 0.120 ± 0.016 μg onto a 1 cm^2 area of the electrospun PCL/CS nanofibers. Collagen functionalization significantly improved the adhesion, spreading, proliferation and osteogenic differentiation of the rat bone marrow-derived stromal cells (rBMSCs). Both osteogenic phenotypic markers, such as alkaline phosphatase (ALP) activity and mineralization, were upregulated on COL-PCL/CS scaffolds. Osteoinductive effect was confirmed by the elevated expression of osteocalcin (OCN), osteopontin (OPN) and ALP genes.

Yet in another study, poly(lactic-co-glycolic acid) was combined with collagen by solvent-induced phase inversion technique for delivery of a bone synthesizing drug, risedronate. Incorporation of collagen resulted in well-defined, continuous pores in the scaffold matrix [14]. Superior adhesion and high proliferation of the viable human bone osteosarcoma cells (Saos-2 cells) were evident on the risedronate-loaded scaffolds. Associated enhancement of the ALP activity with mineralization confirmed the osteogenic potential of the hybrid biomaterial [15]. used an alternate calcium and phosphate (Ca–P) solution dipping method for synthesis of nano-hydroxyapatite (n-HA) on both poly(lactide-co-glycolide) acid (PLGA) and blended PLGA/Col nanofibers. The functional groups of collagen significantly expedited the deposition of n-HA up to ninefold, which in turn remarkably enhanced the specific surface area of the PLGA/Col scaffolds. The resulting PLGA/Col nanofibers were 353 ± 81 nm in diameter, respectively. The nanocrystalline n-HA with a diameter of 50–70 nm was uniformly deposited on both the exterior and interior surfaces of the PLGA/Col scaffolds, resulting in spiky ridges and grooves as evident from Figure 11.5. The amount of n-HA in mineralized PLGA/Col was 73.9% ± 10.7. Human fetal osteoblast cells (hFOB 1.19) exhibited better cell adhesion on the surface and proliferation, which are considered as early stages of osteoblast behavior on n-HA functionalized scaffolds. However, the immediate/late stages associated with proliferation and differentiation were not prominent. Additionally, n-HA facilitated more protein secretion by the osteoblasts, as evident from Figure 11.5.

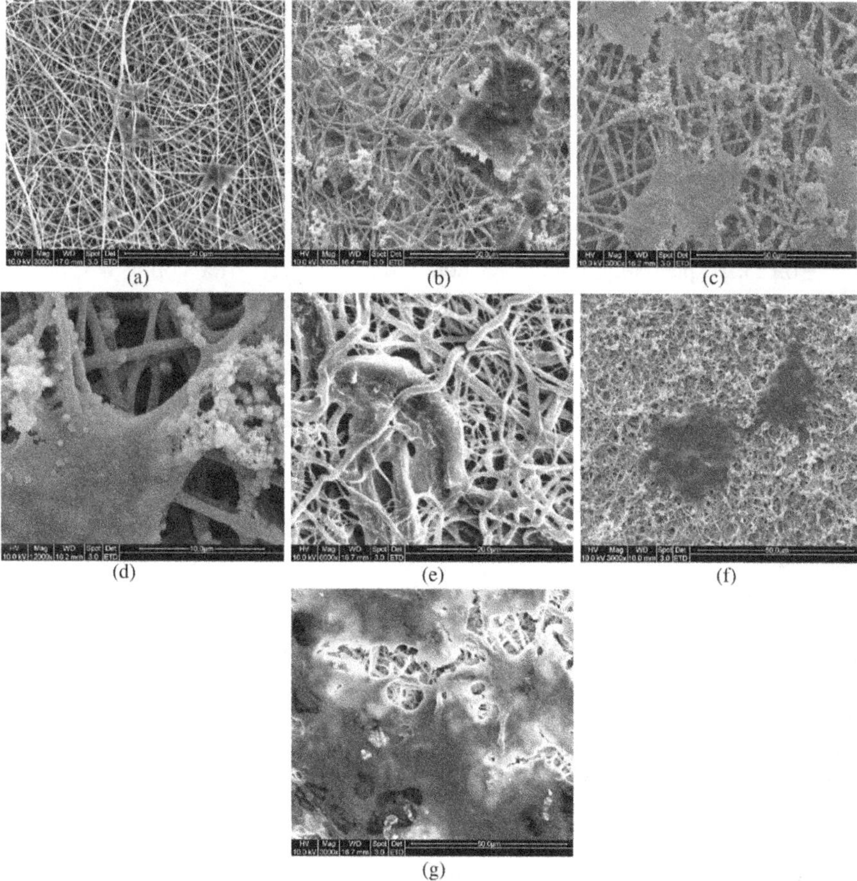

FIGURE 11.5 Osteoblasts on mineralized and non-mineralized nanofibers. (a) PLGA (day 1), (b) PLGA+n-HA (day 1), (c) PLGA+n-HA (day 4), (d) is the enlargement of the central part of (c), (e) PLGA/Col (day 1), (f) PLGA/Col+n-HA (day 1), and (g) PLGA/Col+n-HA (day 4). Reprinted with permission from [15]. Copyright © 2009 Elsevier Inc.

11.2.4 Natural Polymers

Biomedical applications of the scaffolds are largely dependent upon their biocompatibility, which is a critical factor for effective integration with the host tissue [16]. Apart from their mechanical robustness and tolerance to external local forces, the scaffolds must exhibit very low or no immunogenicity [17]. Another important property of the scaffold is its high biodegradability, with non-toxic degradation products that should be effectively metabolized and eliminated from the body [18]. Hence, naturally occurring biopolymers are often used for obtaining desirable topographical features that in turn modulate cellular behavior, adherence, proliferation, and differentiation.

Cellulose-based polysaccharide microspheres made from cellulose acetate (CA) and ethyl cellulose (EC) were sintered together into 3D porous scaffolds [19]. Surface functionalization with collagen type I nanofibers employing a molecular self-assembly strategy was carried out for 24 h with 0.1% (w/v) collagen type I solution at 37°C and pH 5.2. The scaffolds with optimum mechanical strength and pore volume were comprised of microspheres that were 600–700 μm in size. Homogenous distribution of the collagen nanofiber with a diameter of 140 ± 40 nm for CA scaffolds and 120 ± 34 nm for EC scaffolds was noted. Average maximum compressive modulus of the dry scaffolds was 266.75 ± 33.22 MPa, which reduced to 130.53 ± 13.97 MPa under wet conditions. Similarly, the strength (12.15 ± 2.23 MPa), load (225.14 ± 42.09 N) and energy at failure (0.34 ± 0.13 J) changed to 7.15 ± 1.24 MPa, 144.76 ± 24.43 N and 0.36 ± 0.12 J, respectively, under wet conditions. Porosity after collagen functionalization was $33.9\% \pm 5.2\%$, with an average pore diameter of 185.4 ± 8.6 μm. The human osteoblasts (HOB) exhibited enhanced adhesion and phenotype maintenance, apart from higher ALP activity and mineral deposition, when grown on the collagen-functionalized cellulose microsphere scaffolds.

Yet in another very interesting study, a hybrid hydrogel composed of genipin crosslinked collagen/chitosan/lysine-modified hyaluronic acid (ColChHAmod) was fabricated [20]. Hyaluronic acid (HA) was functionalized by lysine attachment via primary amine groups, resulting in HAmod. Stable architecture of the hydrogel was obtained by crosslinking with genipin, which resulted in covalent bond formation with other components of the complex hydrogel. Various physicochemical characteristics of the hydrogel, such as swelling, wettability, and susceptibility to enzymatic degradation, could be modulated by varying the concentration of the HAmod and genipin. The resulting ColChHAmod-based hydrogel with 85%–95% exhibited promising injectability and rheological properties. A 90% weight loss after treatment with collagenase confirmed the high degradability of the hydrogel, although it is largely dependent on the chemical composition. The composite scaffolds promoted adhesion of the MG-63 cell line and facilitated its proliferation and ALP expression, as evident from Figure 11.6. Furthermore, its antibacterial activity against *Escherichia coli* indicated that, apart from rapid healing of bone injuries, it is also efficient against postsurgical bacterial infections.

Another similar study reported that the liquid uptake ability of such a composite scaffold on supplementation with HA is also composition dependent, as it absorbed 2671%–4987% of water after 24 hours of immersion [21]. Scaffolds with a chitosan

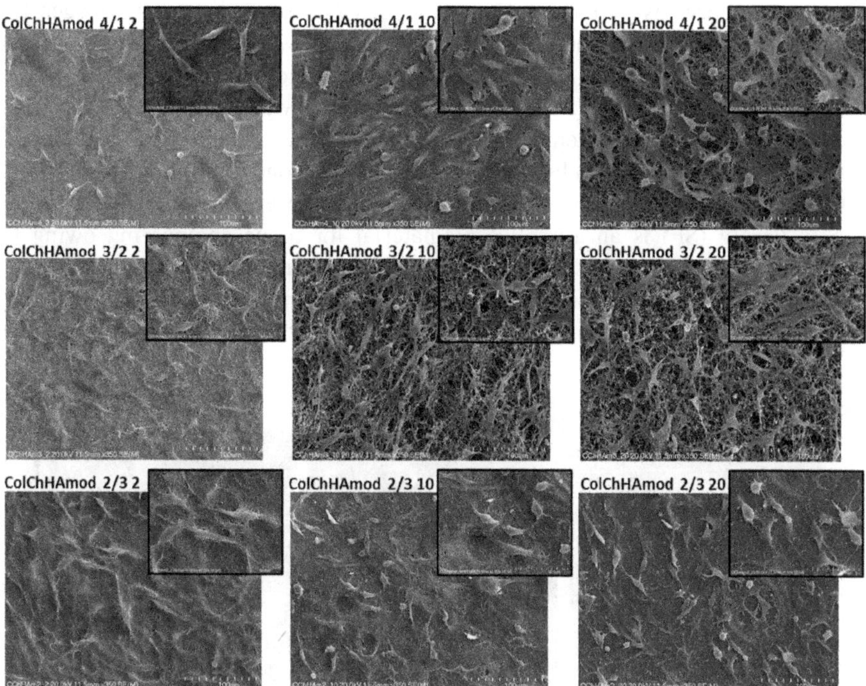

FIGURE 11.6 SEM microphotographs of the MG-63 cell line cultured on the collagen/chitosan/amino-functionalized hyaluronic acid-based hydrogels crosslinked with 2, 10 and 20 mM genipin solutions. Reprinted with permission from [20]. Copyright © 2019 Elsevier B.V.

and collagen mixture supplemented with 2% wt. hyaluronic acid and 80% wt. HA exhibited better surface adherence of human SaOS-2 cells. Furthermore, the in vivo studies with injury on the right side of the subscapular region of New Zealand white rabbits indicated granulation and tissue healing on implantation of the scaffolds. The onset of granulation is primarily attributed to the presence of angioblasts, fibroblasts, and collagen synthesis.

Alginate-based microspheres and fibers are more stable as they do not disintegrate in an aqueous environment, which is mainly attributed to the crosslinking property of alginate in contact with divalent ions such as calcium (Ca^{2+}). Mesenchymal stem cells (MSCs) were loaded into the collagen solution in order to deposit them into a fibrous structure that was simultaneously sheathed with alginate using a core–shell nozzle [22]. An outer syringe was filled with sodium alginate solution at ratios of 2%–5% (% wt) in water, while the inner syringe contained collagen solution. Core–shell-structured collagen-alginate fibers were then injected into a bath containing 50 mM calcium chloride for 5 min using the concentric nozzle. This led to crosslinking and gelation as soon as the outer alginate came into contact with the calcium ions. The continuous fiber in composite scaffolds had a diameter of 700–1000 μm for the core and 200–500 μm for the shell area. The dimension of the fibers varied with the alginate concentration and (2%–5%) the injection rate (20–80 mL/h). High water uptake capacity (98%) rationalized the ability of the core-shell structures to serve as pore channels for the transport of nutrients and oxygen for cellular metabolism. Around 43% of the biomaterial was degraded after 14 days. High viability, proliferation and remarkable osteogenic differentiation of the MSCs encapsulated within the collagen core were associated with the upregulated expression of osteogenic genes such as osteocalcin, bone sialoprotein, and osteopontin. On implantation into rat calvarium defect, notable bone healing was observed, confirming their application as a promising bone tissue-engineered construct.

Silk fibroin (SF) is an attractive biomaterial for tissue engineering owing to its high biocompatibility, superior mechanical properties, low immunogenicity, and ease of processing. The mechanical properties and the porosity of the silk-based scaffolds can be controlled by selecting the ideal fabrication process that

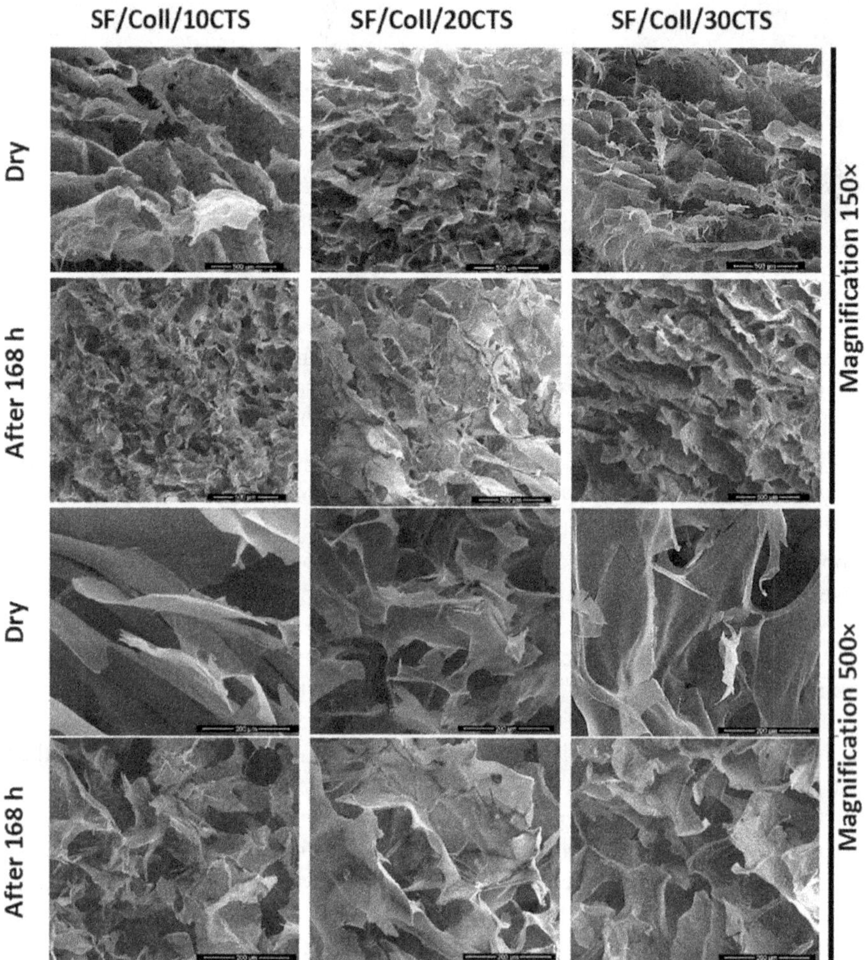

FIGURE 11.7 SEM images (magnifications 500× and 150×) of SF/Coll mixtures with 10%, 20%, and 30% CTS (left to right columns) for dry scaffolds and after 168 hours of immersion in PBS. Reprinted from [23].

includes gas phase forming method, salt immersion method, and electrostatic spinning. Composite scaffolds composed of SF, collagen and chitosan were synthesized employing glyoxal-mediated crosslinking for bone tissue regeneration [23]. The three-component biomaterial was produced by mixing silk/collagen in a 50/50 weight ratio that was further supplemented with 10%, 20%, and 30% chitosan that were designated as SF/Coll/10CTS, SF/Coll/20CTS and SF/Coll/20CTS, respectively. The maximum densities of SF/Coll/10CTS and SF/Coll/20CTS were 21.11 ± 1.56 and 21.25 ± 0.32 mg/cm^3, respectively, while the porosity was between 80% and 90%. Interestingly, the highest moisture content was found for Coll/CTS/10SF scaffolds (14.29 g/100 g), while the lowest was for the SF/CTS/30Coll sample (only 10.84 ± 0.22 g/100g). Easily wettable scaffolds showed extremely high swelling ability, which was mainly attributed to the water-binding functional groups of SF, collagen, and chitosan. Highly porous structures with interconnected pores were observed in SEM images of the scaffolds both before immersion in PBS and after 168 h of immersion, as evident from Figure 11.7. The highest Young's modulus, rigidity and deformation were observed for the SF/CTS/10Coll scaffold, which were equivalent to 46.7 ± 0.3 kPa, 73.1 ± 3.4 kPa, and $3.8\% \pm 0.3\%$, respectively. The composite scaffolds were cytocompatible with the MG-63 osteoblast-like cells and promoted their colonization and proliferation.

In another study, a novel recombinant human-like collagen (RHLC) was blended with silk in an 80:20 ratio at 50°C–60°C, followed by freezing at –20°C. A porous matrix was obtained by freeze-drying the resulting ice/wire composite material [24]. The scaffolds demonstrated compressive strength and modulus up to 662 ± 32 kPa and 7.8 ± 0.64 MPa, apart from high water binding capacity. Neonatal rat osteoblasts (Wistar) exhibited protrusions and a plurality of filamentous feet that helped in their adherence to the scaffold surface. The cells further proliferated significantly and grew into the internal pores of the scaffolds, which is critical for bone tissue engineering and formation of microenvironment for rapid healing and osseointegration.

11.2.5 Metal Nanoparticles

Several metal nanoparticles are used for reinforcement of the collagen-based composite scaffolds. Incorporation of the metal and metal oxide nanoparticles not only enhances the mechanical properties of the scaffolds but also makes them more biocompatible and resistant to microbial infections and degradation. Metallic nanoparticles composed of gold and silver are more attractive due to their established biomedical applications [25–29]. Gold nanoparticles (AuNPs) have more anticancer and antioxidant properties that can synergistically enhance the therapeutic spectrum of the composite scaffolds towards bone cancer, osteoarthritis, and osteoporosis [30–32]. Likewise, silver nanoparticles (AgNPs) are more potent antimicrobial agents that can significantly inhibit pathogenic bacteria and fungi [28,33,34]. Additionally, AgNPs can effectively inhibit and eradicate bacterial biofilms, which are closely associated with critical postsurgical nosocomial infections [29,35].

Collagen-based scaffold composite encapsulating AgNPs and bone morphogenetic protein 2 (BMP-2) was reported to promote healing of infected bone defects [36]. Initially, 10 mM $AgNO_3$ was mixed with 250 mg collagen powder and reacted with NaOH and $NaBH_4$ at room temperature, which resulted in formation of AgNPs of 10–50 nm size suspended in collagen solution, as evident from Figure 11.8a. Further addition of BMP-2 to the reaction cocktail led to the encapsulation of AgNPs and BMP-2 by the collagen, which was then freeze-dried. Figure 11.8b and c reveals the porous network in the collagen scaffolds, which formed a coarse surface after impregnation with the AgNPs. The composite scaffold exhibited notable inhibition of the bacterial pathogen, *Staphylococcus aureus.* Bone marrow-derived mesenchymal stromal cells (BMSCs) could proliferate and remain viable on the scaffold surface with expression of RUNX2, osteopontin and osteonectin genes, which are markers of osteogenic differentiation. ALP activity was also enhanced during the growth of the BMSCs on the composite scaffolds.

Yet in another study, AuNPs were incorporated within collagen-based scaffolds containing HAP using an in situ chemical reduction process for bone tissue engineering [37]. Initially, a collagen solution was mixed with 0.01 M aqueous $HAuCl_4$ solution for 1 hour, followed by dropwise addition of 1.0 M $NaBH_4$ in 0.3 M NaOH. Appearance of pink color after 24 hours confirmed the synthesis of AuNPs. Then HAP was synthesized using a Col-Au nano-matrix by the reaction of $CaCl_2$ and $Na_2HPO_4.12H_2O$ for 1–2 hours under stirring. The particle size was between 3 and 5 nm. The Ca^{2+} ions trapped within the gap near the carboxyl group served as a crystal nucleation point that grew with the concomitant addition of Na_2HPO_4, eventually resulting in the formation of puckered, quarter-moon-like platelet structures. Such materials with superior mechanical properties can be employed for modification of the implant surfaces for enhancement of shelf life and biocompatibility.

More recently, magnetic nanoparticles like iron oxide nanoparticles have gained potential attention due to their ability to be targeted for injury [38]. Very low toxicity, high biocompatibility and ease of bioimaging have made them promising theranostic agents [39–41]. In an innovative attempt, iron oxide

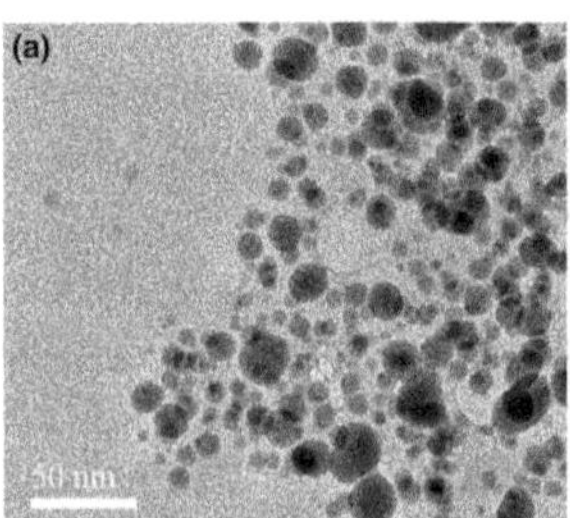

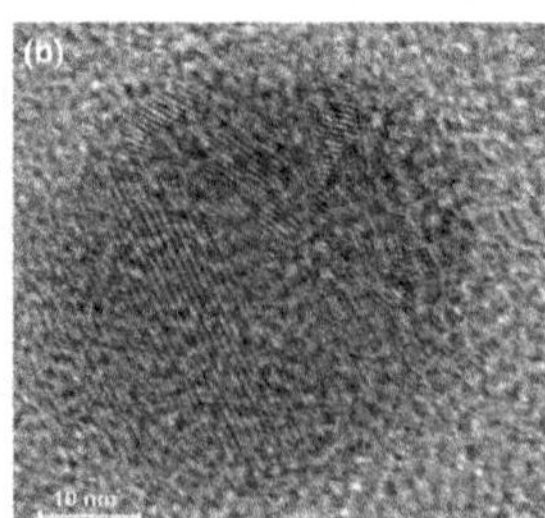

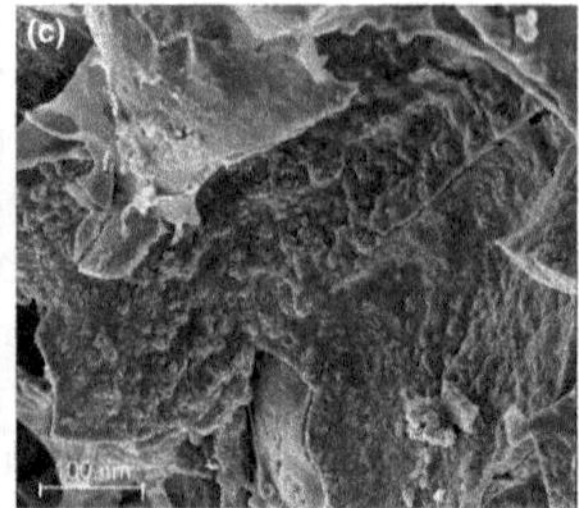

FIGURE 11.8 (a) Typical TEM image of an as-prepared collagen solution containing AgNPs; (b) HR-TEM image of a single AgNP in the collagen solution; (c) SEM image of the surface of BMP-2/AgNPs/collagen scaffolds. Reprinted with permission from [36]. Copyright © 2014 Springer Science+Business Media Dordrecht.

TABLE 11.1
Materials for Reinforcement and Activity Enhancement of Collagen-Based Biocomposites

Materials	Cells/Models	References
Hydroxyapatite	-	[10]
Hydroxyapatite, Fe/Mn	Mouse calvarial 3T3-E1, cells, bone marrow mesenchymal stem cells (BMSCs), mouse calvarial defect model	[11]
45S5 bioactive glass	Simulated body fluid (SBF), Osteoblast-like cells (MG-63)	[12]
Polycaprolactone (PCL)-and chitosan (CS)	Rat bone marrow derived stromal cells (rBMSCs)	[13]
Poly(lactic-co-glycolic acid), risedronate	Human bone osteosarcoma cells (Saos-2 cells)	[14]
Poly(lactide-co-glycolide) acid (PLGA), nano-hydroxyapatite (n-HA)	Human fetal osteoblast cells (hFOB 1.19)	[15]
Cellulose microsphere	Human osteoblasts (HOB)	[19]
Chitosan, lysine-modified hyaluronic acid	MG-63 cell line	[20]
Chitosan, hyaluronic acid, hydroxyapatite	SaOS-2 cells, subscapular injury of New Zealand White rabbits	[21]
Alginate	Mesenchymal stem cells (MSCs), rat calvarium defect	[22]
Silk fibroin, chitosan	MG-63 cell line	[23]
Silk, novel recombinant human-like collagen (RHLC)	Neonatal rat osteoblast (Wistar)	[24]
AgNPs, bone morphogenetic protein 2 (BMP-2)	Bone marrow-derived mesenchymal stromal cells (BMSCs)	[36]
AuNPs, hydroxyapatite	-	[37]
Iron oxide nanospheres, hydroxyapatite, strontium	MC3T3-E1 cells	[42]

nanospheres-hydroxyapatite-strontium@collagen (IONSs-HA-SR@C) composite biomaterials were synthesized by the co-precipitation method [42]. The resulting IONSs-HA-SR@C were more or less spherical, with a uniform size of 63.4 ±2 .78 nm. The release of strontium was highest (81%) at pH 6 during 192 hours, while a burst of <40% was evident in 24 hours. The MC3T3-E1 cells exhibited superior viability, proliferation, and differentiation on treatment with IONSs-HA-SR@C, as indicated by high expression of BMP-2, ALP, OCN, RUNX-2 and COL1 genes (Table 11.1).

11.3 CONCLUSIONS AND FUTURE PERSPECTIVES

Multicomponent scaffolds have emerged as crucial templates for bone tissue engineering and have led to development of effective strategies for rapid wound healing and the prevention of post-surgical complications.

Promising biodegradable polymers are continuously being developed to ensure biocompatibility, cost-effectiveness, omission of removal surgery, and decrease in the number of radiographs taken. New-generation implants with antibiotics incorporated in the polymeric matrix of PLGA are used for assessing the risk of re-infection in appropriate animal models. Likewise, aliphatic polyesters like polyhydroxybutyrate (PHB) of microbial origin can be impregnated with cellular growth factors and signaling molecules for rapid bone healing. Polyhydroxyvalerate (PHV) can be copolymerized with PHB for crystallinity reduction and failure strain enhancement. Hence, implantation site-specific modulation of the mechanical properties can be brought about in the polymers for substantial improvement in the healing process. Polymers such as copolyesterurethane networks, PDLLA-hydroxyapatite composites, and PCL-co-PLLA (PCLA) can be further introduced in scaffolds to effectively mold them into desired shapes [43].

The bone ECM is rich in type I collagen, which rationalizes its use to develop scaffolds that can not only facilitate adhesion and proliferation of the cells but also help in superior promotion of the chemostatic response [44]. Therefore, collagen-based functionalized scaffolds have significant applications due to their biocompatibility and osteogenic potential. Such scaffolds can be effectively designed employing 3D bioprinting technique in order to mimic the tissue microarchitecture [45]. Porosity, elasticity, stiffness, and other parameters identical to the tissue microenvironment can be explicitly controlled by the nature of the biomaterial and the mode of the 3D-bioprinting techniques [46,47].

Another important perspective lies in the rational functionalization of a large variety of RNA, including long noncoding RNA (lncRNA), messenger RNA (mRNA), microRNA (miRNA), and small interfering RNA (siRNA), on the collagen scaffolds for facilitating bone regeneration [48]. Likewise, carbon-based nanostructures like SWCNTs and MWCNTs, GO, GNRs, and others can be incorporated for reinforcement of the collagen scaffolds to obtain appropriate mechanical properties and cellular responses [49–51]. Similarly, osteoinductive cytokines and signaling biomolecules can be rationally cofunctionalized on collagen-based scaffolds for promising osteogenic induction [52]. Hence, collagen-containing biomaterials can be a potential candidate for revolutionizing regenerative nanomedicine for treating bone injuries.

ACKNOWLEDGEMENTS

Dr. Sougata Ghosh acknowledges Kasetsart University, Bangkok, Thailand for a postdoctoral fellowship and funding under the Reinventing University Program (Ref. No. 6501.0207/9219 dated 14th September, 2022). E.M. would like to acknowledge the support from the National Institute of Biomedical Imaging and Bioengineering (5T32EB009035).

REFERENCES

1. Y. Li, Y. Liu, R. Li, H. Bai, Z. Zhu, L. Zhu, C. Zhu, Z. Che, H. Liu, J. Wang, L. Huang, Collagen-based biomaterials for bone tissue engineering, *Materials and Design*. 210 (2021). https://doi.org/10.1016/j.matdes.2021.110049.
2. A. Rahmani Del Bakhshayesh, E. Mostafavi, E. Alizadeh, N. Asadi, A. Akbarzadeh, S. Davaran, Fabrication of three-dimensional scaffolds based on nano-biomimetic collagen hybrid constructs for skin tissue engineering, *ACS Omega*. 3 (2018). https://doi.org/10.1021/acsomega.8b01219.
3. R. Parenteau-Bareil, R. Gauvin, F. Berthod, Collagen-based biomaterials for tissue engineering applications, *Materials*. 3 (2010) 1863–1887. https://doi.org/10.3390/ma3031863.
4. D.M. Ibrahim, E.S. Sani, A.M. Soliman, N. Zandi, E. Mostafavi, A.M. Youssef, N.K. Allam, N. Annabi, Bioactive and elastic nanocomposites with antimicrobial properties for bone tissue regeneration, *ACS Applied Bio Materials*. 3 (2020). https://doi.org/10.1021/acsabm.0c00250.
5. G.A. Rico-Llanos, S. Borrego-González, M. Moncayo-Donoso, J. Becerra, R. Visser, Collagen type I biomaterials as scaffolds for bone tissue engineering, *Polymers (Basel)*. 13 (2021) 1–20. https://doi.org/10.3390/polym13040599.
6. B. Sarker, J. Hum, S.N. Nazhat, A.R. Boccaccini, Combining collagen and bioactive glasses for bone tissue engineering: A review, *Advanced Healthcare Materials*. 4 (2015) 176–194. https://doi.org/10.1002/adhm.201400302.
7. X. Xue, Y. Hu, Y. Deng, J. Su, Recent advances in design of functional biocompatible hydrogels for bone tissue engineering, *Advanced Functional Materials*. 31 (2021). https://doi.org/10.1002/adfm.202009432.
8. W. Zheng, W. Zhang, X. Jiang, Biomimetic collagen nanofibrous materials for bone tissue engineering, *Advanced Engineering Materials*. 12 (2010) B451–B466. https://doi.org/10.1002/adem.200980087.
9. E. Mostafavi, P. Soltantabar, T.J. Webster, Nanotechnology and picotechnology: A new arena for translational medicine, 2018. https://doi.org/10.1016/B978-0-12-813477-1.00009-8.
10. J. Wang, C. Liu, Biomimetic collagen/hydroxyapatite composite scaffolds: Fabrication and characterizations, *Journal of Bionic Engineering*. 11 (2014) 600–609. https://doi.org/10.1016/S1672–6529(14)60071–8.
11. L. Yu, D.W. Rowe, I.P. Perera, J. Zhang, S.L. Suib, X. Xin, M. Wei, Intrafibrillar mineralized collagen-hydroxyapatite-based scaffolds for bone regeneration, *ACS Applied Materials and Interfaces*. 12 (2020) 18235–18249. https://doi.org/10.1021/acsami.0c00275.
12. J. Hum, A.R. Boccaccini, Collagen as coating material for 45S5 bioactive glass-based scaffolds for bone tissue engineering, *International Journal of Molecular Sciences*. 19 (2018). https://doi.org/10.3390/ijms19061807.
13. Y. Cheng, D. Ramos, P. Lee, D. Liang, X. Yu, S.G. Kumbar, Collagen functionalized bioactive nanofiber matrices for osteogenic differentiation of mesenchymal stem cells: Bone tissue engineering, *Journal of Biomedical Nanotechnology*. 10 (2014) 287–298. https://doi.org/10.1166/jbn.2014.1753.
14. N.A. Elkasabgy, A.A. Mahmoud, R.N. Shamma, Determination of cytocompatibility and osteogenesis properties of in situ forming collagen-based scaffolds loaded with bone synthesizing drug for bone tissue engineering, *International Journal of Polymeric Materials and Polymeric Biomaterials*. 67 (2018) 494–500. https://doi.org/10.1080/00914037.2017.1354195.
15. M. Ngiam, S. Liao, A.J. Patil, Z. Cheng, C.K. Chan, S. Ramakrishna, The fabrication of nano-hydroxyapatite on PLGA and PLGA/collagen nanofibrous composite scaffolds and their effects in osteoblastic behavior for bone tissue engineering, *Bone*. 45 (2009) 4–16. https://doi.org/10.1016/j.bone.2009.03.674.

16. S. Ghosh, T.J. Webster, Mesoporous silica based nanostructures for bone tissue regeneration, *Frontiers in Materials*. 8 (2021). https://doi.org/10.3389/fmats.2021.692309.
17. S. Ghosh, T.J. Webster, Metallic nanoscaffolds as osteogenic promoters: Advances, challenges and scope, *Metals (Basel)*. 11 (2021). https://doi.org/10.3390/met11091356.
18. S. Ghosh, S. Sanghavi, P. Sancheti, Metallic biomaterial for bone support and replacement, In: *Fundamental Biomaterials: Metals*, Elsevier, 2018: pp. 139–165. https://doi.org/10.1016/B978-0-08-102205-4.00006-4.
19. A. Aravamudhan, D.M. Ramos, J. Nip, M.D. Harmon, R. James, M. Deng, C.T. Laurencin, X. Yu, S.G. Kumbar, Cellulose and collagen derived micro-nano structured scaffolds for bone tissue engineering, *Journal of Biomedical Nanotechnology*. 9 (2013) 719–731. https://doi.org/10.1166/jbn.2013.1574.
20. A. Gilarska, J. Lewandowska-Łańcucka, K. Guzdek-Zając, A. Karewicz, W. Horak, R. Lach, K. Wójcik, M. Nowakowska, Bioactive yet antimicrobial structurally stable collagen/chitosan/lysine functionalized hyaluronic acid – based injectable hydrogels for potential bone tissue engineering applications, *International Journal of Biological Macromolecules*. 155 (2020) 938–950. https://doi.org/10.1016/j.ijbiomac.2019.11.052.
21. B. Kaczmarek, A. Sionkowska, M. Gołyńska, I. Polkowska, T. Szponder, D. Nehrbass, A.M. Osyczka, In vivo study on scaffolds based on chitosan, collagen, and hyaluronic acid with hydroxyapatite, *International Journal of Biological Macromolecules*. 118 (2018) 938–944. https://doi.org/10.1016/j.ijbiomac.2018.06.175.
22. R.A. Perez, M. Kim, T.H. Kim, J.H. Kim, J.H. Lee, J.H. Park, J.C. Knowles, H.W. Kim, Utilizing core-shell fibrous collagen-alginate hydrogel cell delivery system for bone tissue engineering, *Tissue Engineering - Part A*. 20 (2014) 103–114. https://doi.org/10.1089/ten.tea.2013.0198.
23. S. Grabska-Zielińska, A. Sionkowska, C.C. Coelho, F.J. Monteiro, Silk fibroin/collagen/chitosan scaffolds cross-linked by a glyoxal solution as biomaterials toward bone tissue regeneration, *Materials*. 13 (2020) 1–20. https://doi.org/10.3390/ma13153433.
24. K. Hu, M. Hu, Y.H. Xiao, Y. Cui, J. Yan, G. Yang, F. Zhang, G. Lin, H. Yi, L. Han, L.H. Li, Y. Wei, F. Cui, Preparation recombination human-like collagen/fibroin scaffold and promoting the cell compatibility with osteoblasts, *Journal of Biomedical Materials Research - Part A*. 109 (2021) 346–353. https://doi.org/10.1002/jbm.a.37027.
25. S. Ghosh, A.N. Harke, Gloriosa superba mediated synthesis of silver and gold nanoparticles for anticancer applications, *Journal of Nanomedicine & Nanotechnology*. 7 (2016). https://doi.org/10.4172/2157-7439.1000390.
26. S. Ghosh, S.P. Gurav, A.N. Harke, M.J. Chacko, K.A. Joshi, A. Dhepe, C. Charolkar, V. Shinde, R. Kitture, Dioscorea oppositifolia mediated synthesis of gold and silver nanoparticles with catalytic activity, *Journal of Nanomedicine & Nanotechnology*. 07 (2016). https://doi.org/10.4172/2157-7439.1000398.
27. S. Ghosh, M. Jini Chacko, Barleria prionitis leaf mediated synthesis of silver and gold nanocatalysts, *Journal of Nanomedicine & Nanotechnology*. 7 (2016). https://doi.org/10.4172/2157-7439.1000394.
28. E. Mostafavi, A. Zarepour, H. Barabadi, A. Zarrabi, L.B. Truong, D. Medina-Cruz, Antineoplastic activity of biogenic silver and gold nanoparticles to combat leukemia: Beginning a new era in cancer theragnostic, *Biotechnology Reports*. (2022). https://doi.org/10.1016/j.btre.2022.e00714.
29. M. Saravanan, H. Vahidi, D. Medina Cruz, A. Vernet-Crua, E. Mostafavi, R. Stelmach, T.J. Webster, M. Ali Mahjoub, M. Rashedi, H. Barabadi, Emerging antineoplastic biogenic gold nanomaterials for breast cancer therapeutics: A systematic review, *International Journal of Nanomedicine*. 15 (2020). https://doi.org/10.2147/IJN.S240293.
30. A. Pormohammad, N.K. Monych, S. Ghosh, D.L. Turner, R.J. Turner, Nanomaterials in wound healing and infection control, *Antibiotics*. 10 (2021). https://doi.org/10.3390/antibiotics10050473.

31. G.R. Salunke, S. Ghosh, R.J. Santosh Kumar, S. Khade, P. Vashisth, T. Kale, S. Chopade, V. Pruthi, G. Kundu, J.R. Bellare, B.A. Chopade, Rapid efficient synthesis and characterization of silver, gold, and bimetallic nanoparticles from the medicinal plant Plumbago zeylanica and their application in biofilm control, *International Journal of Nanomedicine.* 9 (2014). https://doi.org/10.2147/IJN.S59834.
32. S. Ghosh, S. Patil, M. Ahire, R. Kitture, A. Jabgunde, S. Kale, K. Pardesi, J. Bellare, D.D. Dhavale, B.A. Chopade, Synthesis of gold nanoanisotrops using Dioscorea bulbifera tuber extract, *Journal of Nanomaterials.* 2011 (2011). https://doi.org/10.1155/2011/354793.
33. B. Ranpariya, G. Salunke, S. Karmakar, K. Babiya, S. Sutar, N. Kadoo, P. Kumbhakar, S. Ghosh, Antimicrobial synergy of silver-platinum nanohybrids with antibiotics, *Frontiers in Microbiology.* 11 (2021). https://doi.org/10.3389/fmicb.2020.610968.
34. K. Kalantari, E. Mostafavi, A.M. Afifi, Z. Izadiyan, H. Jahangirian, R. Rafiee-Moghaddam, T.J. Webster, Wound dressings functionalized with silver nanoparticles: Promises and pitfalls, *Nanoscale.* 12 (2020). https://doi.org/10.1039/c9nr08234d.
35. B.P. Singh, S. Ghosh, A. Chauhan, Development, dynamics and control of antimicrobial-resistant bacterial biofilms: A review, *Environmental Chemistry Letters.* 19 (2021). https://doi.org/10.1007/s10311-020-01169-5.
36. C. Sun, Y. Che, S. Lu, Preparation and application of collagen scaffold-encapsulated silver nanoparticles and bone morphogenetic protein 2 for enhancing the repair of infected bone, *Biotechnology Letters.* 37 (2015) 467–473. https://doi.org/10.1007/s10529-014-1698-8.
37. S. Aryal, K.C. Remant Bahadur, S.R. Bhattarai, P. Prabu, H.Y. Kim, Immobilization of collagen on gold nanoparticles: Preparation, characterization, and hydroxyapatite growth, *Journal of Materials Chemistry.* 16 (2006) 4642–4648. https://doi.org/10.1039/b608300e.
38. S. Ghosh, P. More, A. Derle, R. Kitture, T. Kale, M. Gorain, A. Avasthi, P. Markad, G.C. Kundu, S. Kale, D.D. Dhavale, J. Bellare, B.A. Chopade, Diosgenin functionalized iron oxide nanoparticles as novel nanomaterial against breast cancer, *Journal of Nanoscience and Nanotechnology.* 15 (2015) 9464–9472. https://doi.org/10.1166/jnn.2015.11704.
39. R. Kitture, S. Ghosh, P. Kulkarni, X.L. Liu, D. Maity, S.I. Patil, D. Jun, Y. Dushing, S.L. Laware, B.A. Chopade, S.N. Kale, Fe_3O_4-citrate-curcumin: Promising conjugates for superoxide scavenging, tumor suppression and cancer hyperthermia, *Journal of Applied Physics.* 111 (2012). https://doi.org/10.1063/1.3696001.
40. R. Kitture, S. Ghosh, Hybrid nanostructures for in vivo imaging. In: *Hybrid Nanostructures for Cancer Theranostics*, Elsevier, 2018: pp. 173–208. https://doi.org/10.1016/B978-0-12-813906-6.00010-X.
41. R. Kitture, S. Ghosh, Nanopharmacokinetics: Key role in in vivo imaging, In: *Nano-Pharmacokinetics and Theranostics*, Elsevier, 2021: pp. 233–251. https://doi.org/10.1016/b978-0-323-85050-6.00009-8.
42. X. Wei, X. Zhang, Z. Yang, L. Li, H. Sui, Osteoinductive potential and antibacterial characteristics of collagen coated iron oxide nanosphere containing strontium and hydroxyapatite in long term bone fractures, *Arabian Journal of Chemistry.* 14 (2021). https://doi.org/10.1016/j.arabjc.2020.102984.
43. R.J. Kroeze, M.N. Helder, L.E. Govaert, T.H. Smit, Biodegradable polymers in bone tissue engineering, *Materials.* 2 (2009) 833–856. https://doi.org/10.3390/ma2030833.
44. A.M. Ferreira, P. Gentile, V. Chiono, G. Ciardelli, Collagen for bone tissue regeneration, *Acta Biomater.* 8 (2012) 3191–3200. https://doi.org/10.1016/j.actbio.2012.06.014.
45. S. Ghosh, E. Mostafavi, N. Thorat, T.J. Webster, Nanobiomaterials for three-dimensional bioprinting. In: *Nanotechnology in Medicine and Biology*, Elsevier, 2022: pp. 1–24. https://doi.org/10.1016/b978-0-12-819469-0.00003-4.

46. X. Du, S. Fu, Y. Zhu, 3D printing of ceramic-based scaffolds for bone tissue engineering: An overview, *Journal of Materials Chemistry B*. 6 (2018) 4397–4412. https://doi.org/10.1039/c8tb00677f.
47. S. Saghati, A. Akbarzadeh, A.R. del Bakhshayesh, R. Sheervalilou, E. Mostafavi, Chapter 6: Electrospinning and 3D printing: Prospects for market opportunity, 2018. https://doi.org/10.1039/9781788012942-00136.
48. Q. Leng, L. Chen, Y. Lv, RNA-based scaffolds for bone regeneration: Application and mechanisms of mRNA, miRNA and siRNA, *Theranostics*. 10 (2020) 3190–3205. https://doi.org/10.7150/thno.42640.
49. N. Shadjou, M. Hasanzadeh, B. Khalilzadeh, Graphene based scaffolds on bone tissue engineering, *Bioengineered*. 9 (2018) 38–47. https://doi.org/10.1080/21655979.2017.1373539.
50. H. Zare, S. Ahmadi, A. Ghasemi, M. Ghanbari, N. Rabiee, M. Bagherzadeh, M. Karimi, T.J. Webster, M.R. Hamblin, E. Mostafavi, Carbon nanotubes: Smart drug/gene delivery carriers, *International Journal of Nanomedicine*. 16 (2021). https://doi.org/10.2147/IJN.S299448.
51. S. Mehranfar, I. Abdi Rad, E. Mostafav, A. Akbarzadeh, The use of stromal vascular fraction (SVF), platelet-rich plasma (PRP) and stem cells in the treatment of osteoarthritis: An overview of clinical trials, *Artificial Cells, Nanomedicine and Biotechnology*. 47 (2019). https://doi.org/10.1080/21691401.2019.1576710.
52. S. Preethi Soundarya, V. Sanjay, A. Haritha Menon, S. Dhivya, N. Selvamurugan, Effects of flavonoids incorporated biological macromolecules based scaffolds in bone tissue engineering, *International Journal of Biological Macromolecules*. 110 (2018) 74–87. https://doi.org/10.1016/j.ijbiomac.2017.09.014.

12 Composite Hydrogels for Adipose Tissue Engineering

P.N. Blessy Rebecca
SRM Institute of Science and Technology

D. Durgalakshmi
Anna University
Ethiraj College for Women

R. Ajay Rakkesh
SRM Institute of Science and Technology

CONTENTS

12.1 Introduction 256
12.2 Scope of Adipose Tissue Engineering 256
  12.2.1 Cosmetic Surgery 256
  12.2.2 Reconstructive Surgery 257
  12.2.3 Wound Healing 257
  12.2.4 Bone Healing 257
12.3 Biomaterials for Adipose Tissue Engineering 257
  12.3.1 Natural Polymers 258
  12.3.2 Synthetic Polymers 258
12.4 Hydrogels 258
12.5 Composite Hydrogels 259
  12.5.1 Collagen-Based Composite Hydrogels 259
  12.5.2 Alginate-Based Composite Hydrogels 259
  12.5.3 Hyaluronic Acid-Based Composite Hydrogels 260
  12.5.4 Matrigel-Based Composite Hydrogels 261
  12.5.5 Fibrin-Based Composite Hydrogels 262
  12.5.6 Poly(Lactic-Co-Glycolic Acid) (PLGA)-Based Composite Hydrogels 263
  12.5.7 Poly(Ethylene Glycol)-Based Composite Hydrogels 263
  12.5.8 Other Materials-Based Composite Hydrogels 263
  12.5.9 Naturally Derived Hydrogels 264
12.6 Conclusion 269
References 269

DOI: 10.1201/9781003251767-12

12.1 INTRODUCTION

Adipose tissue is a form of connective tissue that can reserve energy in its fat cells, called adipocytes. Adipose tissue is the predominant tissue in the body and is essential for biological responses such as angiogenesis, metabolic hemostasis, inflammation, and immune regulation (Louis and Matsusaki 2020). Adipocyte cells store energy, maintain body contours, provide protection to the inner organs, and serve as a storehouse for steroid and cholesterol hormones (Klaus 2001). The reconstruction of adipose tissue is essential after tumors or trauma. The damage to the soft tissue affects not only the physique of the patients but also their mentality and emotional well-being. The reconstruction of soft tissue usually involves autologous grafts, liposuction, synthetic prostheses, and commercially available fillers. These procedures have drawbacks such as donor-site morbidity and immune response, are highly invasive, and cause long-term problems such as volume loss. The emerging tissue engineering techniques focus on developing a suitable substitute that can promote regeneration, eliminating the need for organ transplants (Casadei et al. 2012). Generally, tissue engineering involves biomaterial scaffolds, cell sources, and an apt environment for the formation and development of damaged tissues (Choi et al. 2010). A biomaterial should promote cell attachment, differentiation, and proliferation and have suitable characteristics to imitate the nature of the soft tissue. The main important characteristics of the biomaterial used in soft tissue regeneration are adipogenesis and neovascularization (Chiu et al. 2011). Adipogenesis is the differentiation of progenitor cells into adipocytes, which occurs until the end of life and produces body fat. Neovascularization is the formation of new blood vessels, and adipose tissue is a highly vascularized tissue. The vasculature involves supplying oxygen and nutrients, playing a part in metabolism, and emitting soluble factors that control the survival of adipocytes. The formulation of adipose tissue is regulated by many factors, including extracellular matrix (ECM), growth factors, and hormones (Katz et al. 1999; Cinti 2001).

12.2 SCOPE OF ADIPOSE TISSUE ENGINEERING

Adipose tissue is the most important component in the body. It protects the underlying structures and presents a natural appearance. Cancers leave patients with defects and disfiguration, which require tissue (Flynn et al. 2008). Patients prefer autologous adipose tissue as fillers provide general shape and elasticity, but the long-term stability and assessment of the autologous tissue give unpredictable results and pose challenges in medical practice (Louis and Matsusaki 2020). The natural fillers may diminish or be resorbed, and artificial fillers can create an immune response in the host. The following section presents the current applications of adipose tissue engineering in various domains.

12.2.1 Cosmetic Surgery

Adipose tissue engineering in cosmetic surgery focuses on enhancing the facial features and structure of the body. The most common surgery is breast augmentation, a facial reconstruction that mainly includes the nose, lips, cheeks, and fat injections to reduce the wrinkles caused due to aging process. Often, soft tissue augmentation is completed by fat grafting, and the absorption, volume estimation, and longevity of the graft differ (Cook et al. 2004; Mughal et al. 2021). Adipose-derived stem cells (ADSCs) are also used in facial reconstruction as the chondrogenicity of these cells is used in joint and disc repair and reconstruction of the ear and nose (Casadei et al. 2011).

12.2.2 Reconstructive Surgery

The reconstruction of the breasts is among the most widely done reconstructive treatments for patients with breast cancer to enhance beauty. The implantation of the adipose tissue provides natural shape and suppleness. The transfer of tissues from one place to another leads to substantial donor-site morbidity and recipient site morbidity, which leads to volume loss with time (Upadhyaya et al. 2018). The main limitations are the lack of similarity compared to natural soft tissue and volume loss over time, which leads to structure and shape changes (Butterwick et al. 2007).

12.2.3 Wound Healing

Large wounds with damage to the subcutaneous fat tissues need adipose tissue implantation. The ADSCs are pluripotent cells and can be used to renew various types of tissues, including the skin (Zuk et al. 2002). The addition of ADSCs improves the healing process through fibroblast activation and proliferation and collagen synthesis. Chronic leg ulcers in diabetic patients are a common example of adipose tissue regeneration in wound healing (Amos et al. 2010, Holm et al. 2018). Numerous studies also showed that adipose tissue engineering can also be used in the healing of wounds from irradiation and burns (Kim et al. 2007, Lee et al. 2009, Akita et al. 2010).

12.2.4 Bone Healing

During the healing process of the bone, the adipose tissues are absorbed and replaced without any tissue volume being lost by the bone tissues. The bone marrow stem cells (BMSCs) and ADSCs are similar and have the potential to be used in both osteogenic and angiogenic reconstruction (Puissant et al. 2005). Studies show that BMSCs and ADSCs are driven to move toward the damaged site to enhance healing (Lee et al. 2015). Moreover, ADSCs can be used for various tissue regenerations and also for diabetes mellitus to secrete insulin, chronic liver failure (Watanabe et al. 1997), and several autoimmune diseases (Miranville et al. 2004, Ebrahimian et al. 2009, Lindroos et al. 2011).

12.3 BIOMATERIALS FOR ADIPOSE TISSUE ENGINEERING

A biomaterial scaffold should provide an adequate environment for the cells by promoting cell attachment and proliferation and facilitating cell-matrix and cell-cell interactions. The biomaterial should have characteristics to simulate the function and structure of typical tissues, including biocompatibility and biodegradability as the new tissue regenerates (Levenberg and Langer 2004). The amendment of the soft tissue is dependent on the vascularization and the competence of mimicking the natural ECM to assure the feasibility of the regenerated tissue (Katz et al. 1999; Beahm et al. 2003). The biomaterials are chosen based on their chemistry, molecular weight, solubility, surface energy, water absorption rate, and degradation rate. The polymers are widely used because of their large surface-to-volume ratio, high porosity, pore size, biodegradability, biocompatibility, and mechanical properties. Adipose tissue engineering involves a scaffold material that aids the progression of new tissue, cell sources for the formation of fat tissue, and a suitable microenvironment for the regeneration of the adipose tissues (Yang et al. 2021).

12.3.1 Natural Polymers

Natural polymers can be found as part of the natural ECM or formed by biological systems. Natural polymers have active sites for crosslinking, ligand conjugation, and other modifications and have advantages such as biocompatibility and similar mechanical and biological properties that match those of natural tissues. They have better interactions with cells due to their bioactivity, which enhances the regeneration of tissues. The most commonly used natural polymers in soft tissue regeneration are collagen, silk fibroin, hyaluronic acid, gelatin, and fibrin (Singh 2016).

12.3.2 Synthetic Polymers

Synthetic polymers have been widely used as a result of their advantages, including the capability of modification with respect to specific tissues. The structure and characteristics of the synthetic polymer can be controlled during the construction process. For soft tissue, generally exploited polymers are poly(lactic acid) (PLA), poly(glycolic acid) (PGA), and copolymer poly(lactic-co-glycolic) acid (PLGA) (Wang et al. 2011).

12.4 HYDROGELS

Hydrogels are water-soluble, crosslinked polymers that are either degradable or non-degradable depending on the nature and chemistry of the polymer. The utilization of hydrogels in soft tissue engineering has attracted a great deal of attention due to their high biocompatibility and mechanical properties that are identical to those of soft tissues (Lavik and Langer 2004). Hydrogels are injectable materials with control over gelation and are injected into the soft tissue defect site (Patrick 2001). They have advantages such as highwater content, flexibility, biocompatibility, and easy control of the structure and characteristics. The behaviors of the hydrogels, such as stiffness, degradation, and the cellular response, can be modulated by optimizing the number and nature of crosslinking moieties. Since every material has its own advantages and disadvantages, preparing composites from one or two materials along with cells and growth factors is needed (Slaughter et al. 2009).

12.5 COMPOSITE HYDROGELS

Natural polymeric scaffolds have advantages like biocompatibility, bioactivity, and biodegradability, but the rate of degradation cannot be controlled. Synthetic polymers have tunable properties but may cause an immune reaction in the host. These limitations of the polymers can be overcome by developing composite scaffolds (Zhu and Roger 2011). For soft tissue regeneration, the scaffolds are usually seeded with a cell source for the formation of the fat tissue. Hydrogels were also developed into composite hydrogels with other structural polymers like meshes, fibers, and microspheres to mimic the native ECM.

12.5.1 Collagen-Based Composite Hydrogels

The most frequently investigated natural polymer for tissue engineering applications is type I collagen. Type I collagen is used because of its biocompatibility, biodegradability, low immunogenicity, availability, and low cost (Nimmi et al. 1987; Kim et al. 2000). Due to their poor mechanical properties and fast degradation, collagens are mixed with other polymers and prepared as composite hydrogels. Collagen hydrogels with FGF-2 engulfed gelatin microspheres have been found to promote vascularized adipose tissue development with and without ADSCs (Kimura et al. 2003, Vashi et al. 2006). Another study shows the addition of collagen fibers to gels increases cell viability and lipid accumulation (Gentleman et al. 2006). Collagen seeded with ADSCs was implanted in nude mice, and tissue formation, neovascularization, and the appearance of a fibrous capsule around the implant were confirmed (von Heimburg et al. 2001). Collagen, PLA, and silk fibroin were studied in vivo and in vitro with ADSCs and BMSCs and the implantation of scaffolds in a rat model. The results show that the scaffolds undergo degradation and support differentiation and adipogenesis (Mauney et al. 2007). Glutaraldehyde-crosslinked collagen-chitosan hydrogels were developed and seeded with primary rat adipose precursors, and the results showed the formation of cells in in vitro and rat models (Wu et al. 2007). A silver-impregnated and collagen-coated PLGA/PCL scaffold was prepared and evaluated for orofacial tissue reconstruction. The PLGA/PCL scaffold was prepared by electrospinning, followed by the impregnation of silver nanoparticles and the coating of polydopamine and collagen. The intermediate products are used as control scaffolds, and the prepared PP-pDA-Ag-COL scaffold shows enhancement in biocompatibility, osteogenicity and antibacterial properties. Figure 12.1 shows the analysis of composite hydrogel and control scaffolds (Qian et al. 2021).

12.5.2 Alginate-Based Composite Hydrogels

Alginates are natural polymers and are widely used as a substitute for natural ECM. Alginate hydrogels are unable to interact with cells as they promote minimal cell adhesion and have a hydrophilic nature (Rowley et al. 1999). To increase the cellular interaction, alginate is generally modified with RGD-containing peptides. An injectable alginate scaffold with fibroblasts was prepared and investigated in an inbred rat subcutaneous model. Alginate was modified by incorporating the RGD sequence, and

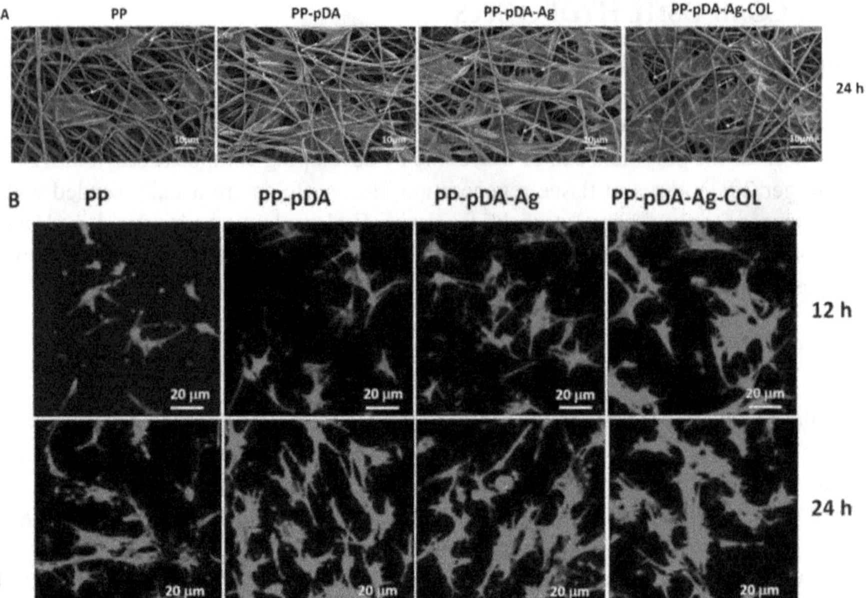

FIGURE 12.1 The MC3T3 cells are cultivated in the scaffolds for 12 or 24 hours. (a) Scanning electron microscopy images of the cultured scaffolds after 24 hours. (b) Fluorescent staining of the cytoskeleton of cells shows the higher cell density in the PP-pDA-Ag-COL scaffold.

Source: Qian et al. 2021.

the results have shown volume loss in the unseeded scaffolds. Fibroblasts were added, and it was observed that the addition increased volume retention in both modified and unmodified controls and increased adipogenesis (Marler et al. 2000). Similarly, injection of alginate hydrogel with RGD sequence in sheep shows the subcutaneous implants support the growth of tissues and vessels without any inflammability in the host (Halberstadt et al. 2002). Hyaluronic acid, laminin, and alginate hydrogel composites were prepared, and the results displayed their prospective use as carriers in adipose tissue engineering (Chen et al. 2015). Composite hydrogels of gelatin with alginate or chitosan have been prepared and evaluated. The scaffolds were implanted with ADSCs and investigated for cell adherence and proliferation. The results showed that cell proliferation is greater in composite hydrogels (Ye et al. 2021). Alginate–GelMA hydrogels with gingival-derived mesenchymal stem cells (GMSCs) were prepared and evaluated for wound rejuvenation and soft tissue reconstruction. Figure 12.2 shows the wound closure competency of the prepared composite hydrogel (Ansari et al. 2021).

12.5.3 Hyaluronic Acid-Based Composite Hydrogels

Hyaluronic acid is found in the ECM and is actively angiogenic. The study shows that the hyaluronic acid hydrogel injected into patients as a facial intradermal implant for lip augmentation and therapy for wrinkles and folds is effective for therapy of soft tissues of the face (Duranti et al. 1998). A scaffold made of crosslinked hyaluronan and decellularized human placenta with ADSCs was prepared and analyzed for understanding

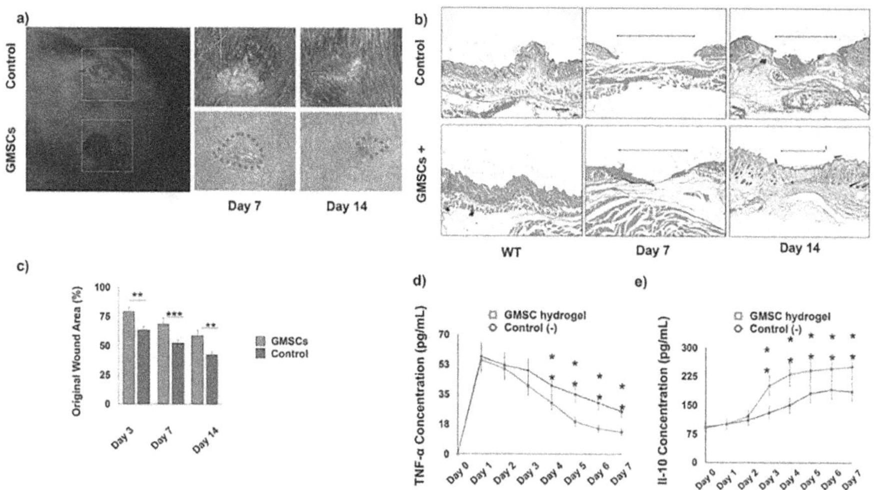

FIGURE 12.2 (a) The alginate–GelMA hydrogels without cells (control) and with cells in a rat model after 7 and 14 days. (b) Histological assessment of the retrieved sections of the control and GMSCs at different intervals. (c) Evaluation of the wound closure percentage over time after implanting hydrogel. (d) Analysis of TNF-α and IL-10 productions.

Source: Ansari et al. 2021.

the effect of the scaffold environment on the stem cells. The results showed that differentiation of adipocytes was induced (Flynn et al. 2007). Hyaluronan was chemically modified by dodecyl-amidation of the carboxyl groups of the glucuronic acid components with the adipocyte precursor, showing regeneration of adipose tissue (Rhodes et al. 2008). Human adipocyte precursors seeded on hyaluronic acid as a soft tissue filler were prepared, and the results have shown the adipocytes differentiation (Halbleib et al. 2003). Hyaluronan/gelatin composite scaffolds were prepared, crosslinked with lithium phenyl-2,4,6-trimethylbenzoylphosphinate, and incorporated with ADSCs. The adipocytes matured after 7 days, and proliferation was observed in 28 days with good cell viability (Kessler et al. 2017). Gellan gum and hyaluronic acid-spongy hydrogels were constructed with human adipose stem cells and human microvascular endothelial cells. The composite structure of the sponge and the hydrogels enables cell encapsulation, attachment, and proliferation. The prepared scaffolds were then transplanted into wounded mice, and the observed results, as shown in Figure 12.3, show increased neovascularization, re-epithelialization, and wound remodeling (Cerqueira et al. 2014).

12.5.4 Matrigel-Based Composite Hydrogels

Matrigel is a commercially available product composed of collagen IV, laminin, entactin and perlecan. Matrigel with FGF-2 is injected into 6-week-old mice, and the results show that neovascularization was induced and the preadipocytes were recruited and differentiated (Kawaguchi et al. 1998). Another study with matrigel and FGF in a specialized silicone housing showed adipogenesis and volume maintenance of the formed tissues (Walton et al. 2004). Despite being an effective matrix for adipose tissue engineering, the matrigel is limited because of the origin of murine sarcoma.

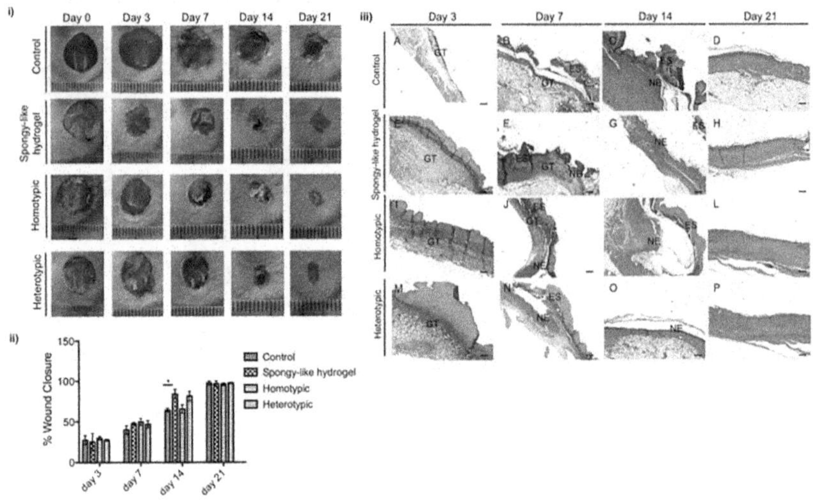

FIGURE 12.3 (i) The composite hydrogels as control, acellular, homotypic, and heterotypic Gellan gum-HA spongy hydrogels, and with cells in a mouse model after 3, 7, 14, and 21 days. (ii) Histological assessment of the retrieved section of the control and composite hydrogels at days 3, 7, 14, and 21. (iii) Analysis of the wound closure percentage over time after the implantation of hydrogels.

Source: Cerqueira et al. 2014.

Another drawback of matrigel is that the formation of new tissues is reduced without the presence of growth factors or adipocytes (Choi et al. 2005, Hemmrich and von Heimburg 2006, Piasecki et al. 2007). Another material, myogel, has been extracted from the skeletal muscles of animal species as an alternative to matrigel. The in vivo results showed preadipocyte differentiation and vascularized adipose tissue formation (Abberton et al. 2008). Since myogel is also prepared from animal sources, its suitability as a matrix for in vivo applications is still unknown.

12.5.5 Fibrin-Based Composite Hydrogels

Fibrin influences neovascularization and the regeneration of new tissue, encouraging its applications in tissue engineering. An intramuscular capsule for producing a cavity to implant a scaffold was prepared by implanting a silicone tube in a rat model. After the formation of the capsule, the tube is removed, and preadipocytes immobilized in fibrin are infused into the cavity. The results showed well-organized adipose tissue formation within 4 weeks (Schoeller et al. 2001). FGF-2 loaded in fibrin glue and PGA matrix with or without preadipocytes was also found to generate adipose tissue (Hofer et al. 2003). Injectable fibrin with PGA-PLA incorporated with ADSCs and FGF was developed and studied. The results showed that the implant maintained the original volume for 6 weeks and caused the formation of adipose tissue in the fibrin gel (Cho et al. 2005). Fibrin hydrogels with poly(caprolactone)-based polyurethane scaffolds were developed, and the scaffolds exhibited volume stability. The ADSCs were added, and the scaffolds were observed for adipogenic differentiation. Further in vivo study shows vascularized adipose tissue formation after 5 weeks (Wittmann et al. 2016). The production of fibrin from one's own blood can reduce the possibility of a foreign body reaction, making it a promising hydrogel for adipose tissue engineering (Torio-Padron et al. 2007).

12.5.6 Poly(Lactic-Co-Glycolic Acid) (PLGA)-Based Composite Hydrogels

A study has shown that injectable PLGA with preadipocytes forms new adipose tissue. The porous PLGA scaffolds added with adipose-derived stromal cells aid the growth and differentiation of adipose tissue (Choi et al. 2005). PLGA seeded with primary rat adipose seeded cells was implanted in the rats, and the differentiation was seen within 5 weeks. The long-term study showed complete resorption of adipose tissue by 5 months (Patrick et al. 1999). Another study with PLGA-PEG composites with insulin, insulin-like growth factor-1, and basic fibroblast growth factor showed that incorporating scaffolds with growth factors enhanced the free fat graft weight and volume (Neubauer et al. 2005).

12.5.7 Poly(Ethylene Glycol)-Based Composite Hydrogels

Poly(ethylene glycol) (PEG)-based hydrogels are synthetic polymers. Molecules can be incorporated into PEG based on specific biological signals, and optimized polymerization conditions lead to selective functionality. PEG hydrogels can be prepared with the ability to permit adipose tissue formation in response to signals (Stosich et al. 2007). PEG incorporated with laminin-111 peptide and cell-degradable crosslinks provides a suitable habitat for preadipocytes to differentiate. Preadipocytes in PEG improve adipose formation. Porous PEG with FGF-2 and adipocytes or mesenchymal cells also improves adipose formation (Patel et al. 2005). PEG hydrogels were prepared, and results showed the mechanical properties were similar to those of native adipose tissue. ADSCs were cultured in the prepared hydrogels, and the results showed good cell differentiation of adipose tissue (Vaicik et al. 2015).

12.5.8 Other Materials-Based Composite Hydrogels

Several other polymers are being explored for adipose tissue regeneration. Poly(ethylene glycol)-diacrylate hydrogels (PEGDA) hydrogels encapsulated with human mesenchymal stem cells were reported, and the in vivo results showed that the scaffolds maintained their structure, facilitated the formation of adipose tissues, and had 100% volume retention after 4 weeks in vivo (Alhadlaq et al. 2005). Silk fibroin incorporated into cells adipocytes and endothelial cells resulted in the formation of adipose tissues (Altmann et al. 2003). Biomimetic scaffolds made of thio-norbornene crosslinked gelatin, and the outcomes showed that the developed scaffolds have properties consistent with the native adipose tissue (Van Damme et al. 2021). Low-acyl gella gum hydrogels were prepared and modified with hemicellulose nanofibers, which were found nontoxic to the rat ADSCs and promoted angiogenesis

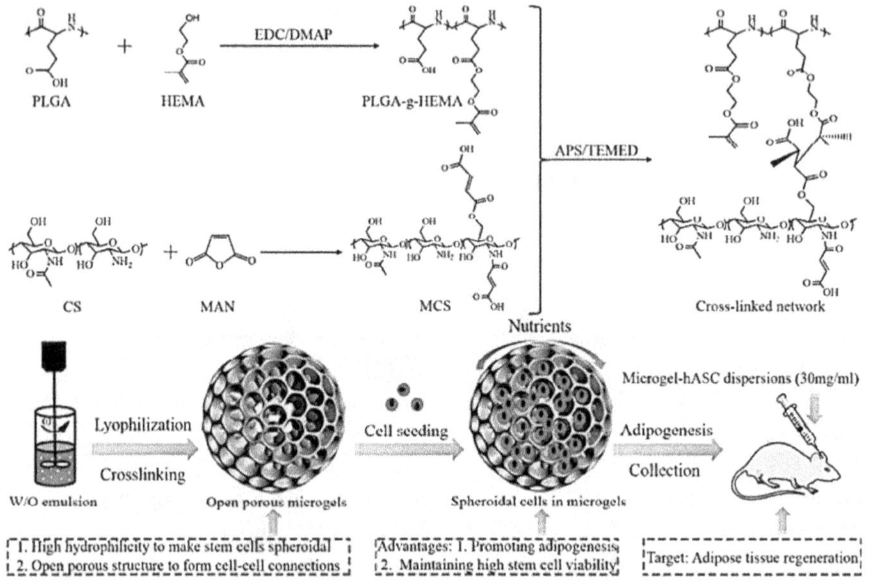

FIGURE 12.4 An illustration of preparation and application of an open-pore microgel to evaluate adipose tissue formation.

Source: Xia et al. 2017.

(Ning et al. 2019). Poly-(l-glutamic acid)-g-2-hydroxyethyl methacrylate with maleic anhydride-modified chitosan composite hydrogel was prepared and studied for adipose tissue restoration. The injected gels showed high cell viability and formation of new adipose tissues and blood vessels. Figure 12.4 shows a schematic representation of the development of composite open-pore microgels. The prepared gels were seeded with cells and evaluated (Xia et al. 2017).

12.5.9 Naturally Derived Hydrogels

Most of the engineered biomaterials do not have the specific characteristics of the adipose ECM. Decellularization helps prepare bioscaffolds with complex ECM composition and can be prepared from any type of tissue in the body (Uriel et al. 2009). The composition and properties of the developed hydrogels depend on the tissue source. The hydrogels derived from tissues aid integrin-mediated interactions with cells (Cheng et al. 2010). Subcutaneous adipose tissue-derived hydrogels promote vessel assembly and the differentiation of preadipocytes. The hydrogel derived from the dermis and adipose tissue induces neovascularization (Uriel et al. 2008, Shridhar et al. 2017). Human decellularized adipose tissue with methacrylated glycol chitosan and methacrylated chondroitin sulfate hydrogels is prepared and studied, and the outcome shows that the prepared composite hydrogels promote the differentiation of ADSCs (Cheung et al. 2014). The methacrylated chondroitin sulfate-formed hydrogel composite with decellularized adipose tissue encapsulating the ADSCs and cryo-milled ECM provides the pro-adipogenic environment for the ADSCs (Brown et al. 2015, Shridhar et al. 2019). Naturally derived placental decellular matrix with

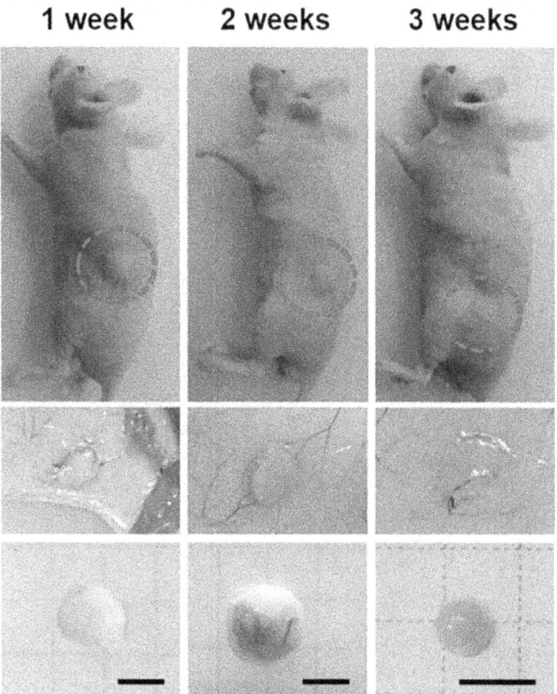

FIGURE 12.5 The implantation of the naturally derived ECM and methylcellulose hydrogels in the nude mouse models and the tissue formation at 1, 2 and 3 weeks after the injection.

Source: Kim et al. 2017.

crosslinked hyaluronan gels was prepared and studied with primary ADSCs. The results have shown that the scaffolds promoted cell attachment, proliferation and migration and supported the differentiation of adipocytes. The prepared scaffolds were also examined in a mouse model, and the results have shown that the formation of adipocytes and volume were maintained throughout the study (Flynn et al. 2006, 2009). Adult rat and human omenta were decellularized to be used as scaffolds, and the preliminary analysis of the scaffolds with ADSCs shows the scaffold can be exploited for adipose tissue regeneration (Porzionato et al. 2011). Adipose decellularized ECM hydrogels with poly(l-lactide-co-caprolactone) were prepared and studied for adipogenesis and angiogenesis. The results show that the prepared scaffolds have mechanical properties similar to the native adipose tissue, and the 12-week study showed both angiogenesis and adipogenesis were promoted and apoptosis was suppressed (Kim et al. 2021). Naturally derived adipose-derived soluble ECM was developed with methylcellulose as a cell-free scaffold for the regeneration of adipose tissue. The in vivo results presented showed that the hydrogel formed increased the number of ADSCs and adipose tissue macrophages. Figure 12.5 shows the implantation of the hydrogels into the back of the mouse and the development of the tissues (Kim et al. 2017) Table 12.1 presents information on different composite hydrogels employed in adipose tissue engineering, the types of cells utilized in experiments, and the corresponding observed outcomes.

TABLE 12.1
Composite Hydrogels Used in Adipose Tissue Engineering

Composite Hydrogel	Cell Type Used	Observation	References
Collagen hydrogels with FGF-2 encapsulated gelatin microspheres	-	Promote vascularization	Kimura et al. (2003)
Collagen hydrogels with FGF-2 encapsulated gelatin microspheres	ADSCs	Promote vascularization	Vashi et al. (2006)
Collagen gels with collagen fibers	Preadipocytes	Increase cell viability and lipid accumulation	Gentleman et al. (2006)
Collagen with cells	ADSCs	Adipose tissue formation and neovascularization	Von Heimburg et al. (2001)
Collagen, PLA along with silk fibroin hydrogel	ADSCs and BMSCs	Differentiation and adipogenesis	Mauney et al. (2007)
Glutaraldehyde-crosslinked collagen-chitosan hydrogels	Primary rat adipose precursor cells	Formation of cells	Wu et al. (2007)
A silver-impregnated/collagen-coated PLGA/PCL scaffold	-	Enhances biocompatibility, osteogenic and antibacterial property	Qian et al. (2021)
Alginate with RGD sequence scaffold	Fibroblasts	Increased adipogenesis	Marler et al. (2000)
Alginate hydrogel with RGD sequence	-	Neovascularization	Halberstadt et al. (2002)
Hyaluronic acid, Laminin and Alginate hydrogel	-	Adipogenic differentiation	Chen et al. (2015)
Gelatin hydrogel with alginate or chitosan	ADSCs	Cell proliferation	Ye et al. (2021)
Alginate - GelMA hydrogels	Gingival-derived mesenchymal stem cells	Wound healing and soft tissue reconstruction	Ansari et al. (2021)
Crosslinked hyaluronan and decellularized human placenta	ADSCs	Adipocyte differentiation	Flynn et al. (2007)
Hyaluronan was chemically modified by dodecyl-amidation of the carboxyl groups of the glucuronic acid	Adipocyte precursor	Adipose tissue regeneration	Rhodes et al. (2008)

(Continued)

TABLE 12.1 (*Continued*)
Composite Hydrogels Used in Adipose Tissue Engineering

Composite Hydrogel	Cell Type Used	Observation	References
Hyaluronic acid with cells	Human adipocyte precursors	Adipocyte differentiation	Halbleib et al. (2003)
Hyaluronan/gelatin composite scaffolds crosslinked with lithium phenyl-2,4,6-trimethyl benzoyl phosphinate	ADSCs	Maturation and proliferation of adipocytes	Kessler et al. (2017)
Gellan gum-hyaluronic acid spongy like hydrogels	Human adipose stem cells and human microvascular endothelial cells	Neovascularization, re-epithelialization and wound remodeling	Cerqueira et al. (2014)
Matrigel with FGF-2	-	Neovascularization and recruitment and differentiation of preadipocytes	Kawaguchi et al. (1998)
Matrigel and FGF in a specialized silicone housing	-	Adipogenesis and volume maintenance	Walton et al. (2004)
Myogel	-	Preadipocyte differentiation and vascularization	Abberton et al. (2008)
Fibrin	Preadipocytes	Adipose tissue formation	Schoeller et al. (2001)
FGF-2 loaded in fibrin glue and PGA matrix with or without preadipocytes	-	Adipose tissue formation	Hofer et al. (2003)
Injectable fibrin with PGA-PLA incorporated with ADSCs and FGF	ADSCs	Volume maintenance and adipose tissue formation	Cho et al. (2005)
Fibrin hydrogel with poly(caprolactone)-based polyurethane scaffold	ADSCs	Vascularized adipose tissue formation	Wittmann et al. (2016)
PLGA seeded with primary rat adipose seeded cells	Primary rat adipose cells	Frowth and differentiation of adipose tissue	Patrick et al. (1999)

(Continued)

TABLE 12.1 (*Continued*)
Composite Hydrogels Used in Adipose Tissue Engineering

Composite Hydrogel	Cell Type Used	Observation	References
PLGA-PEG composite with insulin, insulin-like growth factor-1 and basic fibroblast growth factor	-	Enhanced free fat graft weight and volume	Neubauer et al. (2005)
PEG incorporated with laminin-111 peptide with FGF2	Adipocyte or mesenchymal cells	Differentiation of preadipocyte	Patel et al. (2005)
Poly (ethylene glycol)-diacrylate (PEGDA) hydrogels	Human mesenchymal stem cells	Adipose tissue formation and 1000% volume retention	Alhadlaq et al. (2005)
Silk fibroin	adipocytes and endothelial cells	Formation of adipose tissue	Altmann et al. (2003)
Thio-norbornene crosslinked gelatin	-	Properties of native adipose tissue	Van Damme et al. (2021)
Low-acyl gella gum hydrogels modified with hemicellulose nanofibers	Rat ADSCs	Promote angiogenesis	Ning et al. (2019)
Poly-(l-glutamic acid)-g-2-hydroxyethyl methacrylate with maleic anhydride-modified chitosan composite hydrogel	-	High cell viability, formation of adipose tissue and neovascularization	Xia et al. (2017)
Human decellularized adipose tissue with methacrylated glycol chitosan and methacrylated chondroitin sulfate hydrogels	ADSCs	Promote differentiation of ADSCs	Cheung et al. (2014)
The methacrylated chondroitin sulfate-formed hydrogel composite with decellularized adipose tissue	ADSCs	Provide pro-adipogenic environment for ADSCs	Brown et al. (2015)
Naturally derived placental decellular matrix with crosslinked hyaluronan gels	ADSCs	Adipocytes formation and volume maintenance	Flynn et al. (2006, 2009)

(Continued)

TABLE 12.1 (*Continued*)
Composite Hydrogels Used in Adipose Tissue Engineering

Composite Hydrogel	Cell Type Used	Observation	References
Adipose decellularized extracellular matrix hydrogel with poly(l-lactide-co-caprolactone)	-	Angiogenesis and adipogenesis	Kim et al. (2021)
Naturally derived adipose-derived soluble ECM with methylcellulose	-	Increased ADSCs and adipose tissue	Kim et al. (2017)

12.6 CONCLUSION

The focus on adipose tissue engineering is increasing, and several therapies are becoming more available for the rejuvenation of the soft tissue. To date, many biomaterial scaffolds have been constructed and investigated both in vitro and in vivo for the regeneration of adipose tissues. To develop a suitable hydrogel for soft tissue regeneration, the mechanical strength and biodegradation rate must match the natural soft tissue. Even with advancements in tissue engineering, the ideal microenvironment for fat formation over an extended period of time remains unresolved. The long-term cell survival of the engineered cells was also a limitation for the reconstructed tissues. Regeneration using scaffolds seeded with cells has been widely used, and several studies have shown that the seeded scaffolds are better for the revitalizaiton of the soft tissues than the unseeded scaffolds. The potential of using ADSCs with various biomaterials could be used in several modalities. Overall, adipose tissue engineering is an emerging field, and long-term and stable regeneration of the soft tissues may be possible in the near future.

REFERENCES

Abberton K.M., Bortolotto S.K., Woods A.A., Findlay M., Morrison W.A., Thompson E.W., Messina A. 2008. Myogel, a novel, basement membrane-rich, extracellular matrix derived from skeletal muscle, is highly adipogenic in vivo and in vitro. *Cell Tissues Organs*. 188(4):347–58.

Akita S., Akino K., Hirano A., Ohtsuru A., Yamashita S. 2010. Noncultured autologous adipose-derived stem cells therapy for chronic radiation injury. *Stem Cells Int*. 2010:1–8.

Alhadlaq A., Tang M., Mao J.J. 2005. Engineered adipose tissue from human mesenchymal stem cells maintains predefined shape and dimension: Implications in soft tissue augmentation and reconstruction. *Tissue Eng*. 11(3–4):556–66.

Altman G.H., Diaz F., Jakuba C., Calabro T., Horan R.L., Chen J., Lu H., Richmond J., Kaplan D.L. 2003. Silk-based biomaterials. *Biomaterials*. 24(3):401–16.

Amos P.J., Kapur S.K., Stapor P.C., Shang H., Bekiranov S., Khurgel M., Rodeheaver G.T., Pierce S.M., Katz A.J. 2010. Human adipose derived stromal cells accelerate diabetic wound healing: Impact of cell formulation and delivery. *Tissue Eng Part A*. 16(5):1595–1606.

Ansari S., Pouraghaei Sevari S., Chen C., Sarrion P., Moshaverinia A. 2021. RGD-modified alginate–GelMA hydrogel sheet containing gingival mesenchymal stem cells: A unique platform for wound healing and soft tissue regeneration. *ACS Biomater Sci Eng*. 7(8): 3774–82.

Beahm E.K., Walton R.L., Patrick Jr. C.W. 2003. Progress in adipose tissue construct development. *Clin Plast Surg*. 30(4):547–58.

Brown C.F.C., Yan J., Han T.T.Y., Marecak D.M., Amsden B.G., Flynn L.E. 2015. Effect of decellularized adipose tissue particle size and cell density on adipose-derived stem cell proliferation and adipogenic differentiation in composite methacrylated chondroitin sulphate hydrogels. *Biomed. Mater*. 10(4):045010.

Butterwick K.J., Nootheti P.K., Hsu J.W., Goldman M.P. 2007. Autologous fat transfer: An in-depth look at varying concepts and techniques. *Facial Plast Surg Clin North Am*. 15(1):99–111.

Casadei A., Agolli E., Vicari Sottosanti M.C., Bovani B., Cinti S. 2011. Clinical use of ADSC in plastic surgery: Case report. *Proceedings of the International Conference on Adipose Tissue*, December 2011, Venice, Italy.

Casadei A., Epis R., Ferroni L., Touch I., Gardin C., Bressan E., Sivolella S., Vindigni V., Pinton P., Mucci G., Zavan B. 2012. Adipose tissue regeneration: A state of the art. *J Biomed Biotechnol*. 2012:1–12.

Cerqueira M.T., da Silva L.P., Santos T.C., Pirraco R.P., Correlo V.M., Reis R.L., Marques A.P. 2014. Gellan gum-hyaluronic acid spongy-like hydrogels and cells from adipose tissue synergize promoting neoskin vascularization. *ACS Appl Mater Interfaces*. 6(22):19668–79.

Chen Y.S., Chen Y.Y., Hsueh Y.S., Tai H.C., Lin F.H. 2015. Modifying alginate with early embryonic extracellular matrix, laminin, and hyaluronic acid for adipose tissue engineering. *J Biomed Mater Res Part A*. 104(3):669–77.

Cheng M.H., Uriel S., Moya M.L., Francis-Sedlak M., Wang R., Huang J.J., Chang S.Y., Brey E.M. 2010. Dermis-derived hydrogels support adipogenesis in vivo. *J Biomed Mater Res*. 92(3):852–8.

Cheung H.K., Han T.T.Y., Marecak D.M., Watkins J.F., Amsden B.G., Flynn L.E., et al. 2014. Biomaterials composite hydrogel scaffolds incorporating decellularized adipose tissue for soft tissue engineering with adipose-derived stem cells. *Biomaterials*. 35(6):1914–23.

Chiu Y.C., Cheng M.H., Uriel S., Brey E.M. 2011. Materials for engineering vascularized adipose tissue. *J Tissue Viability*. 20(2):37–48.

Cho S.W., Kim S.S., Rhie J.W., Cho H.M., Choi C.Y., Kim B.S. 2005. Engineering of volume-stable adipose tissues. *Biomaterials*. 26(17):3577–85.

Choi J.H., Gimble J.M., Lee K., Marra K.G., Rubin J.P., Yoo J.J., Vunjak-Novakovic G., Kaplan D.L. 2010. Adipose tissue engineering for soft tissue regeneration. *Tissue Eng Part B: Reviews*. 16(4):413–26.

Choi Y.S., Park S.N., Suh H. 2005. Adipose tissue engineering using mesenchymal stem cells attached to injectable PLGA microspheres. *Biomaterials*. 26(29):5855–63.

Cinti S. 2001. The adipose organ: Morphological perspectives of adipose tissues. *Proc Nutr Soc*. 60(3):319–28.

Cook T., Nakra T., Shorr N., Douglas R.S. 2004. Facial recontouring with autogenous fat. *Facial Plast Surg* 20(2):145–7.

Duranti F., Salti G., Bovani B., Calandra M., Rosati M.L. 1998. Injectable hyaluronic acid gel for soft tissue augmentation. *Dermatol Surg*. 24(12):1317–25.

Ebrahimian T.G., Pouzoulet F., Squiban C., et al. 2009. Cell therapy based on adipose tissue-derived stromal cells promotes physiological and pathological wound healing. *Arterioscler Thromb Vasc Biol*. 29(4):503–10.

Flynn L., Semple J.L., Woodhouse K.A. 2006. Decellularized placental matrices for adipose tissue engineering. *J Biomed Mater Res A*. 79(2):359–69.

Flynn L., Prestwich G.D., Semple J.L., Woodhouse K.A. 2007. Adipose tissue engineering with naturally derived scaffolds and adipose-derived stem cells. *Biomaterials*. 28(26):3834–42.

Flynn L., Woodhouse K.A. 2008. Adipose tissue engineering with cells in engineered matrices. *Organogenesis*. 4(4):28–235.

Flynn L., Prestwich G.D., Semple J.L., Woodhouse K.A. 2009. Adipose tissue engineering in vivo with adipose-derived stem cells on naturally derived scaffolds. *J Biomed Mater Res A*. 89(4):929–41.

Gentleman E., Nauman E.A., Livesay G.A., Dee K.C. 2006. Collagen composite biomaterials resist contraction while allowing development of adipocytic soft tissue in vitro. *Tissue Eng*. 12(6):1639–49.

Halberstadt C., Austin C., Rowley J., Culberson C., Loebsek A., Wyatt S., Coleman S., Blacksten L., Burg K., Mooney D., Holder Jr. W. 2002. A hydrogel material for plastic and reconstructive applications injected into the subcutaneous space of a sheep. *Tissue Eng*. 8(2):309–19.

Halbleib M., Skurk T., Luca C., Heimburg D., Hauner H. 2003. Tissue engineering of white adipose tissue using hyaluronic acid-based scaffolds. I: In vitro differentiation of human adipocyte precursor cells on scaffolds. *Biomaterials*. 24(18):3125–32.

Hemmrich, K., von Heimburg D. 2006. Biomaterials for adipose tissue engineering. *Expert Rev Med Devices*. 3(5):635–45.

Hofer S.O., Knight K.M., Cooper-White J.J. et al. 2003. Increasing the volume of vascularized tissue formation in engineered constructs: An experimental study in rats. *Plast Reconstr Sur*. 111(3):1186–92.

Holm J.S., Toyserkani N.M., Sorensen J.A. 2018. Adipose-derived stem cells for treatment of chronic ulcers: Current status. *Stem Cell Res Ther*. 9(1):142.

Katz A.J., Llull R., Hedrick M.H., Futrell J.W. 1999. Emerging approaches to the tissue engineering of fat. *Clin Plast Surg*. 26:587–603.

Kawaguchi N., Toriyama K., Nicodemu-Lena E., Inou K., Torii S., Kitagawa Y. 1998. De novo adipogenesis in mice at the site of injection of basement membrane and basic fibroblast growth factor. *Proc. Natl. Acad. Sci*. 95:1062–6.

Kessler L., Gehrke S., Winnefeld M., Huber B., Hoch E., Walter T., Wyrwa R., Schnabelrauch M., Schmidt M., Kückelhaus M., Lehnhardt M., Hirsch T., Jacobsen F. 2017. Methacrylated gelatin/hyaluronan-based hydrogels for soft tissue engineering. *J Tissue Eng*. 8. doi: 10.1177/2041731417744157.

Kim B.S., Baez C.E., Atala A. 2000. Biomaterials for tissue engineering. *World J Urol*. 18:2–9.

Kim J.S., Choi J.S., Cho Y.W. 2017. Cell-free hydrogel system based on a tissue-specific extracellular matrix for in situ adipose tissue regeneration. *ACS Appl Mater Interfaces*. 9(10):8581–8.

Kim S.H., Kim D., Cha M., Kim S.H., Jung Y. 2021. The regeneration of large-sized and vascularized adipose tissue using a tailored elastic scaffold and dECM hydrogels. *Int J Mol Sci*. 22(22): 12560.

Kim W.S., Park B.S., Sung J.H., Yang J.M., Park S.B., Kwak S.J., Park J.S. 2007. Wound healing effect of adipose-derived stem cells: A critical role of secretory factors on human dermal fibroblasts. *J Dermatol Sci*. 48(1):15–24.

Kimura Y., Ozeki M., Inamoto T., Tabata Y. 2003. Adipose tissue engineering based on human preadipocytes combined with gelatin microspheres containing basic fibroblast growth factor. *Biomaterials*. 24:2513–21.

Klaus S. 2001. Overview: Biological significance of fat and adipose tissues. *Bioscience* 2001; 1–10.

Lavik E., Langer R. 2004. Tissue engineering: Current state and perspectives. *Appl Microbiol Biotechnol*. 65:1.

Lee E.Y., Xia Y., Kim W.S., et al. 2009. Hypoxia-enhanced woundhealing function of adipose-derived stem cells: Increase in stem cell proliferation and up-regulation of VEGF and bFGF. *Wound Repair Regen*. 17(4):540–7.

Lee S.W., Jeon T.J., Biswal S. 2015. Fracture healing effects of locally-administered adipose tissue-derived cells. *Yonsei Med J.* 56:1106–13.

Levenberg S., Langer R. 2004. Advances in tissue engineering. *Curr Top Dev Biol.* 61:113.

Lindroos B., Suuronen R., Miettinen S. 2011. The potential of adipose stem cells in regenerative medicine. *Stem Cell Rev Rep.* 7(2):269–91.

Louis F., Matsusaki M. 2020. Adipose tissue engineering. *Biomaterials for Organ and Tissue Regeneration*, 393–423. doi: 10.1016/B978-0-08-102906-0.00008-8.

Marler J.J., Guha A., Rowley J., Koka R., Mooney D., Upton J., Vacanti J.P. 2000. Soft tissue augmentation with injectable alginate and syngeneic fibroblasts. *Plast Reconstr Surg* 105:2049–58.

Mauney J.R., Nguyen T., Gillen K., Kirker-Head C., Gimble J.M., Kaplan D.L. 2007. Engineering adipose-like tissue in vitro and in vivo utilizing human bone marrow and adiposederived mesenchymal stem cells with silk fibroin 3D scaffolds. *Biomaterials.* 28(35):5280–90.

Miranville A., Heeschen C., Sengenes C., Curat C.A., Busse R., Bouloumie A. 2004. Improvement of postnatal neovascularization by human adipose tissue-derived stem cells. *Circulation.* 110(3):349–55.

Mughal M., Sindali K., Man J., Roblin P. 2021. 'Fat chance': A review of adipose tissue engineering and its role in plastic and reconstructive surgery. *Ann R Coll Surg Engl.* 103(4): 245–9.

Neubauer M., Hacker M., Bauer-Kreisel P., Weiser B., Fischbach C., Schulz M.B., Goepferich A., Blunk T. 2005. Adipose tissue engineering based on mesenchymal stem cells and basic fibroblast growth factor in vitro. *Tissue Eng.* 11:1840–51.

Nimni M.E., Cheung D., Strates B., Kodama M., Sheikh K. 1987. Chemically modified collagen: A natural biomaterial for tissue replacement. *J Biomed Mater Res.* 21:741–71.

Ning H., Wu X., Wu Q., Yu W., Wang H., Zheng S., Chen Y., Li Y., Su J. 2019. Microfiber-reinforced composite hydrogels loaded with rat adipose-derived stem cells and BMP-2 for the treatment of medication-related osteonecrosis of the jaw in a rat model. *ACS Biomater Sci Eng.* 5(5):2430–43.

Patel P.N., Gobin A.S., West J.L., Patrick Jr. C.W. 2005. Poly(ethylene glycol) hydrogel system supports preadipocyte viability, adhesion, and proliferation. *Tissue Eng.* 11:1498–505.

Patrick C.W. 2001. Tissue engineering strategies for adipose tissue repair. *Anat Rec.* 263(4):361–6.

Patrick Jr. C.W., Chauvin P.B., Hobley J., Reece G.P. 1999. Preadipocyte seeded PLGA scaffolds for adipose tissue engineering. *Tissue Eng.* 5:139–51.

Piasecki J.H., Gutowski K.A., Lahvis G.P., Moreno K.I. 2007. An experimental model for improving fat graft viability and purity. *Plast Reconstr Surg.* 119:1571–83.

Porzionato A., Sfriso M.M., Macchi V., et al. 2011. Decellularization of rat and human omentum to develop novel scaffolds to be recellularized with adipose derived stem cells. *Ital J Anat Embryol.* 116(1):149.

Puissant B., Barreau C., Bourin P., et al. 2005. Immunomodulatory effect of human adipose tissue-derived adult stem cells: Comparison with bone marrow mesenchymal stem cells. *Br J Haematol.* 129(1):118–29.

Qian Y.Z., Zhou X., Zhang F.M., Diekwisch T.G.H., Luan X., Yang J. 2019. Triple PLGA/PCL scaffold modification including silver-impregnation, collagen-coating, and electrospinning significantly improve biocompatibility, antimicrobial, and osteogenic properties for oro-facial tissue regeneration. *ACS Appl Mater Interfaces*, 11(41):37381–396.

Rhodes N., Di Bartolo C., Bellini D. 2008. Induction of adipose tissue regeneration by chemically-modified hyaluronic acid. *Int J Nano Biomater.* 1(3):250–62.

Rowley J.A., Madlambayan G., Mooney D.J. 1999. Alginate hydrogels as synthetic extracellular matrix materials. *Biomaterials.* 20(1):45–53.

Schoeller T., Lille S., Wechselberger G., Otto A., Mowlavi A., Piza-Katzer H. 2001. Histomorphologic and volumetric analysis of implanted autologous preadipocyte cultures suspended in fibrin glue: A potential new source for tissue augmentation. *Aesthetic Plast. Surg*. 25(1):57–63.

Shridhar A., Amsden B.G., Gillies E.R., Flynn L.E. 2019. Investigating the effects of tissue-specific extracellular matrix on the adipogenic and osteogenic differentiation of human adipose-derived stromal cells within composite hydrogel scaffolds. *Front Bioeng Biotechnol*. 7:402.

Shridhar A., Gillies E., Amsden B.G., Flynn L.E. 2017. Composite bioscaffolds incorporating decellularized ECM as a cell-instructive component within hydrogels as in vitro models and cell delivery systems. *Methods Mol Biol*. 1577:183–208.

Singh M.R. 2016. Natural polymer-based hydrogels as scaffolds for tissue engineering. In: A.M. Grumezescu (ed.) *Nanobiomaterials in Soft Tissue Engineering*. Elsiver, Amsterdam. pp. 231–60.

Slaughter B.V., Khurshid S.S., Fisher O.Z. 2009. Hydrogels in regenerative medicine. *Adv Mater*. 21:3307–29.

Stosich M.S., Bastian B., Marion N.W., Clark P.A., Reilly G., Mao J.J. 2007. Vascularized adipose tissue grafts from human mesenchymal stem cells with bioactive cues and microchannel conduits. *Tissue Eng*. 13(12):2881–90.

Torio-Padron N., Baerlecken N., Momeni A., Stark G.B., Borges J. 2007. Engineering of adipose tissue by injection of human preadipocytes in fibrin. *Aesthetic Plast Surg*. 31:285–93.

Upadhyaya S.N., Bernard S.L., Grobmyer S.R., Yanda C., Tu C., Valente S.A. 2018. Outcomes of autologous fat grafting in mastectomy patients following breast reconstruction. *Ann Surg Oncol*. 25:3052–6.

Uriel S., Huang J.J., Moya M.L., Francis M.E., Wang R., Chang S.Y., et al. 2008. The role of adipose protein derived hydrogels in adipogenesis. *Biomaterials*. 29:3712–9.

Uriel S., Labay E., Francis-Sedlak M., Moya M.L., Weichselbaum R.R., Ervin N., et al. 2009. Extraction and assembly of tissue-derived gels for cell culture and tissue engineering. *Tissue Eng Part C Methods*. 15(3):309–21.

Vaicik M.K., Morse M., Blagajcevic A., Rios J., Larson J., Yang F., Cohen R.N., Papavasiliou G., Brey E.M. 2015. Hydrogel-based engineering of beige adipose tissue. *J Mater Chem B*. 3(40):7903–11.

Van Damme L., Van Hoorick J., Blondeel P., Van Vlierberghe S. 2021. Toward adipose tissue engineering using thiol-norbornene photo-crosslinkable gelatin hydrogels. *Biomacromolecules*. 22(6): 2408–18.

Vashi A.V., Abberton K.M., Thomas G.P., Morrison W.A., O'Connor A.J., Cooper-White J.J., Thompson E.W. 2006. Adipose tissue engineering based on the controlled release of fibroblast growth factor-2 in a collagen matrix. *Tissue Eng*. 12:3035.

Von Heimburg D., Zachariah S., Heschel I., Kuhling H., Schoof H., Hafemann B., Pallua N. 2001. Human preadipocytes seeded on freeze-dried collagen scaffolds investigated in vitro and in vivo. *Biomaterials*. 22:429–38.

Walton R.L., Beahm E.K., Wu L. 2004. De novo adipose formation in a vascularized engineered construct. *Microsurgery*. 24:378–84.

Wang S., Dhandayuthapani B., Yoshida Y., Maekawa T., Kumar D.S. 2011. Polymeric scaffolds in tissue engineering application: A review. *Int J Polym Sci*. 2011:290602.

Watanabe F.D., Mullon C.J.P., Hewitt W.R., et al. 1997. Clinical experience with a bioartificial liver in the treatment of severe liver failure: A phase I clinical trial. *Ann Surg*. 225(5):484–94.

Wittmann K., Storck K., Muhr C., Mayer H., Regn S., Staudenmaier R., Wiese H., Maier G., Bauer-Kreisel P., Blunk T. 2016. Development of volume-stable adipose tissue constructs using polycaprolactone-based polyurethane scaffolds and fibrin hydrogels. *J Tissue Eng Regen Med*. 10(10):409–18.

Wu X., Black L., Santacana-Laffitte G., Patrick Jr. C.W. 2007. Preparation and assessment of glutaraldehyde-crosslinked collagen-chitosan hydrogels for adipose tissue engineering. *J Biomed Mater Res A*. 81:59–65.

Xia P., Zhang K., Gong Y., Li G., Yan S., Yin J. 2017. Injectable stem cell-laden open porous microgels that favour adipogenesis: In vitro and in vivo evaluation. *ACS Appl Mater Interfaces*. 9(40):34751–61.

Yang J., Zhou C., Fu J., Yang Q., He T., Tan Q., Lv Q. 2021. In situ adipogenesis in biomaterials without cell seeds: Current status and perspectives. *Front Cell Dev Biol*. 9: 647149.

Ye J., Yang G., Zhang J., Xiao Z., He L., Zhang H., Liu Q. 2021. Preparation and characterization of gelatin-polysaccharide composite hydrogels for tissue engineering. *PeerJ* 9:e11022.

Zhu J., Roger E.M. 2011. Design properties of hydrogel tissue-engineering scaffolds. *Expert Rev Med Devices*. 8(5):607–26.

Zuk P.A., Zhu M., Ashjian P., et al. 2002. Human adipose tissue is a source of multipotent stem cells. *Mol Biol Cell*. 13(12):4279–95.

13 Recent Progress in Organic-Inorganic Hybrids for Bone Tissue Reconstruction

Toshiki Miyazaki
Kyushu Institute of Technology

CONTENTS

13.1 Need for Bone-Repairing Materials.......275
13.2 Bioactive Ceramics.......276
13.3 Evaluation of Bioactivity Using Simulated Body Fluid.......276
13.4 Needs for Bone-Repairing Composites.......277
13.5 Ceramics-Metal Composites.......277
13.6 Ceramics-Polymer Composites.......278
13.7 Ceramic-Polymer Nanocomposites.......281
13.8 Self-Setting Ceramics-Polymer Composites.......282
13.9 Conclusions.......284
References.......284

13.1 NEED FOR BONE-REPAIRING MATERIALS

The human body is made up of a combination of multiple bones, and the number is 300 or more for babies and about 200 for adults. Bones are connected by joints, and bones and muscles are connected by tendons to form the musculoskeletal system of the human body. The musculoskeletal system plays various roles, such as shaping the human body, supplying nutrition, regulating the endocrine system, and enabling the movement of the human body.

If a small part of the bone is lost due to disease or injury, it will be repaired by the healing abilities of the human body. However, when the defect exceeds the repair capacity of the human body, bone grafting is performed to fill the defect. Bone grafts include autografts and allografts. The problems with the autograft are that it is necessary to injure a healthy part in order to collect the patient's bone and that there are restrictions on the part, amount, and size to be collected. Although the allograft has few problems with the autograft, they can cause infections when transplanted. If bone repair can be achieved using artificial materials, the problem of bone grafting can be solved. However, the problem of foreign body reactions still

DOI: 10.1201/9781003251767-13

remains. For example, when sintered alumina ceramics and polymethyl methacrylate (PMMA) bone cement are implanted in bone defects, they are covered with a fibrous tissue of collagen and isolated from the bone [1,2]. This is a defensive reaction for the living body to protect itself.

13.2 BIOACTIVE CERAMICS

Ceramics have advantages for bone repair, such as high mechanical strength and hardness in comparison with other inorganic materials. Among them, some ceramics are known to directly bond to living bone without the foreign body reaction. They are called bioactive ceramics. Bioglass [3,4], sintered hydroxyapatite [5] and glass-ceramic A-W, where fluorapatite and wollastonite are precipitated in a glassy matrix [5] are known as bioactive ceramics.

They bond to bone via a low-crystalline apatite layer with composition and structure similar to those of bone minerals. The apatite layer is formed by consumption of Ca^{2+} and PO_4^{3-} ions in the surrounding body fluid. The body fluid is already supersaturated with respect to the apatite. When the apatite layer is formed, the leukocytes responsible for immunity misrecognize the apatite layer as broken bone and instruct undifferentiated cells (mesenchymal cells) to produce osteoblasts instead of fibroblasts. Consequently, bone formation is enhanced on the apatite layer to integrate with the bone tissue. It has been reported that calcite-type calcium carbonate [6], β-tricalcium phosphate [7], and δ-alumina [8] also bond to bone, but no apatite layer formation is observed at the interface with bone.

Bioactive ceramics have the advantage of having the potential to prevent slippage and loosening in the body and achieve stable fixation over a long period of time due to their spontaneous bone-bonding ability.

13.3 EVALUATION OF BIOACTIVITY USING SIMULATED BODY FLUID

Ultimately, the bone-bonding phenomenon needs to be evaluated *in vivo*, but it requires a large amount of money for animal experiments. In order to conventionally reproduce the apatite formation on the surfaces of bioactive ceramics at the laboratory level, simulated body fluid (SBF) having inorganic ion concentrations nearly equal to human plasma has been proposed [9–11]. SBF has the composition shown in Table 13.1 and can be prepared by dissolving predetermined amounts of chemical reagents in distilled water in a predetermined order and then adjusting the pH of the solution. SBF does not contain cells or proteins. Therefore, it should be noted that SBF is intended to reproduce only the chemical reaction of apatite formation. The preparation procedure for SBF has been listed in ISO23317 since 2007 [12]. However, the concentrations of HCO_3^- and Cl^- ions are still different from those of human blood plasma. Therefore, a revised SBF with the ion concentrations described above closer to the body fluids has also been proposed [13].

TABLE 13.1
Ion Concentrations of SBF and Human Blood Plasma

	Concentration/mM	
Ion	**SBF**	**Human Blood Plasma**
Na^+	142.0	142.0
K^+	5.0	5.0
Mg^{2+}	1.5	1.5
Ca^{2+}	2.5	2.5
Cl^-	148.8	103.0
HCO_3^-	4.2	27.0
HPO_4^{2-}	1.0	1.0
SO_4^{2-}	0.5	0.5

13.4 NEEDS FOR BONE-REPAIRING COMPOSITES

Bioactive ceramics are attractive for bone repair. However, the ceramics still have problems with their mechanical properties. Namely, fracture toughness is lower and Young's modulus is higher in comparison with the bone tissue. The mechanical properties of representative biomaterials are shown in Table 13.2. Therefore, it is effective to make a composite in order to cover the disadvantages of the ceramics. The design of bone-repairing composites using a combination of bioactive ceramics and various materials is reviewed below.

13.5 CERAMICS-METAL COMPOSITES

Bioactive ceramics cannot be used in areas where a large load is applied, such as the femur, tibia, and tooth root, due to their low fracture toughness. Metallic materials are widely used for the repair of such portions. Several metals such as Ti, Ta, Nb, and Hf are histologically observed to directly contact bone without inclusions, a process called osseointegration [14]. However, the bonding strength is not high. Therefore, novel biomaterials having both bone tissue affinity and high fracture toughness are expected to be obtained by combining them with bioactive ceramics.

For example, Ti-hydroxyapatite composites are developed by conventional sintering [15]. Generally, the sintering of Ti requires an inert atmosphere and a temperature of 1300°C or higher, but the hydroxyapatite is thermally decomposed in this temperature range. Therefore, it is shown that a sintered body with a bending strength of 100 MPa or more can be obtained by hot pressing at 1100°C.

However, since both Ti and hydroxyapatite have a higher Young's modulus than natural bone, stress shielding is likely to occur. This is a phenomenon in which the implanted material bears most of the load, and consequently, the load on the bone is

TABLE 13.2
Mechanical Properties of Representative Biomaterials in Comparison with Human Bone

Material	Tensile Strength/MPa	Young's Modulus/GPa
Pure Ti (Grade 1)	290–410	105–110
Ti-6Al-4V	920–950	100–110
Bioglass	42[a]	35
Glass-ceramics A-W	215[a]	118
Ultra high molecular weight polyethylene	30–40	0.45–1.3
Poly-L-lactic acid	15–150	2.7–4.1
Human cortical bone	50–150	7–30
Human cancellous bone	10–20	0.5–0.05

[a] Bending strength.

reduced. Bone is encouraged to grow by applying a moderate load. This is due to the piezoelectric effect caused by the specific orientation of bone, and the strain on osteocytes caused by the load activates the cellular pathway that promotes bone regeneration and reduces bone resorption [16]. This stress shielding may cause embrittlement of the surrounding bone. This is similar to the phenomenon in which the bones of a bedridden person weaken. Therefore, the development of next-generation bone-repairing materials with Young's modulus analogous to natural bone is desired. Although Young's modulus can be reduced by using a porous composite, it should be noted that mechanical strength also decreases at high porosity.

Some β-type Ti alloys are closer to bone than pure Ti and clinically used Ti-6Al-4V [17]. Composites of Ti-Nb-Sn alloy and hydroxyapatite are obtained by high-frequency induction- heated sintering and have a Young's modulus of 22 GPa, similar to that of human cortical bone, and a compressive strength of 877 MPa [18]. Therefore, this technique is quite effective for reducing the stress shielding of the surrounding bone.

Fabrication of the composites by coating is also widely attempted. Bioactivity can be imparted by plasma spraying of hydroxyapatite onto Ti [19]. The hydroxyapatite layer exhibits an adhesive strength of 80 MPa or more to the substrate. Hydroxyapatite can also be coated on Ti by sputtering [20] or electrodeposition [21].

The above-described SBF can also be used as a coating solution for the apatite. For example, if Ti metal is subjected to NaOH and heat treatment, a bone-like apatite layer is formed on the surface in SBF [22]. Such an apatite layer can be coated on Ti in SBF after anodic oxidation or H_2O_2 treatment [23]. Furthermore, the apatite layer can be coated with surface-modified Ta [24], Zr [25] and Hf [26].

13.6 CERAMICS-POLYMER COMPOSITES

Natural bone is an organic-inorganic composite consisting of inorganic apatite and organic collagen fibers [27]. Inspired by this specific structure, various ceramic-polymer composites have been developed for the purpose of bone repair. The most typical method for producing such a composite is the heat kneading of fine ceramic particles and thermoplastic polymer. In this method, a conventional extrusion molding apparatus can be utilized. In the case of polymers with low heat resistance, such as collagen, fine particles of the apatite precipitate in an aqueous solution, and collagen is freeze-dried [28]. Synthetic polymers such as polyethylene [29], poly(vinyl alcohol) [30], polylactic acid [31], and poly(ε-caprolactone) [32] and natural polymers such as collagen, chitosan [33], and cellulose [34] are combined with the hydroxyapatite to fabricate a composite.

The mechanical properties of the composites largely depend on the ratio of organic and inorganic components. In addition, Young's modulus of a composite changes depending on the distribution of each component, as shown in Figure 13.1, even at the same composition.

If each component receives constant stress, Young's modulus is expressed as follows:

$$E_c = \frac{1}{\frac{\bar{V}_a}{E_a} + \frac{1-\bar{V}_a}{E_p}} \tag{13.1}$$

If each component receives constant strain, Young's modulus is as follows:

$$E_c = E_a\bar{V}_a + E_p(1 - v_a) \tag{13.2}$$

Here, E_c, E_a, and E_p are Young's modulus of the composite, hydroxyapatite, and polyethylene, respectively, and V_a is the volume fraction of hydroxyapatite in the composite. Actual Young's modulus of the composite is between the minimum and maximum values, as shown in Figure 13.2.

The mechanical properties of the composites prepared by mixing various bioactive ceramics with high molecular weight polyethylene are shown in Figure 13.3 [29,35,36].

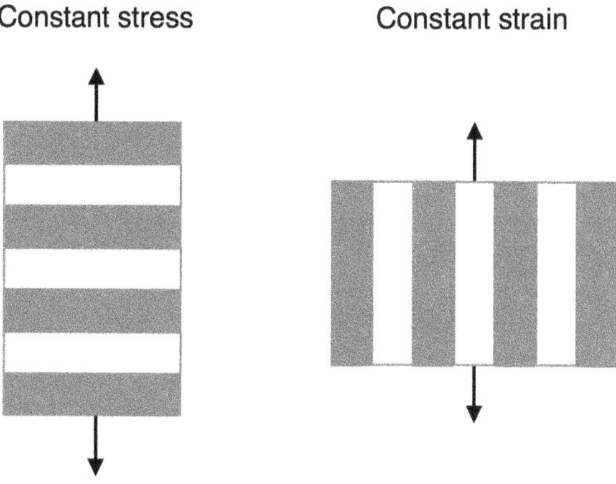

FIGURE 13.1 Differences in deformation modes of the composites.

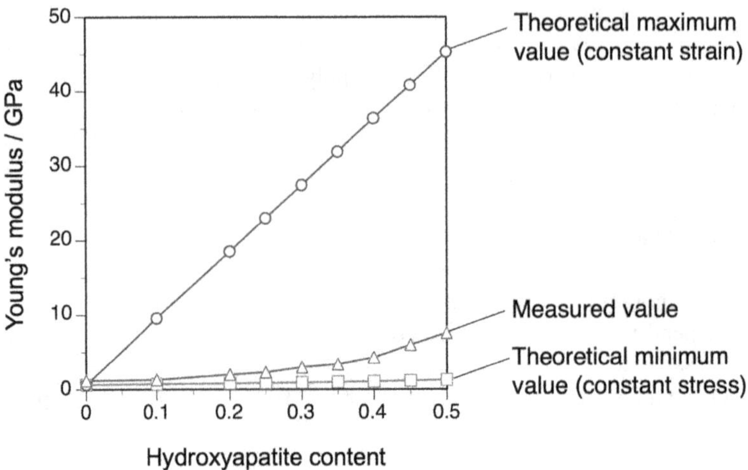

FIGURE 13.2 Compositional dependence of Young's modulus of hydroxyapatite/polyethylene composites as well as their theoretical value.

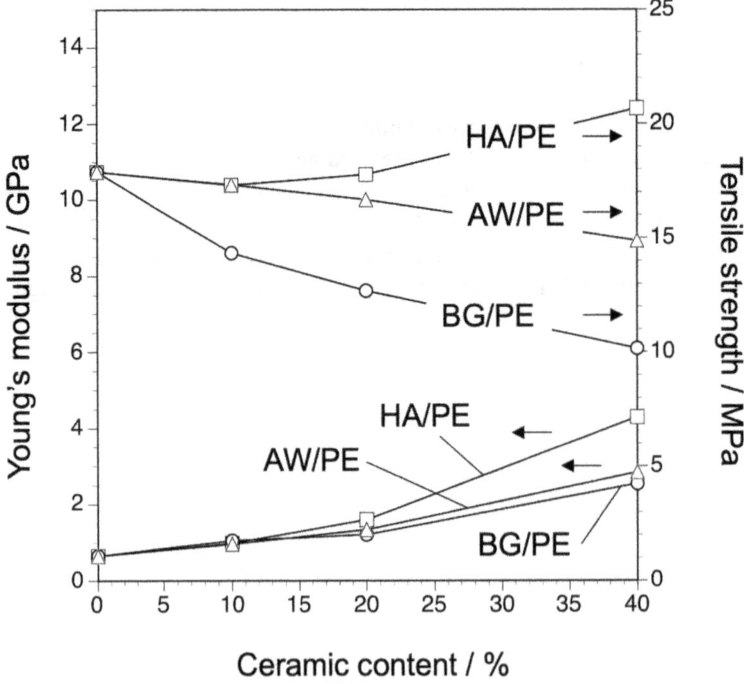

FIGURE 13.3 Compositional dependence of mechanical properties of various bioactive composites. HA/PE, AW/PE and BG/PE means hydroxyapatite/polyethylene, glass-ceramic A-W/polyethylene and bioglass/polyethylene composites, respectively.

Young's modulus almost corresponds to the ceramic content, but strength does not necessarily correlate. Namely, the strength of the ceramics is higher than that of the polyethylene, but the strength of AW/PE and BG/PE rather decreases as ceramic content increases. This is considered to be because the strength depends not only on the ceramic content but also on the bonding between the ceramic particles and the organic matrix. If the interface bonding is weak, the strength of the composite is not improved, even if it contains a large amount of ceramic. Especially in the case of tensile and bending tests, the interfacial influence appears more clearly than in the compressive test. Modification with silane coupling agents is effective for reinforcement of the interface [37]. The silane coupling agents have both hydrophilic silicate and hydrophobic organic functional groups. Therefore, the bonding between the hydrophilic ceramics and the hydrophobic polymer can be reinforced. The added silane coupling agents are reported to promote penetration of polymer into cavities in each ceramic filler to reinforce ceramic-polymer interface [38]. Recently, phosphonic acid-based coupling agents with higher water resistance than silane coupling agents have also become commercially available [39]. It is reported that pre-treatment of hydroxyapatite filler with 2-carboxyethylphosphonic acid enhances the tensile strength of hydroxyapatite-poly (ethylene-co-vinyl alcohol) nanocomposite [40].

13.7 CERAMIC-POLYMER NANOCOMPOSITES

If the organic component and the inorganic component are mixed at nanometer level, development of highly homogeneous materials is expected. However, the limit of mechanical pulverization of ceramic powder is submicron level, even by wet pulverization using a bead mill. Therefore, nanocomposites can be obtained by a bottom-up approach in which inorganic and organic components are dispersed in a solution in the form of ions, molecules and colloids.

It is believed that the presence of Ca^{2+} and silicates is important for bioactive glass to exhibit apatite formation in the body environment [3,4]. Based on these findings, a method for producing bioactive ceramic-polymer composites from alkoxysilane, calcium salt, and organic polymer by the sol-gel method has been proposed. Bioactive nanocomposites containing synthetic polymers such as ploymer of hydroxyethylmethacrylate (HEMA) [41], poly(tetramethylene oxide) [42], polydimethylsiloxane [43], poly(vinyl alcohol) [44], and poly(ε-caprolactone) [45], and natural polymers such as starch [46] and chitin [47] have been developed.

In addition to silicate, titanate [48] and tantalate [49] can also be used as inorganic components. Appearance of the titanate-HEMA nanocomposites is shown in Figure 13.4.

The obtained nanocomposite is highly flexible. Hara et al. prepared a transparent composite film from triethoxysilyl-terminated polyethylene glycol and titanium tetraisopropoxide by the sol-gel method [50]. When it was immersed in SBF for 14 days, calcium titanate was formed in addition to the apatite. It was speculated that the apatite formation was promoted by the calcium titanate formed by the reaction of titania in the film and SBF.

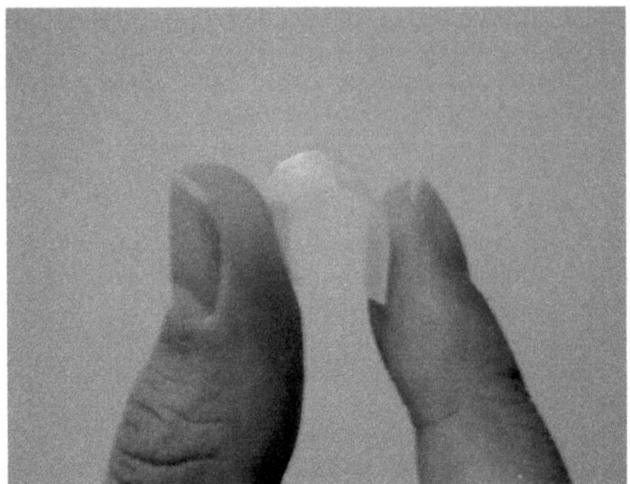

FIGURE 13.4 Appearance of the titanate-HEMA nanocomposites.

13.8 SELF-SETTING CERAMICS-POLYMER COMPOSITES

In addition to bulk bone-repairing materials, the concept of composites can be applied to self-setting bone cements. In artificial joint replacement, PMMA bone cement is popularly used for fixation of the artificial joint to the bone [51]. It has a history of more than half a century since it was first used by Charnley for hip prosthesis replacement surgery. Bone cement is composed of liquid and powder. The powder portion contains PMMA and a polymerization initiator of MMA, and the liquid portion is composed of MMA and a polymerization accelerator. After mixing the powder and the liquid, MMA is polymerized while penetrating into the PMMA powder to form a hardened polymer.

However, since it does not show bioactivity, there is a risk that the artificial joint will loosen after a long implantation period. Therefore, attempts have been made to add bioactive ceramics such as hydroxyapatite [52], bioactive glass and glass-ceramics [53], and titanium oxide [54] to PMMA cement. Bioactivity of this type of cement is achieved by the added ceramic particles coming into contact with surrounding body fluid and forming bone-like apatite on their surfaces. However, in a typical composite, the polymer matrix covers the ceramic filler. Therefore, in order for the ceramic particles to be exposed on the surface and exhibit bioactivity, a large amount of addition is required. This may reduce operability of the cement.

The concept of nanocomposites can also be applied to the production of bioactive bone cement. Bioactive cement is obtained by adding a water-soluble calcium salt to the powder and 3-methacryloxypropyltrimethoxysilane (MPS), a kind of alkoxysilane, to the liquid [55]. Since MPS has a polymerizable vinyl group, it is considered that an MPS-MMA copolymer is formed in the cement. Furthermore, novel bone cements having antibacterial properties in addition to bioactivity can be obtained by adding a vinyl compound with an amino group to these cements [56]. Its chemical structure is shown in Figure 13.5.

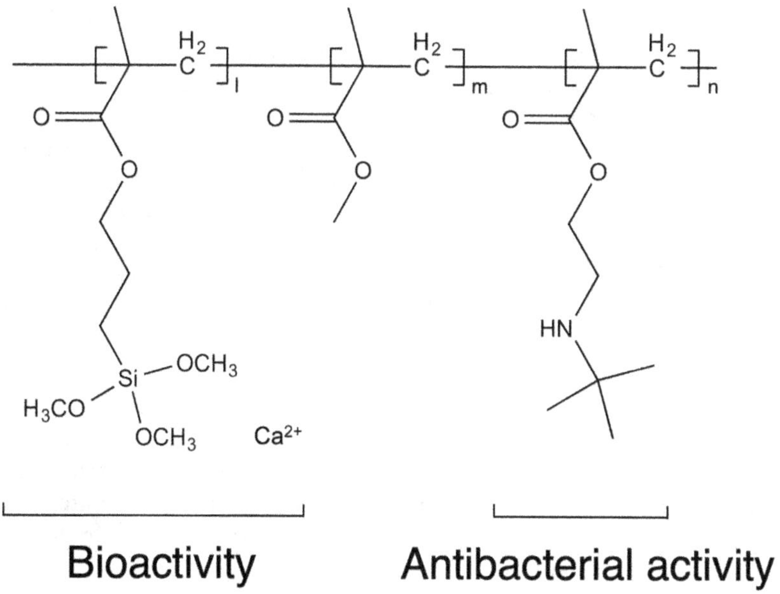

Bioactivity Antibacterial activity

FIGURE 13.5 Chemical structure of bone cement with bioactivity and antibacterial properties.

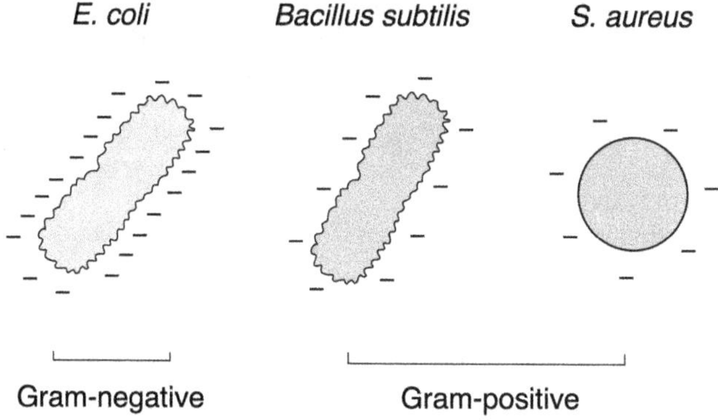

FIGURE 13.6 Schematic illustration of different bacteria.

Antibacterial properties changed in the order: *E. coli*>*Bacillus subtilis*>*S. aureus*. *E. coli* is a gram-negative bacterium, and its surface is more negatively charged than that of *Bacillus subtilis* and *S. aureus*, the gram-positive bacteria. Therefore, it is considered that *E. coli* is easily combined with the positively charged amino group in the cement. Furthermore, comparing *Bacillus subtilis* and *S. aureus*, the former has a wavy shape, whereas the latter has a spherical shape. Differences in these properties are schematically illustrated in Figure 13.6.

Therefore, the cement would show a higher antibacterial effect against *Bacillus subtilis* because of its large specific surface area.

Bone cements composed of calcium phosphate powder and various aqueous solutions have been clinically applied. When these powders and liquids are mixed, apatite is precipitated and hardened by the dissolution-reprecipitation reaction. The bone defect can be repaired by a simple injection of cement, so minimally invasive treatment is expected. Composites have been developed by adding polymers to this cement. For example, Ishikawa et al. found that the addition of alginic acid to the cement can prevent its decay through contact with body fluid [57]. It is also revealed that the addition of cationic polymers such as poly(ethyleneimine) and poly(allylamine hydrochloride) significantly improved the compressive strength of the cement [58]. This is attributed to the densification of the cement by the polymer modification.

13.9 CONCLUSIONS

Material design based on composites is useful for adjusting and improving the biological and mechanical affinities of bone-repairing materials. In the future, development of bone-repairing materials with excellent long-term durability in the body is desired by utilizing composites.

REFERENCES

1. Hench L.L., Wilson J. Introduction. In: Hench L.L., Wilson J., editors. *An Introduction to Bioceramics*. Singapore: World Scientific; 1993. pp. 1–24.
2. Cimatti B., Santos M.A.D., Brassesco M.S., Okano L.T., Barboza W.M., Nogueira-Barbosa M.H., Engel E.E. Safety, osseointegration, and bone ingrowth analysis of PMMA-based porous cement on animal metaphyseal bone defect model. *J Biomed Mater Res B Appl Biomater.* 2018;106:649–658. doi: 10.1002/jbm.b.33870.
3. Hench L.L. Bioceramics: From concept to clinic. *J Am Ceram Soc.* 1991;74:1487–1510. doi: 10.1111/j.1151-2916.1991.tb07132.x.
4. Hench L.L. Bioceramics. *J Am Ceram Soc.* 1998;81:1705–1728. doi: 10.1111/j.1151-2916.1998.tb02540.x.
5. Neo M., Kotani S., Nakamura T., Yamamuro T., Ohtsuki C., Kokubo T., Bando Y. A comparative study of ultrastructure of the interfaces between four kinds of surface-active ceramic and bone. *J Biomed Mater Res.* 1992;26:1419–1432. doi: 10.1002/jbm.820261103.
6. Fujita Y., Yamamuro T., Nakamura T., Kotani S., Ohtsuki C., Kokubo T. The bonding behavior of calcite to bone. *J Biomed Mater Res.* 1991;25:991–1003.
7. Neo M., Nakamura T., Ohtsuki C., Kokubo T., Yamamuro T. Apatite formation on three kinds of bioactive material at an early stage in vivo: A comparative study by transmission electron microscopy. *J Biomed Mater Res.* 1993;27:999–1006. doi: 10.1002/jbm.820270805.
8. Kobayashi M., Kikutani T., Kokubo T., Nakamura T. Direct bone formation on alumina bead composite. *J Biomed Mater Res.* 1997;37:554–565. doi: 10.1002/(sici)1097-4636(19971215)37:4<554::aid-jbm15>3.0.co;2-8.
9. Kokubo T., Kushitani H., Sakka S., Kitsugi T., Yamamuro T. Solutions able to reproduce in vivo surfacestructure changes in bioactive glassceramic AW. *J Biomed Mater Res.* 1990;24:721–734. doi: 10.1002/jbm.820240607.
10. Cho S.B., Nakanishi K., Kokubo T., Soga N., Ohtsuki C., Nakamura T., Kitsugi T., Yamamuro T. Dependence of apatite formation on silica gel on its structure: Effect

of heat treatment. *J Am Ceram Soc.* 1995;78:1769–1774. doi: 10.1111/j.1151-2916.1995.tb08887.x.

11. Kokubo T., Takadama H. How useful is SBF in predicting in vivo bone bioactivity? *Biomaterials.* 2006;27:2907–2915. doi: 10.1016/j.biomaterials.2006.01.017.
12. International Organization for Standardization (ISO). Implants for surgery — in vitro evaluation for apatite-forming ability of implant materials. Geneve: ISO; 2014. Standard No. ISO 23317:2014.
13. Oyane A., Kim H.M., Furuya T., Kokubo T., Miyazaki T., Nakamura T. Preparation and assessment of revised simulated body fluids. *J Biomed Mater Res.* 2003;65A:188–195. doi: 10.1002/jbm.a.10482.
14. Matsuno H., Yokoyama A., Watari F., Uo M., Kawasaki T. Biocompatibility and osteogenesis of refractory metal implants, titanium, hafnium, niobium, tantalum and rhenium. *Biomaterials.* 2001;22:1253–1262. doi: 10.1016/s0142-9612(00)00275-1.
15. Arifin A., Sulong A.B., Muhamad N., Syarif J., Ramli M.I. Material processing of hydroxyapatite and titanium alloy (HA/Ti) composite as implant materials using powder metallurgy: A review. *Mater Des.* 2014;55:165–175. doi: 10.1016/j.matdes.2013.09.045.
16. Carter A., Popowski K., Cheng K., Greenbaum A., Ligler F.S., Moatti A. Enhancement of bone regeneration through the converse piezoelectric effect, a novel approach for applying mechanical stimulation. *Bioelectricity.* 2021;3:255–271. doi: 10.1089/bioe.2021.0019.
17. Sakaguchi N., Niinomi M., Akahori T., Takeda J., Toda H. Relationships between tensile deformation behavior and microstructure in Ti–Nb–Ta–Zr system alloys. *Mater Sci Eng C.* 2005;25:363–369. doi: 10.1016/j.msec.2004.12.014.
18. Wang X., Chen Y., Xu L., Xiao S., Kong F., Woo K.D. Ti–Nb–Sn–hydroxyapatite composites synthesized by mechanical alloying and high frequency induction heated sintering. *J Mech Behav Biomed Mater.* 2011;4:2074–2080. doi: 10.1016/j.jmbbm.2011.07.006.
19. Lacefield W.R. Hydroxyapatite coatings. In: Hench L.L., Wilson J., editors. *An Introduction to Bioceramics.* Singapore: World Scientific; 1993. pp. 223–238.
20. Wan T., Aoki H., Hikawa J., Lee J.H. RF-magnetron sputtering technique for producing hydroxyapatite coating film on various substrates. *Bio-Med Mater Eng.* 2007;17:291–297.
21. Wei M., Ruys A., Swain M., Kim S., Milthorpe B., Sorrell C. Interfacial bond strength of electrophoretically deposited hydroxyapatite coatings on metals. *J Mater Sci Mater Med.* 1999;10:401–409. doi: 10.1023/a:1008923029945.
22. Kim H.M., Miyaji F., Kokubo T., Nakamura T. Preparation of bioactive Ti and its alloys via simple chemical surface treatment. *J Biomed Mater Res.* 1996;32:409–417. doi: 10.1002/(SICI)1097-4636(199611)32:3<409::AID-JBM14>3.0.CO;2-B.
23. Wang X.X., Hayakawa S., Tsuru K., Osaka A. A comparative study of in vitro apatite deposition on heat-, H(2)O(2)-, and NaOH-treated titanium surfaces. *J Biomed Mater Res.* 2001;54:172–178. doi: 10.1002/1097-4636(200102)54:2<172::aid-jbm3>3.0.co;2-#.
24. Miyazaki T., Kim H.M., Miyaji F., Kokubo T., Nakamura T. Bioactive tantalum metal prepared by NaOH treatment. *J Biomed Mater Res.* 2000;50:35–42. doi: 10.1002/(sici)1097-4636(200004)50:1<35::aid-jbm6>3.0.co;2-8.
25. Uchida M., Kim H.M., Miyaji F., Kokubo T., Nakamura T. Apatite formation on zirconium metal treated with aqueous NaOH. *Biomaterials.* 2002;23:313–317. doi: 10.1016/s0142-9612(01)00110-7.
26. Miyazaki T., Sueoka M., Shirosaki Y., Shinozaki N., Shiraishi T. Development of hafnium metal and titanium-hafnium alloys having apatite-forming ability by chemical surface modification. *J Biomed Mater Rest B Appl Biomater.* 2018;106B:2519–2523. doi: 10.1002/jbm.b.34068.
27. Park J.B., Lakes R.S. *Biomaterials: An Introduction.* Second Edition. New York: Plenum Press; 1992.

28. Kikuchi M., Itoh S., Ichinose S., Shinomiya K., Tanaka J. Self-organization mechanism in a bone-like hydroxyapatite / collagen nanocomposite synthesized in vitro and its biological reaction in vivo. *Biomaterials.* 2001;22:1705–1711. doi: 10.1016/s0142-9612(00)00305-7.
29. Bonfield W. Design of bioactive ceramic-polymer composites. In Hench L.L., Wilson J., editors. *An Introduction to Bioceramics.* Singapore: World Scientific; 1993. pp. 299–303.
30. Poursamar S.A., Azami M., Mozafari M. Controllable synthesis and characterization of porous polyvinyl alcohol/hydroxyapatite nanocomposite scaffolds via an in situ colloidal technique. *Colloids Surf B: Biointerfaces.* 2011;84:310–316. doi: 10.1016/j.colsurfb.2011.01.015.
31. Shikinami Y., Okuno M. Bioresorbable devices made of forged composites of hydroxyapatite (HA) particles and poly L-lactide (PLLA). Part II: practical properties of miniscrews and miniplates. *Biomaterials.* 2001;22:3197–3211. doi: 10.1016/s0142-9612(01)00072-2.
32. Zavřel F., Novák M., Kroupová J., Beveridge C., Štěpánek F., Ruphuy G. Development of hot-melt extrusion method to produce hydroxyapatite/polycaprolactone composite filaments. *Adv Eng Mater.* Published online. doi: 10.1002/adem.202100820.
33. Yamaguchi I., Tokuchi K., Fukuzaki H., Koyama Y., Takakuda K., Monma H., Tanaka J. *J Biomed Mater Res.* 2001;55:20–27. doi: 10.1002/1097-4636(200104)55:1<20::AID-JBM30>3.0.CO;2-F.
34. Yoshida A., Miyazaki T., Ishida E., Ashizuka M. Bioactivity and mechanical properties of cellulose/carbonate hydroxyapatite composites prepared in situ through mechanochemical reaction. *J Biomater Appl.* 2006;21:179–194. doi: 10.1177/0885328206059796.
35. Wang M., Kokubo T., Bonfield W. A-W glass-ceramic reinforced polyethylene for medical applications. In Kokubo T., Nakamura T., Miyaji F., editors. *Bioceramics,* Vol. 9. Elsevier: Oxford; 1996. pp. 387–390.
36. Huang J., DiSilvio L., Wang M., Rehman I., Ohtsuki C., Bonfield W. Evaluation of in vitro bioactivity and biocompatibility of Bioglass®-reinforced polyethylene composite. *J Mater Sci Mater Med.* 1997;8:809–813. doi: 10.1023/a:1018581100400.
37. Pleuddemann E.P. *Silane Coupling Agents.* New York: Plenum Press; 1982.
38. Wang M., Bonfield W. Chemically coupled hydroxyapatite–polyethylene composites: structure and properties. *Biomaterials.* 2001;22:1311–1320. doi: 10.1016/S0142-9612(00)00283-0.
39. Hanson E.L., Schwartz J., Nickel B., Koch N., Danisman M.F. Bonding self-assembled, compact organophosphonate monolayers to the native oxide surface of silicon. *J Am Chem Soc.* 2003;125:16074–16080. doi: 10.1021/ja035956z.
40. Pramanik N., Mohapatra S., Bhargava P., Pramanik P. Chemical synthesis and characterization of hydroxyapatite (HAp)-poly (ethylene co vinyl alcohol) (EVA) nanocomposite using a phosphonic acid coupling agent for orthopedic applications. *Mater Sci Eng C.* 2009;29:228–236. doi: 10.1016/j.msec.2008.06.013.
41. Miyazaki T., Ohtsuki C., Tanihara M. Synthesis of bioactive organic-inorganic nanohybrid for bone repair through sol-gel processing. *J Nanosci Nanotech.* 2003;3:511–515. doi: 10.1166/jnn.2003.221.
42. Miyata N., Fuke K., Chen Q., Kawashita M., Kokubo T., Nakamura T. Preparation of PTMO-modified CaO-TiO_2 hybrids via sol-gel processing: their apatite-forming ability and mechanical properties. *J Ceram Soc Japan.* 2003;111:555–559. doi: 10.2109/jcersj.111.555.
43. Tsuru K., Ohtsuki C., Osaka A., Iwamoto T., Mackenzie J.D. Bioactivity of sol-gel derived organically modified silicates, Part I: In vitro examination. *J Mater Sci Mater Med.* 1997;8:157–161. doi: 10.1023/A:1018523203667.

44. You C., Miyazaki T., Ishida E., Ashizuka M., Ohtsuki C., Tanihara M. Fabrication of poly(vinyl alcohol)-apatite hybrids through biomimetic process. *J Eur Ceram Soc.* 2007;27:1585–1588. doi: 10.1016/j.jeurceramsoc.2006.04.055.
45. Rhee S.H. Bone-like apatite-forming ability and mechanical properties of poly(epsilon-caprolactone)/silica hybrid as a function of poly(epsilon-caprolactone) content. *Biomaterials.* 2004;25:1167–1175. doi: 10.1016/j.biomaterials.2003.08.004.
46. Miyazaki T., Yasunaga S., Ishida E., Ashizuka M., Ohtsuki C. Effects of cross-linking agent on apatite-forming ability and mechanical property of organic-inorganic hybrids based on starch. *Mater Trans.* 2007;48:317–321. doi: 10.2320/matertrans.48.317.
47. Miyazaki T., Ohtsuki C., Ashizuka M. Synthesis of osteoconductive organic-inorganic nanohybrids through modification of chitin with alkoxysilane and calcium chloride. *J Biomater Appl* 2007;22:71–81. doi: 10.1177/0885328206070447.
48. Miyazaki T., Akita H., Ishida E., Ashizuka M., Ohtsuki C. Synthesis of bioactive organic-inorganic hybrids from tetraisopropyl titanate and hydroxyethylmethacrylate. *J Ceram Soc Japan.* 2006;114:87–91. doi: 10.2109/jcersj.114.87.
49. Kamitakahara M., Kawashita M., Miyata N., Kokubo T., Nakamura T. Preparation of bioactive flexible poly(tetramethylene oxide) (PTMO)–CaO–Ta_2O_5 hybrids. *J Mater Sci Mater Med.* 2007;18:1117–1124. doi:10.1007/s10856-007-0147-9.
50. Hara S., Aisu J., Nishizaki Y., Kato H., Sanae G., Kurebayashi S., Shimizu S., Ikake H. Bulk structure of poly (ethylene glycol)/titania hybrid system and the evaluation of their influence on apatite growth using simulated body fluid (SBF). *Polymer Test.* 2021;94:106984. doi: 10.1016/j.polymertesting.2020.106984.
51. Kühn K.D. *Bone Cements.* Berlin (Germany): Springer; 2000.
52. Dalby M.J., Di Silvio L., Harper E.J., Bonfield W. In vitro evaluation of a new polymethylmethacrylate cement reinforced with hydroxyapatite. *J Mater Sci Mater Med.* 1999;10:793–796. doi: 10.1023/a:1008907218330.
53. Shinzato S., Kobayashi M., Mousa W.F., Kamimura M., Neo M., Kitamura Y., Kokubo T., Nakamura T. Bioactive polymethyl methacrylate-based bone cement: Comparison of glass beads, apatite- and wollastonite-containing glass-ceramic, and hydroxyapatite fillers on mechanical and biological properties. *J Biomed Mater Res.* 2000;51:258–272. doi: 10.1002/(sici)1097-4636(200008)51:2<258::aid-jbm15>3.0.co;2-s.
54. Goto K., Tamura J., Shinzato S., Fujibayashi S., Hashimoto M., Kawashita M., Kokubo T., Nakamura T. Bioactive bone cements containing nano-sized titania particles for use as bone substitutes. *Biomaterials.* 2005;26:6496–6505. doi: 10.1016/j.biomaterials.2005.04.044.
55. Miyazaki T., Ohtsuki C., Kyomoto M., Tanihara M., Mori A., Kuramoto K. Bioactive PMMA bone cement prepared by modification with methacryloxypropyltrimethoxysilane and calcium chloride. *J Biomed Mater Res A.* 2003;67:1417–1423. doi: 10.1002/jbm.a.20042.
56. Wang H., Maeda T., Miyazaki T. Preparation of bioactive and antibacterial PMMA-based bone cement by modification with quaternary ammonium and alkoxysilane. *J Biomater Appl.* 2021;36:311–320. doi: 10.1177/08853282211004413.
57. Ishikawa K., Miyamoto Y., Kon M., Nagayama M., Asaoka K. Non-decay type fast-setting calcium phosphate cement: Composite with sodium alginate. *Biomaterials.* 1995;16:527–532. doi: 10.1016/0142-9612(95)91125-i.
58. Mickiewicz R.A., Mayes A.M., Knaack D. Polymer-calcium phosphate cement composites for bone substitutes. *J Biomed Mater Res.* 2002;61:581–592. doi: 10.1002/jbm.10222.

14 Biomaterials and Microfluidics Systems Used for Modeling Pathological Tissues

Baeckkyoung Sung
KIST Europe Forschungsgesellschaft mbH
University of Science & Technology (UST)

CONTENTS

14.1 Introduction ... 290
14.2 Microfluidic Phenomena and Devices ... 291
  14.2.1 Physical Basis of Microfluidics ... 291
  14.2.2 Design and Fabrication of Microfluidic Devices ... 291
  14.2.3 Device Operation and Flow Control ... 292
14.3 Biomaterials Coupled with Microfluidic Devices ... 293
  14.3.1 Engineering Principles of Biomaterials ... 293
  14.3.2 Materials for Microfluidic Device Frame ... 294
  14.3.3 Microfluidic Chip-Integrated Biomaterials ... 294
  14.3.4 Miniaturized Biomaterials and Tissue Engineering ... 295
14.4 On-Chip Tissue Mimicry ... 296
  14.4.1 Microfluidic Platforms for Cell Culture ... 296
  14.4.2 Microphysiological Systems ... 296
14.5 Microfluidic Pathological Modeling ... 298
  14.5.1 Bioengineered Disease Models In Vitro ... 298
  14.5.2 Organ-on-Chips for Pathological Modeling ... 298
  14.5.3 Cardiovascular Diseases on Chip ... 299
  14.5.4 Musculoskeletal Diseases on Chip ... 300
  14.5.5 Endocrine Diseases on Chip ... 300
  14.5.6 Liver and Kidney Diseases on Chip ... 301
  14.5.7 Brain and Lung Diseases on Chip ... 302
  14.5.8 Other Pathological Tissue Models on Chip ... 303
14.6 Concluding Remarks ... 304
Acknowledgments ... 304
References ... 304

DOI: 10.1201/9781003251767-14

14.1 INTRODUCTION

Microfluidics, which lies at the intersection between fluid dynamics and microtechnology, deals with all types of transport and surface phenomena occurring at the micrometer scale (Manz et al., 2020). The scope of microfluidics includes applications in life and environmental sciences, chemical and biomedical engineering, pharmaceutical technology, and (pre-)clinical research. The origin of microfluidics traces back to George Keith Batchelor, who coined the term microhydrodynamics in the 1960s (Batchelor, 1967). However, its modern concept was born as a consequence of the advancement of microelectromechanical systems (MEMS) in the late 1980s, under the name "micro total analysis system (μTAS)" (Manz, 1990). Since 1990, microfluidics has been a core technology for fundamental and applied studies of soft and biological systems. The concept of μTAS has evolved to "lab-on-a-chip," emphasizing the microsystems aspect (Dittrich & Manz, 2006).

Combined with the progress in biomaterials science in the 2000s, the use of microfluidic devices has become particularly popular in the biomedical field (Baker, 2011). Advances in microfabrication technology and bioengineering have fueled the development of healthcare lab-on-a-chip platforms that require only a minimal amount of specimens/reagents and provide controllable flow/mixing abilities, together with precisely defined channel geometry and circuitry (Dittrich & Manz, 2006). Moreover, biomicrofluidic platforms have experienced a prominent evolution in the last decade with the integration of a wide range of biomaterials, such as gels and elastomers, which transformed simple microchannel-micropump devices into biosensing or biomimetic chips.

In particular, biomaterial-integrated microfluidic devices have recently been adopted as ideal *in vitro* platforms for simulating native tissue physiology and pathology (Huh et al., 2011, 2012; Bhatia & Ingber, 2014; Ingber, 2016, 2022). Considering the critical roles of biophysical factors in homeostatic mechanisms in cells, tissues, and organs, the embedment of individually controllable variables in an optically accessible platform is the most important feature of microfluidic biomimicry. Compared with conventional cell culture models, cells-on-chip platforms provide dynamic and tunable microenvironments that closely resemble native tissues. Moreover, the advent of stem cell and organoid technologies has increased the robustness of on-chip living-system modeling.

In this chapter, we focus on pathological tissue modeling using miniaturized biomaterial-based microfluidic platforms. We begin with the fundamental background of microfluidics, microdevice fabrication, and the physicochemical properties of the associated biomaterials. We then briefly introduce the concept of physiologically relevant microsystems. Finally, we summarize how such microphysiological systems are used to simulate various pathological conditions in *in vitro* disease models. Throughout this chapter, special emphasis will be given to describing how fluid dynamic and biomechanical aspects of biomaterial-integrated microfluidic chips are related to specific pathological tissue mimics.

14.2 MICROFLUIDIC PHENOMENA AND DEVICES

14.2.1 Physical Basis of Microfluidics

Simple fluids (liquids and gases, for example) are characterized by free deformability without affecting the macroscopic properties of the fluid (Batchelor, 1967). When external forces are exerted on such a fluid, the relative motion of fluid elements results in typical fluid dynamic behaviors (Batchelor, 1967). At the submillimeter scale, where microfluidic phenomena emerge, the dynamics of fluids are dominated by viscous forces rather than inertial forces, which are quantified by a low Reynolds number (Manz et al., 2020). In contrast, turbulent flow is generated at a high Reynolds number when inertial forces are dominant, which rarely occurs under microfluidic conditions. In the standard flow velocity range (in the order of 1 cm/s), microfluidics falls into the laminar flow regime (Atencia & Beebe, 2005; Manz et al., 2020), where the fluid flow can be considered as a stack of mutually sliding fluid layers without lateral mixing, with a decreasing layer velocity as it approaches to the channel wall. Because of the dominant laminar flow, diffusive mass transport is the main mechanism for microfluidic mixing. Furthermore, interfacial effects (hydrophilicity, miscibility, surface tension/charge, etc.) are critical in microfluidics because of the small dimensions of the fluid channels and chambers. Enhanced heat transfer can be achieved in microfluidic devices, which enables lower power consumption for device operation. Physical principles of microfluidic devices are summarized in Figure 14.1.

14.2.2 Design and Fabrication of Microfluidic Devices

The design and fabrication principles for microfluidic devices have been largely inspired and adapted from those of microelectronic chip technology (Duncombe et al., 2015). The typical layout of microfluidic chips consists of an array of unit geometries such as channels of straight/curved lines, spirals, splitters, and funnels (Manz et al., 2020). The design process is performed using computer-aided design tools under consideration of the specific function of each unit, with a particular focus on achieving smooth transitions between blocks of different channel dimensions and sections; for instance, funnels are used for the connection between narrow and wide channels, and Y-bends and fractal structures are used for fluid convergence/divergence (Manz et al., 2020).

After the layout design, the conventional patterning procedure is conducted through the following steps: (i) photolithography with or without masks on a photoresist material, (ii) dry or wet etching to transfer the patterns from a photoresist layer to the substrate layer and (iii) bonding of the patterned substrate (usually made of elastomers) to another substrate (usually glass or elastomer materials) to form closed channel sections (Manz et al., 2020). Before the bonding step, the inner surface of a channel can be radicalized using gas plasma treatments and/or functionalized with biomolecules,

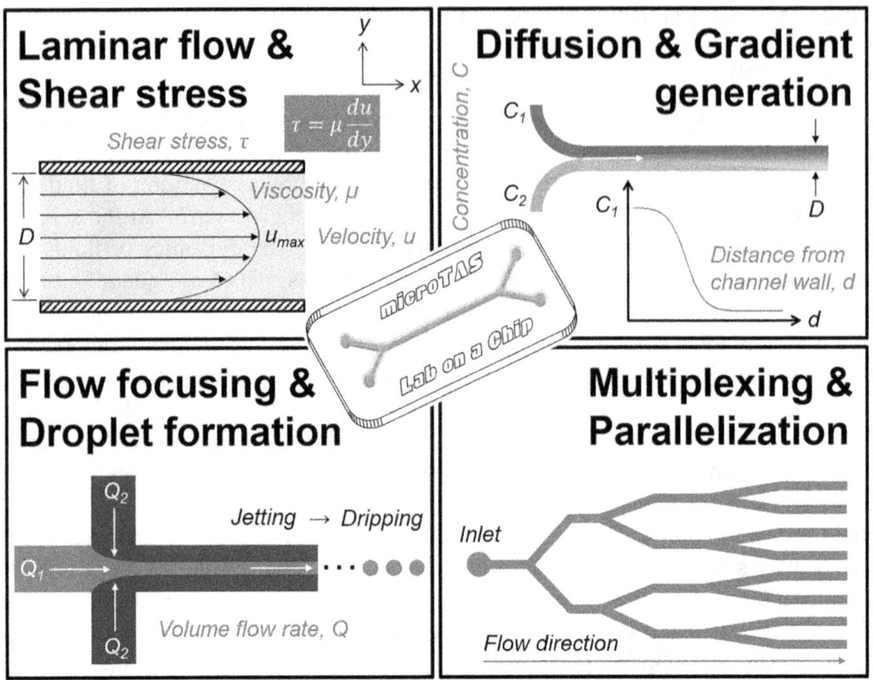

FIGURE 14.1 Schematic of the physical principles of microfluidcs: (i) laminar flow and shear stress (Manz et al., 2020), (ii) diffusive transport and gradient generation (Wolfram et al., 2016), (iii) flow focusing and droplet formation (Manz et al., 2020), and (iv) multiplexing and parallelization (Manz et al. 2020).

micro-/nanoparticles or synthetic polymers (Dittrich & Manz, 2006). Microcontact printing can be used to include extracellular matrix (ECM) proteins in a device for cell growth scaffolding (Low & Tagle, 2017). Depending on the chip design strategy, valves, pumps, and other complex components can be patterned and integrated into the device architecture (Dittrich & Manz, 2006). To enable cell monitoring and related microanalyses, various readout options can be considered in this step, such as platform-embedded biosensors and built-in multielectrode arrays (Low & Tagle, 2017).

14.2.3 Device Operation and Flow Control

Because microfluidic transport predominantly relies on laminar flow and diffusion processes, on-chip pressure control and channel geometry determine the general flow behavior (Manz et al., 2020). Microfluidic flows can remain highly ordered over relatively long distances under precise flow-pattern control through passive or active built-in components (Duncombe et al., 2015). Various channel configurations (such as the V, H, and Y shapes) can be designed to control fluid mixing, filtering, and focusing (Manz et al., 2020). In order to enable extended flow-pattern control, for example, scaling the channels by micrometers in height and millimeters in width and length could support maintaining long-range laminar flows (Atencia & Beebe, 2005). In addition, a pyramidal network of microchannels with multiple splitting and combining of laminar flow streams can be used to create complex concentration profiles across a wide collecting channel (Atencia & Beebe, 2005).

The pump-driven pressure difference between the flow inlet and outlet of a chip is applied to the entire channel structure, and the pressure distribution and flow resistance determine the local flow patterns (Manz et al., 2020). The pumping mode can be either constant or peristaltic actuation, and the flow direction can be controlled through a microvalve structure embedded in the chip (Dittrich & Manz, 2006). Micromixing can typically be achieved by adopting lamination and intersecting channels, repeating convergence-divergence channels, and serpentine channels (Manz et al., 2020). Furthermore, microfluidic chips can be designed to generate microdroplets inside a channel (Dittrich & Manz, 2006). Most microfluidic biodevices have been developed to exhibit characteristic channel dimensions and flow rates observed in the human circulatory system (Duncombe et al., 2015). Tunable molecular diffusion is achieved by forming and on-demand controlling the local concentration gradients across soft matrices integrated in the microfluidic chip, which are adjusted to be relevant to physiological or pathological transport phenomena (Xie et al., 2020).

14.3 BIOMATERIALS COUPLED WITH MICROFLUIDIC DEVICES

14.3.1 Engineering Principles of Biomaterials

A biomaterial is defined as any substance used to produce healthcare devices or biomedical implants aimed at recreating the function of cells, tissues, or organs in a safe and reliable manner (Park & Lakes, 2007). Biomaterials are manufactured from various types of base materials, including gels, polymers, metals, ceramics, and organic/inorganic composites, which should be tailored for fully confirmed biocompatibility and non-toxicity. The surface and mechanical properties are the most fundamental aspects to be considered for the biomaterial design: the surface must be functionalized to support cell attachment, migration, and growth. Furthermore, biomaterials must exhibit specific tissue-compatible mechanical characteristics. Mechanobiological relevance to subcellular, cellular, and tissue-level signaling pathways is a critical aspect to be considered in engineering advanced materials for biomedical applications (Shao & Fu, 2014). The physicochemical and biophysical functionalities of biomaterial platforms should be carefully designed to improve the self-regulation of reconstituted biological systems in an in vivo-like manner. In addition, MEMS-based and nanoengineered biomaterials can be integrated into miniaturized biomimetic platforms to enable multiparametric system control (Shao & Fu, 2014). Depending on the application purpose, the ultrasonic, optical, electric or magnetic properties of such platforms can be tailored to define the biological functionality of the material. Controllable degradability is another key factor to be considered for the proper selection of platform-integrated biomaterials. An in-depth introduction to functional biomaterial engineering is provided in Chapter 1 of this volume.

14.3.2 Materials for Microfluidic Device Frame

The basic materials comprising the main frame of a microfluidic device are typically glass, silicon, and polymeric materials such as polydimethylsiloxane (PDMS), poly(methyl methacrylate) (PMMA), polycarbonate (PC), and polystyrene (PS) (Dong et al., 2019). Among them, the most widely used material for microfluidic biodevices is the PDMS elastomer. PDMS is a polymeric organosilicon compound (commonly called silicone) composed of an inorganic siloxane backbone and organic methyl groups attached to the silicon (Leester-Schädel et al., 2016). When crosslinked, PDMS, originally in the liquid phase at room temperature, is converted to a rubber-like elastomer that is chemically and thermally stable and transparent (Leester-Schädel et al., 2016). Borosilicate glass is optically transparent and mechanically robust, and can be easily micropatterned with cell-compatible surface modifications (Dittrich & Manz, 2006). Silicon is a solid semiconductor material whose mechanical and electrical properties are well defined and fully compatible with current micromachining techniques. It can be precisely processed through chemical etching and electron beam lithography to provide facile structuring of microchannels, nozzles, and passive valves based on MEMS technology (Leester-Schädel et al., 2016). In microfluidics, metallic materials such as gold, copper, aluminum, and titanium are usually used as auxiliary options to enhance device performance, for example, for surface plasmon sensing, electrochemical electrode implementation, and field focalization (Dittrich & Manz, 2006). All the materials mentioned above are generally considered biocompatible.

14.3.3 Microfluidic Chip-Integrated Biomaterials

Soft materials, such as polymers, gels, and membranes, can be integrated into microfluidic devices to function as interfaces between the device frame materials and biological components (biomolecules, cells, and micro-tissues). A polymer is a long chain of repeating monomers that exhibits a thermally fluctuating random coil conformation in a solvent (Piazza, 2011). Upon exposure to external stimuli (e.g., changes in temperature, pH or ionic strength), certain types of polymers may undergo a reversible coil-globule transition (Sung et al., 2021). Polymer chains, mostly synthetic polymers, can be grafted onto the microfluidic channel surface (e.g., in the form of a polymer brush) to perform smart biosensing (Chaterji et al., 2007) or to prevent interactions between the channel surface and biomacromolecules dispersed in the fluid (Eichler et al., 2016).

A gel matrix is an elastic 3D network of crosslinked polymer chains that may exhibit a reversible transition between swollen and collapsed states, analogous to stimuli-responsive polymers (Chaterji et al., 2007; Sung et al., 2021). When water is the solvent for a gel matrix, the gel is termed a hydrogel (Sung et al., 2021), which is relevant for biomedical applications. These hydrated 3D polymeric networks, particularly when made of biopolymers, have been extensively utilized as ECM substitutes for tissue engineering and regeneration owing to their excellent biocompatibility and biodegradability, thereby supporting cell attachment, survival, migration, and self-organization (Guttenplan et al., 2021). The mechanical properties of a hydrogel can be tunable by varying the polymer concentration, type of crosslinking, and/or crosslinking density (Sung & Kim, 2017; Xie et al., 2020). Hybridization of hydrogels with nanomaterials can be considered as a strategy for improving the desired physicochemical functionality (Xie et al., 2020; Sung et al., 2021).

A membrane is typically a flat or curved thin film with tiny holes, usually suspended in a liquid phase (Piazza, 2011). Membranes act as selective barriers for filtration or osmosis, which are limited by hole size. In microfluidics, chip-integrated membranes are used to control particle concentrations and as cell culture inserts (Chen & Shen, 2017). Typical biomaterials used for the microfluidic membranes include thin film assemblies of synthetic biocompatible or naturally occurring polymers, such as polyethylene glycol (Kobel & Lutolf, 2011) and chitosan (Domachuk et al., 2010; Koev et al., 2010). For example, porous films can be placed on-chip to separate two parallel channels to culture two different cell types on opposite sides, allowing emulation of the vascular-parenchymal interface (Bhatia & Ingber, 2014). Moreover, integrating stretchable membranes in the microchannels may help capture the in vivo-like mechanical functions of vascular-epithelial interfaces (Zhang et al., 2018). From a different viewpoint, hydrogel platforms with perfusable microchannels can be used as biomimetic vascularized tissue constructs (Xie et al., 2020).

14.3.4 Miniaturized Biomaterials and Tissue Engineering

Submillimeter-scale biomaterials have been developed for tissue engineering applications to create, repair, and/or replace micro-tissues (Coutinho et al., 2011). The most commonly known bottom-up strategies for these applications include seeding single-type cells on a microscale scaffold and forming a miniaturized tissue mimic in vitro (Ning et al., 2016). For instance, chip-sized hydrogel scaffolds can be utilized to create vascularized channel networks, either based on self-organized endothelial lumens or perfusable microchannel structures implemented by MEMS techniques (Low et al., 2021).

Representative scaffolding materials include hydrogel particles, porous ceramic or polymeric structures, and micro/nanofiber assemblies (Gentsch & Börner, 2010; Smith & Ma, 2011). One of the recently highlighted soft materials for bio-scaffolding is microscale hydrogels, referred to as microgels, which are hydrogel particles with diverse shapes, such as spheres, discs, rods, and cubes (Le Goff et al., 2015; Sung & Kim, 2017; Sung et al., 2021). Owing to their high surface-to-volume ratio, the diffusive transport of gases, ions, and small molecules across gel matrices is significantly faster than that of their macroscopic counterparts (i.e., bulk-scale gels) (Sung et al., 2021). Furthermore, similar to macroscopic hydrogels, the mechanical stiffness and biochemical functionalization can be finely tuned by controlling gel crosslinking and ligand conjugation in/on the matrices (Le Goff et al., 2015). These properties allow the use of cell-embedded microgels as miniaturized tissue mimics optimized for microfluidic chips (Sung & Kim, 2017). Alternatively, cells can be attached to the microgel surface instead of being encapsulated in the gel to function as an artificial tissue interface (Zhang et al., 2018).

Other types of small-size porous scaffolds or fibrous assembly structures can also be integrated into in vitro tissue microsystems (Zhang et al., 2018), depending on the specific bioengineering purpose. In these cases, the seed cells usually adhere to the surfaces of the microcavities and fibers and are then guided for growth and proliferation. Biologically functional microgels, in the form of colloidal particles, thin films, or channel-filled matrices, are key components in the development of biomedical gel-in-microfluidics assays (Shao & Fu, 2014).

14.4 ON-CHIP TISSUE MIMICRY

14.4.1 Microfluidic Platforms for Cell Culture

Since the establishment of animal cell culture techniques in the 1940s, standard in vitro cell biology has long been based on simple and homogeneous surfaces under static culture conditions (Tavana et al., 2008). However, this conventional method does not provide in vivo-like biophysical microenvironments, such as vascular and interstitial flows, or their biomechanical interactions with cells and ECMs (Tavana et al., 2008). Microfluidics can be an ideal tool for overcoming such fundamental limitations using MEMS-driven bioanalytical approaches (Baker, 2011). On this platform, the appropriate choice of chip-embedded biomaterials can support controllable and prolonged cell (co-)cultures and robust tissue modeling. By integrating the cell culture system in a microfluidic tool, several advantages have been obtained, such as (i) physiologically relevant and highly tunable biofluid dynamics; (ii) fully controlled geometric, topographic, and mechanical properties of the chip-integrated 2D/3D microenvironments; (iii) locally and on-demand controlled concentration gradients of protons, gases, and chemicals; and (iv) the ability to isolate single cells, analyze them, and handle them (Tavana et al., 2008; Tian et al., 2019; Sung, 2022).

Microfluidic co-culture techniques may exploit compartmentalization methods using microgels, microchannels, microgrooves, microvalves, or microporous membranes (Sakthivel et al., 2019). Droplet microfluidics-based co-culture systems are also a popular strategy for the study of heterotypic cellular interactions (Sakthivel et al., 2019). Microfluidic platforms can closely mimic the complexity of in vivo tissues by enabling the individual control of multiple physiological parameters (Solanki & Pandey, 2016). Therefore, microfluidic cell culture systems can also be applied for high-throughput drug discovery (Dittrich & Manz, 2006; Dong et al., 2019). In particular, cell-laden microgels fabricated and manipulated using droplet microfluidics have been highlighted as novel building blocks for in vitro 3D tissue regeneration (Gurkan et al., 2012).

Main challenges involved in integrating the cell culture system into a microfluidic device may include (i) small volumes of culture media that could limit buffering/oxygenation and chemical analyses, (ii) complex device control and chip design, (iii) hydrophobicity of the device surface (especially for PDMS-based chips) that requires additional coating procedures, and (iv) non-standard culture protocols (Halldorsson et al., 2015; van Duinen et al., 2015).

14.4.2 Microphysiological Systems

The combination and hybridization of microfluidic devices and bioengineered materials have focused on the development of microphysiological systems, which are often termed "organ-on-chips" (Huh et al., 2011; Low et al., 2020). Organ-on-chips are miniaturized artificial tissue compartments supported by interactive microfluidic dynamics, which are created using MEMS techniques where continuously perfused tissue microchambers are contained (Bhatia & Ingber, 2014), as exemplified in Figure 14.2. They are also an optimal platform for implementing 3D tissue modeling systems, where ECM architectures and heterotypic 3D cell niches are designed for more in vivo-like cell-matrix and cell-cell interactions (Low et al., 2020). Microfluidic biomaterial platforms allow the 3D arrangement of multiple cell types in submillimeter-size confinement (Low & Tagle, 2017). Advances in organoid and stem cell technology have further enabled the realistic recapitalization of human tissue responses (Low et al., 2020). Furthermore, the integration of cells and ECMs into an MEMS-based chip facilitates high adaptation into sensing and imaging systems, which opens the possibility of monitoring real-time outcomes of artificial tissues in a noninvasive manner (Low et al., 2020).

Organ-on-chip platforms ultimately support the implementation of multicompartmental microphysiological systems, where different organ mimics are integrated on a chip and microfluidically connected to each other. For example, they enable the time-resolved measurement of cyclic hormonal effects on interconnected 3D tissues as well as the collection of biofluids for further enzymatic assays (Low & Tagle, 2017).

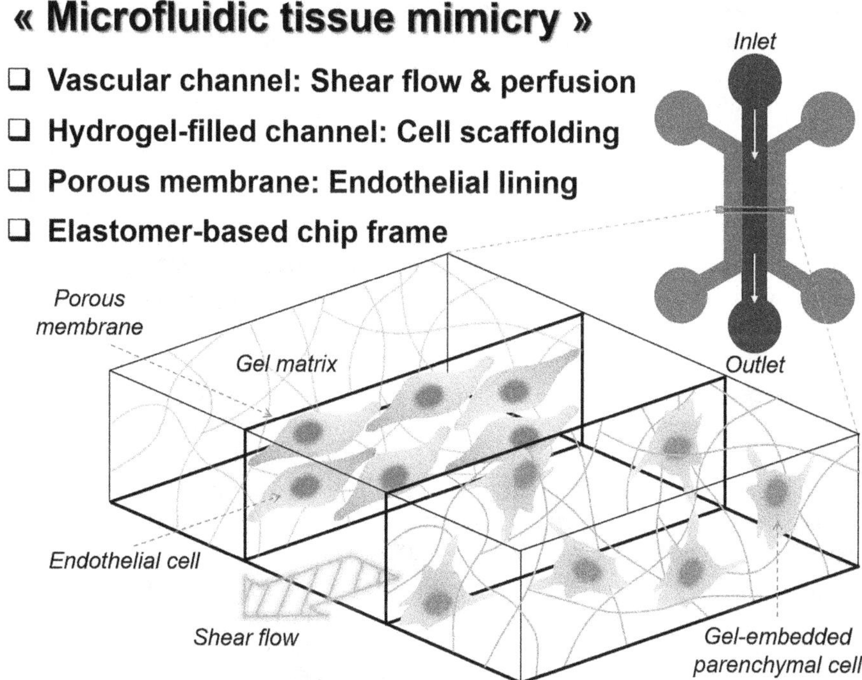

FIGURE 14.2 A microfluidic tissue model comprising a microvessel-mimicking perfusion channel and adjacent parallel channels filled with parenchymal cell-embedded gels. A porous membrane interfaces the vascular and parenchymal compartments, and an endothelial layer is formed on each side of the perfusion channel.

Microfluidic bioprinting techniques can lead to further advances in the manufacture of organ-on-chips, as 3D bioprinting on a microfluidic platform can be used to construct biomimetic heterogeneous ECMs and complex 3D microscaffolds through direct cell printing or patterning in microchips (Yu & Choudhury, 2019).

14.5 MICROFLUIDIC PATHOLOGICAL MODELING

14.5.1 Bioengineered Disease Models In Vitro

Compared with the huge complexity encountered in clinical disease studies, highly simplified in vitro cell systems could allow more direct mechanistic approaches to reveal pathological processes and their outcomes (Benam et al., 2015). Various 3D disease models, associated with advanced biomaterials, have been developed to better represent native pathophysiology, which cannot be fully achieved using standard 2D cell culture platforms (Tonti et al., 2021). Diverse tissue types, including cardiac, pulmonary, intestinal, renal, hepatic, and dermal tissues, can be engineered to simulate pathological states in 2D and 3D ECM-like architectures (Tonti et al., 2021). Bioengineered in vitro systems are constructed based on tissue-specific cell sources, including primary cells, cell lines, and stem cells, in combination with various choices of biocompatible or bio-derived soft materials (Wittmann & Fischbach, 2017). In these systems, recapitulation of cell-cell and cell-ECM interactions, in addition to intracellular signaling, can be realized by mimicking specific features of target diseases. This strategy contributes to obtaining mechanistic information on pathological morphogenesis and functionality at the tissue and organ levels.

14.5.2 Organ-on-Chips for Pathological Modeling

Organ-on-a-chip (OoC) models, also known as tissue chips or microphysiological systems, reflect the structural and functional aspects of human pathological tissues by integrating clinically relevant cell phenotypes, engineered ECMs, and vascular- or interstitial-like microflows (Yu & Choudhury, 2019). For the mimicry of tissue-level pathologies, biomaterials-based microfluidic systems provide well-characterized biophysical and biochemical features, such as cell microenvironments, tissue-like architectures, fluid dynamic cues, biomechanical forces, and vascular perfusion with immune cell circulation (Nawroth et al., 2019). Organ-on-a-chip systems are representative platforms for microfluidic disease modeling, which can emulate the pathophysiological environment and functionality on a microfabricated and biomaterial-integrated chip (Ma et al., 2021). These devices may also reproduce complex organ-level responses to pathogens and inflammatory cytokines (Nawroth et al., 2019), as well as drug-induced toxicities (Ma et al., 2021). The monitoring of pathological ECM remodeling and related recruitment of immune cells during inflammation is one of the benefits that can be achieved by organ-on-a-chip platforms (Nawroth et al., 2019). Organ-on-a-chip devices are particularly well-suited not only to investigate the basic mechanisms that are related to acute pathophysiological processes but also to mechanistically test the efficacy and adverse effects of therapeutics using disease models in vitro (Bhatia & Ingber, 2014; Low et al., 2021).

14.5.3 Cardiovascular Diseases on Chip

Cardiovascular disease mimicry on-chip is typically implemented by using heart- or vessel-like tissue scaffolds integrated into a microfluidic cell culture platform (Simon & Masters, 2019). Cardiomyocytes and other disease-specific cells have been encapsulated in hydrogel-based 3D culture platforms to regenerate miniaturized cardiac tissue mimics (Simon & Masters, 2019). The hydrogel platform is mostly composed of collagen fibers and is designed to provide mechanical support, collagen alignment cues, and ECM-associated biochemical signals to seeded cardiac myocytes (Ariyasinghe et al., 2018). In many cardiac diseases, extensive remodeling occurs in the cellular and ECM components of the myocardium (Ariyasinghe et al., 2018), which can be recreated using engineered 3D tissue platforms coupled with microfluidic architectures to incorporate greater microenvironmental complexity (Bhatia & Ingber, 2014).

Pathophysiologically relevant mechanical stresses and/or hypoxic conditions can be induced and applied to the integrated 2D/3D cells in the device (Simon & Masters, 2019). For example, microfluidic models of atherosclerosis and myocardial infarction can be realized by tuning the microchannel constrictions to induce dysfunction of the channel-lining endothelial cells and subsequent adhesion of inflammatory cells, which may result in hypoxia of the gel-embedded cardiomyocytes (Bhatia & Ingber, 2014; Simon & Masters, 2019). Furthermore, endothelial cell-lined valve-like conduits are expected to be fabricated in fluid channels to model aortic valve structures (Nugent & Edelman, 2003). It is likely that the elasticity of artificial valves can be tuned to simulate that of the ECM in injured valve leaflets to monitor hemodynamic alterations under pathological conditions.

Small vasculatures (diameter less than 100 μm) are the most optimal organ that can be recapitulated by microfluidic techniques, based on the fact that the dimension of microchannels is intrinsically appropriate to characterize and predict flow behaviors in laminar regimes (Lust et al., 2021). Moreover, microfluidic platforms can easily reproduce the native hemodynamic factors (i.e., shear rate and residence time in an organ) and the geometric features of local vasculatures and their interconnected networks (Prabhakarpandian et al., 2011). Pathogenesis in the vessels often results in pathological vascular remodeling, the outcome of which can be either vascular occlusion (caused by inward remodeling) or vessel wall weakening (caused by outward remodeling) (Lust et al., 2021). Such a change in diameter alters the blood flow patterns, which may in turn affect the vascular endothelial cells, which are highly sensitive to fluid mechanical cues, including shear force (Lust et al., 2021). Microfluidic models of vasculatures, combined with human cell lines and miniaturized biomaterial scaffolds, can be simple and useful analogs that represent the dynamic aspects of vascular pathophysiology (Lust et al., 2021).

A major challenge in developing cardiovascular OoC platforms is the limited ability to support multi-organ co-cultures for a longer period of time, which is essential for reproducing chronic aspects of cardiovascular diseases on-chip (Paloschi et al., 2021).

14.5.4 Musculoskeletal Diseases on Chip

Bone tissues and skeletal muscles are characterized by remarkably organized architectures and dynamic regulatory functions. The structural unit of compact bone tissues, called the osteon, is a dense mineralized matrix of collagen, where the collagen fibrils are aligned in parallel to form a concentric lamellar structure (Sung & Kim, 2018). Moreover, osteocytes, which are the major cellular component of bone tissues, exhibit prominent mechanosensitivity, and they transduce external mechanical stimuli to coordinate bone remodeling in a dynamic manner (Whelan et al., 2021). In a different aspect, skeletal muscles have a highly organized structure where the muscle fibers are aligned in parallel to be surrounded by connective tissues as a bundle (Arrigoni et al., 2019). Skeletal muscle tissues comprise heterogeneous cell types, such as myoblasts, endothelial cells, fibroblasts, and satellite cells (Arrigoni et al., 2019).

Vasculatures and/or innervation play central roles in the pathophysiology of both tissues. In bone remodeling, vascular invasion is a critical step for endochondral ossification (Whelan et al., 2021). For skeletal muscles, connection to vascular tissues is essential to meet the strong demand for metabolic supply (Arrigoni et al., 2019). Neuromuscular junctions (NMJs) are key regulators of muscle contractile function (Arrigoni et al., 2019). The small scale of NMJ structures and blood flow-related microenvironments is optimal for investigation using microfluidic in vitro tissue platforms (Arrigoni et al., 2019). Microfluidic ECM mimics can be utilized to investigate the migration behavior of muscle cells in pathological states by stably maintaining the concentration gradient of chemotactic agents (Roveimiab et al., 2019). More complex organs in the human skeletal system, such as joints (articulation), may also be recreated using microfluidic devices. The joint is a specific organ where biomechanical interplay between elastic tissues (cartilage, synovial membrane, ligament, tendon, and muscle) and a viscous fluid (synovial fluid) occurs. Therefore, it is a suitable organ system to be realized on a microfluidic chip where dynamic flow patterns and mechanical stimuli are simulated (Piluso et al., 2019).

Current OoC model systems for the mimicry of musculoskeletal diseases have diverse complexity levels in biological and technological aspects and are required to be highly automated, reproducible, and standardized in future developments (Arrigoni et al., 2020).

14.5.5 Endocrine Diseases on Chip

For in vitro endocrine disease models, microfluidic cell culture systems are particularly advantageous in the sense that either continuous or pulsatile flows and exposure in vivo can be replicated on-chip (Bodke & Burdette, 2021). Tissue mimics grown in microfluidic devices can be stimulated by mechanical cues (e.g., fluid shear stress, tension, and compression) as well as biochemical cues (e.g., spatiotemporally controlled gradients of steroids) (Bodke & Burdette, 2021). Pancreas-on-a-chip platforms focus on the endocrine pathophysiology of the pancreas and enable standardized and real-time assessments to evaluate islet potency and quality (Abadpour et al., 2020). Here, the microfluidic islet devices are designed to have trapping sites for islet immobilization and culture under flowing media so that islet viability, composition, and hormonal secretion can be tested on-chip (Abadpour et al., 2020). In particular, the perfusion system acts as a core regulator in the pancreas-on-a-chip such that the perfused fluids maintain the viability of the trapped islets, remove metabolic products, and stimulate the islets with hormones and nutrients (such as glucose) (Abadpour et al., 2020). Precise flow control of the device is crucial for minimizing potential flow-induced damage to islets and for analyzing complex hormone kinetics (Abadpour et al., 2020). The diabetes-on-chip configuration can be based on the mimicry of liver-pancreas (or adipose tissue-pancreas) communications to model how β-cells interact with hepatocytes through blood circulation in terms of glycogen storage and glucose release in response to insulin secretion (Lewis & Wells, 2021).

Microfluidic cell culture devices can mimic the pathophysiology of the human reproductive system (Nawroth et al., 2018). These devices are capable of recreating the complex spatiotemporal patterns of endocrine signaling within and between different organ mimics to simulate remodeling processes during the menstrual cycle and pregnancy (Nawroth et al., 2018). Biomaterials for 3D cell culture empower organ-on-a-chip systems to mimic uterine tissue remodeling, hormone cycling, and cell migration during the menstrual cycle and in endometriosis (Nawroth et al., 2018). The fallopian tube-on-a-chip can be designed to respond to estrogen signals from a connected ovary mimic (Nawroth et al., 2018). Moreover, placenta-on-a-chip platforms can model human placental dysfunctions with a major focus on the understanding of cell-cell and cell-ECM interactions during inflammatory responses caused by bacterial infections to simulate pathological pregnancy (Tutar & Çelebi-Saltik, 2022). 3D bioprinting methods may contribute to the fabrication of placenta-on-a-chip systems with more complex and organized architectures (Yu & Choudhury, 2019). In addition, breast cancer-on-a-chip emulates the tree-like mammary ductal system (size decreases with a higher degree of branching) and recreates ductal carcinoma in vitro to help investigate signaling pathways between tumor cells and endothelial cells (Nawroth et al., 2018).

One of the main limitations in implementing endocrine OoCs is that it is technically challenging to harbor multiple media in a microfluidic perfusion system. Because the optimal culture medium for each cell type is distinct, it is often not straightforward to evaluate whether endocrine, endothelial, and mesenchymal cells function properly in an interconnected culture platform on a chip (Bakhti et al., 2019).

14.5.6 Liver and Kidney Diseases on Chip

The liver is the primary metabolic organ fundamentally related to human pathology and toxicology. Therefore, liver tissue mimicry has been actively implemented based on microfluidic cell culture systems (Zhang et al., 2018). In most liver-mimicking systems, parenchymal cells (hepatocytes and cholangiocytes) and non-parenchymal cells (such as endothelial cells, stellate cells, and Kupffer cells) are integrated into the microfabricated chips (Bhushan et al., 2013) to construct microfluidic architectures similar to the liver sinusoids and associated microenvironments (Yesil-Celiktas et al., 2018). A typical configuration is a two-compartment chip where a layer of parenchymal cells and a non-parenchymal cell-embedded microgel chamber are separated by a porous membrane (Del Piccolo et al., 2021). This approach enables the remodeling of diverse pathological states, including nonalcoholic fatty liver, cancer metastasis to the liver, and infectious diseases caused by viral and parasitic origins (Yesil-Celiktas et al., 2018; Del Piccolo et al., 2021).

Microfluidic platforms for culturing human kidney epithelial cells can mimic the functionality of the kidney proximal tubules under fluid mechanical cues (Peloso et al., 2015). These kidney tubule-on-a-chip devices can maintain the morphology of proximal cells close to in vivo conditions, exhibiting augmented cellular functional responses such as albumin uptake capability (Peloso et al., 2015). The implantation of renal proximal tubular cells in perfused microchannels may improve waste excretion, glucose reabsorption, and molecular clearance, and the application of laminar flows can stimulate cell polarization and related functions (Ashammakhi et al., 2018). Additionally, kidney glomerulus-on-a-chip can be fabricated by seeding glomerular epithelial cells in a microfluidic cell culture device and culturing the kidney endothelium simultaneously (Peloso et al., 2015). Such devices can be designed to maintain transcellular electrochemical and osmotic pressure gradients (Ashammakhi et al., 2018). These miniaturized artificial kidney systems can also be used to investigate the mechanism of kidney stone formation (Peloso et al., 2015).

For microfluidic chip-based liver mimicry, (i) reproduction of liver zonation and (ii) implementation of a collection channel for bile efflux have been generally limited, and the balance between operational simplicity and biological complexity needs to be improved for promoting commercial uses (Moradi et al., 2020). For the fabrication of kidney-on-a-chips, integration of lymphatic/nervous systems with tissue-tissue interactions remains as the main challenge (Ashammakhi et al., 2018).

14.5.7 Brain and Lung Diseases on Chip

The brain and lung are presumed to be the most challenging organs to model using microfluidic biomaterial platforms because of their complex cellular organizations and sophisticated functional dynamics. For on-chip brain mimicry, research has focused on implementing the architecture of the blood-brain barrier (BBB), which is a tightly controlled interface between the blood and brain parenchyma, in a dynamic and physiologically relevant manner (Jackson et al., 2019; Hajal et al., 2021). BBB capillaries, polarized neurons, and supporting cells constitute a neurovascular unit (NVU), and dysfunction of hemodynamics, cell-cell junctions, and barrier permeability of the NVU may cause several brain diseases (Hajal et al., 2021; Del Piccolo et al., 2021). To reconstruct the MEMS-assisted BBB on-a-chip, cells are typically compartmentalized by membrane(s) in microgel-filled chambers and vascular multichannels, where microflows and shear stresses are finely controlled to provide real-time readouts of BBB permeability, transendothelial electrical resistance, cell migration/protrusion, and angiogenesis (Jackson et al., 2019; Hajal et al., 2021; Del Piccolo et al., 2021). In microfluidic chips, the reconstituted pathological states of the BBB (e.g., Alzheimer's disease) can provide mechanistic information on the metabolic pathways between the vasculature and brain parenchymal tissues (Hajal et al., 2021). Moreover, in vivo-like metastatic patterns can be simulated by inducing extravasation of cancer cells into the gel-filled brain parenchymal chamber (Del Piccolo et al., 2021). Neuroinflammation studies are another area that can be supported by BBB-on-chip technology (Bhatia & Ingber, 2014).

Lung-on-a-chip platforms are designed to recreate highly defined functional units of the lung, including the interface between the alveolar epithelium and blood capillaries and the mucociliary barrier of the airways (Nawroth et al., 2019). Microengineered systems can be fabricated to implement the alveolar-capillary boundary on-chip by longitudinally dividing a chamber into two parallel channels and using an ECM-coated porous membrane to simulate the alveolar interstitium (Nawroth et al., 2019). In this design, the human lung epithelial cells are exposed to air on one side, and the pulmonary vascular endothelial cells undergo the influence of microflows to finally form a dynamic in vitro model of the air-liquid interface (Schilders et al., 2016). Flexible membranous materials, together with the device housing elastomers, can be adopted to exert linear or cyclic stretching on the microfluidic chip to recreate the breathing lung motion, which may influence the physiological responses of embedded cells (Nawroth et al., 2019). Such lung-on-a-chip configurations have been widely considered to model the pathology of human airways, such as pro-inflammatory conditions in respiratory diseases provoked by viral or other microbial infections (Yesil-Celiktas et al., 2018; Nawroth et al., 2019).

In spite of prominent progress in the development of brain-on-a-chip systems, regeneration of entire brain tissue, including vasculogenesis and angiogenesis, in a microdevice has been largely limited (Jahromi et al., 2019). Similarly, reconstruction of physiological airflows with aerosol transport mechanics on lung-on-a-chip platforms remains as a major challenge (Artzy-Schnirman et al., 2019).

14.5.8 Other Pathological Tissue Models on Chip

A plethora of other disease models can be recreated using microfluidic biomaterial platforms, depending on the cell co-culture and scaffolding techniques and device microfabrication strategies. One of the emerging in vitro systems is the gut-on-a-chip, which allows the culturing of intestinal epithelial cells in contact with gastric juice flows (Low & Tagle, 2017). Fat-on-a-chip systems are also of major interest in in vitro obesity models (Li & Easley, 2018; McCarthy et al., 2020). Fibrosis-on-a-chip platforms emulate scar tissue formation and its associated pathological morphogenesis, where the accumulation of fibroblasts and deposition of ECM fibers at injury sites induce significant dysfunction in various organs (Hayward et al., 2021). Microfluidic human microbiome cultivation systems for exploring complex host-microbe interactions are highlighted as the frontier of in vitro pathological modeling owing to the central role of microbiomes in a plethora of disease states associated with the lung, gut, skin, and oral cavity (Tan & Toh, 2020). Microfluidics can potentially be used to improve the pathophysiological relevance of current in vitro skin and oral mucosa models (Kinikoglu et al., 2015; Sierra-Sánchez et al., 2021) by miniaturizing tissue-engineered substitutes. Microfluidic placental barrier models are another main area of research that is closely related to clinical pathology (Arumugasaamy et al., 2020).

14.6 CONCLUDING REMARKS

Initially developed as a biomedical microfluidic system inspired by microelectronic chips in the 1990s, the tissue-mimicking biochip devices have now become the most powerful toolkit for implementing a wide range of microphysiological systems for *in vitro* modeling. Depending on the proper choice of biomaterials and their miniaturized 3D architectures, microdevices can efficiently recreate various pathological dynamics on-chip with low consumption of platform-operational energy and by saving expensive experimental resources (such as specially designed cellular specimens and biochemical assays). When multiplexed, the biochips for disease modeling are expected to reflect multi-organ functionalities through improved methods of scaling, vascularization, and innervation (Park et al., 2020). Nevertheless, connecting multiple tissue chips through a microfluidic system is a challenging task for reverse engineering interlinked organ networks on a microfabricated platform (Low et al., 2021). Furthermore, synergetic coupling between induced pluripotent stem cells and patient-derived primary cells is required for advancements in tissue-mimicking biochip systems, especially with respect to applications in personalized therapeutics (Low et al., 2021). One of the main goals of 3D biomaterial chips for pathological modeling is to fill the data gap between traditional *2D in vitro* testing and laboratory animal models with enhanced prediction capability (Guttenplan et al., 2021). However, to better reflect the physiological and pathological conditions of the *in vivo* ECM environments, there is a strong need to fully integrate mechanical and topographical cues in the artificial tissue compartments of biochips by locally tuning the matrix compliance and introducing higher-order anisotropy in the nanoscale architecture of miniaturized ECM mimics (Sung & Kim, 2018). Facilitated clinical translation, driven by pathological tissue-on-chip technology, could contribute to the future evolution of precision medicine.

ACKNOWLEDGMENTS

The author deeply appreciates Professor Andreas Manz (KIST Europe & Saarland University) for his valuable advice and comments on the manuscript.

REFERENCES

Abadpour S., Aizenshtadt A., Olsen P.A., Shoji K., Wilson S.R., Krauss S., Scholz H., Pancreas-on-a-chip technology for transplantation applications. *Curr. Diabet. Rep.* **20**: 72 (2020).

Arrigoni C., Lopa S., Candrian C., Moretti M., Organs-on-a-chip as model systems for multifactorial musculoskeletal diseases. *Curr. Opin. Biotechnol.* **63**: 79–88 (2020).

Arrigoni C., Petta D., Bersini S., Mironov V., Candrian C., Moretti M., Engineering complex muscle-tissue interfaces through microfabrication. *Biofabrication* **11**: 032004 (2019).

Ariyasinghe N.R., Lyra-Leite D.M., McCain M.L., Engineering cardiac microphysiological systems to model pathological extracellular matrix remodeling. *Am. J. Physiol. Heart Circ. Physiol.* **315**: H771–H789 (2018).

Artzy-Schnirman A., Hobi N., Schneider-Daum N., Guenat O.T., Lehr C.-M., Sznitman J., Advanced in vitro lung-on-chip platforms for inhalation assays: from prospect to pipeline. *Eur. J. Pharmaceut. Biopharmaceut.* **144**: 11–17 (2019).

Arumugasaamy N., Rock K.D., Kuo C.-Y., Bale T.L., Fisher J.P., Microphysiological systems of the placental barrier. *Adv. Drug Deliv. Res.* **161–162**: 161–175 (2020).

Ashammakhi N., Wesseling-Perry K., Hasan A., Elkhammas E., Zhang Y.S., Kidney-on-a-chip: Untapped opportunities. *Kidney Int.* **94**: 1073–1086 (2018).

Atencia J., Beebe D.J., Controlled microfluidic interfaces. *Nature* **437**: 648–655 (2005).

Baker M., A living system on a chip. *Nature* **471**: 661–665 (2011).

Bakhti M., Böttcher A., Lickert H., Modelling the endocrine pancreas in health and disease. *Nat. Rev. Endocrinol.* **15**: 155–171 (2019).

Batchelor G.K., *An Introduction to Fluid Dynamics* (Cambridge University Press, Cambridge, 1967).

Benam K.H., Dauth S., Hassell B., Herland A., Jain A., Jang K.-J., Karalis K., Kim H.J., MacQueen L., Mahmoodian R., Musah S., Torisawa Y., van der Meer A.D., Villenave R., Yadid M., Parker K.K., Ingber D.E., Engineered in vitro disease models. *Annu. Rev. Pathol.: Mechanisms Disease* **10**: 195–262 (2015).

Bhatia S.N., Ingber D.E., Microfluidic organs-on-chips. *Nat. Biotechnol.* **32**: 760–772 (2014).

Bhushan A., Senutovitch N., Bale S.S., McCarty W.J., Hegde M., Jindal R., Golberg I., Usta O.B., Yarmush M.L., Vernetti L., Gough A., Bakan A., Shun T.Y., DeBiasio R., Taylor D.L., Towards a three-dimensional microfluidic liver platform for predicting drug effi cacy and toxicity in humans. *Stem Cell Res. Ther.* **4**: S16 (2013).

Bodke V.V., Burdette J.E., Advancements in microfluidic systems for the study of female reproductive biology. *Endocrinology* **162**: 1–14 (2021).

Chaterji S., Kwon I.K., Park K., Smart polymeric gels: Redefining the limits of biomedical devices. *Prog. Polym. Sci.* **32**: 1083–1122 (2007).

Chen X., Shen J., Review of membranes in microfluidics. *J. Chem. Technol. Biotechnol.* **92**: 271–282 (2017)

Coutinho D., Costa P., Neves N., Gomes M.E., Reis R.L., Micro- and nanotechnology in tissue engineering. In: Pallua N., Suschek C.V. (eds.), *Tissue Engineering* (Springer, Berlin, 2011).

Del Piccolo N., Shirure V.S., Bi Y., Goedegebuure P., Gholami S., Hughes C.C.W., Fields R.C., George S.C., Tumor-on-chip modeling of organ-specific cancer and metastasis. *Adv. Drug Deliv. Rev.* **175**: 113798 (2021).

Dittrich P.S., Manz A., Lab-on-a-chip: Microfluidics in drug discovery. *Nat. Rev. Drug Discov.* **5**: 210–218 (2006).

Dong R., Liu Y., Mou L., Deng J., Jiang X., Microfluidics-based biomaterials and biodevices. *Adv. Mater.* **31**: e1805033 (2019).

Duncombe T.A., Tentori A.M., Herr A.E., Microfluidics: Reframing biological enquiry. *Nat. Rev. Mol. Cell Biol.* **16**: 554–567 (2015).

Domachuk P., Tsioris K., Omenetto F.G., Kaplan D.L., Bio-microfluidics: Biomaterials and biomimetic designs. *Adv. Mater.* **22**: 249–260 (2010).

Eichler M., Klages C.-P., Lachmann K., Surface functionalization of microfluidic devices. In: Dietzel A. (ed.), *Microsystems for Pharmatechnology* (Springer, Cham, 2016).

Gentsch R., Börner H.G., Designing three-dimensional materials at the interface to biology. *Adv. Polym. Sci.* **240**: 163–192 (2011).

Guttenplan A.P.M., Birgani Z.T., Giselbrecht S., Truckenmüller R.K., Habibović P., Chips for biomaterials and biomaterials for chips: Recent advances at the interface between microfabrication and biomaterials research. *Adv. Healthcare Mater.* **10**: 2100371 (2021).

Gurkan U.A., Tasoglu S., Kavaz D., Demirel M.C., Demirci U., Emerging technologies for assembly of microscale hydrogels. *Adv. Healthcare Mater.* **1**: 149–158 (2012).

Hajal C., Le Roi B., Kamm R.D., Maoz B.M., Biology and models of the blood-brain barrier. *Annu. Rev. Biomed. Eng.* **23**: 359–84 (2021).

Halldorsson S., Lucumi E., Gómez-Sjöberg R., Fleming R.M.T., Advantages and challenges of microfluidic cell culture in polydimethylsiloxane devices. *Biosens. Bioelectron.* **63**: 218–231 (2015)

Hayward K.L., Kouthouridis S., Zhang B., Organ-on-a-chip systems for modeling pathological tissue morphogenesis associated with fibrosis and cancer. *ACS Biomater. Sci. Eng.* **7**: 2900–2925 (2021)

Huh D., Hamilton G.A., Ingber D.E., From 3D cell culture to organs-on-chips. *Trends Cell Biol.* **21**: 745–754 (2011).

Huh D., Torisawa Y., Hamilton G.A., Kim H.J., Ingber D.E., Microengineered physiological biomimicry: Organs-on-chips. *Lab Chip* **12**: 2156–2164 (2012).

Ingber D.E., Reverse engineering human pathophysiology with organs-on-chips. *Cell* **164**: 1105–1109 (2016).

Ingber D.E., Human organs-on-chips for disease modelling, drug development and personalized medicine. *Nat. Rev. Genet.* (2022). doi: 10.1038/s41576-022-00466-9.

Jackson S., Meeks C., Vézina A., Robey R.W., Tanner K., Gottesman M.M., Model systems for studying the blood-brain barrier: Applications and changes. *Biomaterials* **214**: 119217 (2019).

Jahromi M.A.M., Abdoli A., Rahmanian M., Bardania H., Bayandori M., Basri S.M.M., Kalbasi A., Aref A.R., Karimi M., Hamblin M.R., Microfluidic brain-on-a-chip: Perspectives for mimicking neural system disorders. *Mol. Neurobiol.* **56**: 8489–8512 (2019)

Kinikoglu B., Damour O., Hasirci V., Tissue engineering of oral mucosa: A shared concept with skin. *J. Artif. Organs* **18**: 8–19 (2015).

Kobel S., Lutolf M.P., Biomaterials meet microfluidics: Building the next generation of artificial niches. *Curr. Opin. Biotechnol.* **22**: 690–697 (2011).

Koev S.T., Dykstra P.H., Luo X., Rubloff G.W., Bentley W.E., Payne G.F., Ghodssi R., Chitosan: An integrative biomaterial for lab-on-a-chip devices. *Lab Chip* **10**: 3026–3042 (2010).

Leester-Schädel M., Lorenz T., Jürgens F., Richter C., Fabrication of microfluidic devices. In: Dietzel A. (ed.), *Microsystems for Pharmatechnology* (Springer, Cham, 2016).

Le Goff G.C., Srinivas R.L., Hill W.A., Doyle P.S., Hydrogel microparticles for biosensing. *Eur. Polym. J.* **72**: 386–412 (2015).

Lewis P.L., Wells J.M., Engineering-inspired approaches to study β-cell function and diabetes. *Stem Cells* **39**: 522–535 (2021).

Li X., Easley C., Microfluidic systems for studying dynamic function of adipocytes and adipose tissue. *Anal. Bioanal. Chem.* **410**: 791–800 (2018).

Low L.A., Tagle D.A., Tissue chips - innovative tools for drug development and disease modeling. *Lab Chip* **17**: 3026–3036 (2017).

Low L.A., Sutherland M., Lumelsky N., Selimovic S., Lundberg M.S., Tagle D.A., Organs-on-a-Chip. In: Oliveira J.M., Reis R.L. (eds.), *Biomaterials- and Microfluidics-Based Tissue Engineered 3D Models* (Springer, Cham, 2020).

Low L.A., Mummery C., Berridge B.R., Austin C.P., Tagle D.A., Organs-on-chips: into the next decade. *Nat. Rev. Drug Discov.* **20**: 345–361 (2021).

Lust S.T., Shanahan C.M., Shipley R.J., Lamata P., Gentleman E., Design considerations for engineering 3D models to study vascular pathologies in vitro. *Acta Biomaterialia* **132**: 114–128 (2021).

Ma C., Peng Y., Li H., Chen W., Organ-on-a-chip: A new paradigm for drug development. *Trends Pharmacol. Sci.* **42**:119–133 (2021).

Manz A., Miniaturized total chemical analysis systems: A novel concept for chemical sensing. *Sensors Actuators B* **1**: 244–248 (1990).

Manz A., Neužil P., O'Connor J.S., Simone G., *Microfluidics and Lab-on-a-Chip* (Royal Society of Chemistry Publishing, London, 2020).

McCarthy M., Brown T., Alarcon A., Williams C., Wu X., Abbott R.D., Gimble J., Frazier T., Fat-on-a-chip models for research and discovery in obesity and its metabolic comorbidities. *Tissue Eng. Part B Rev*. **26**: 586–595 (2020).

Moradi E., Jalili-Firoozinezhad S., Solati-Hashjin M., Microfluidic organ-on-a-chip models of human liver tissue. *Acta Biomaterialia* **116**: 67–83 (2020).

Nawroth J., Rogal J., Weiss M., Brucker S.Y., Loskill P., Organ-on-a-chip systems for women's health applications. *Adv. Healthcare Mater*. **7**: 1700550 (2018).

Nawroth J., Barrile R., Conegliano D., van Riet S., Hiemstra P.S., Villenave R., Stem cell-based lung-on-chips: The best of both worlds? *Adv. Drug Deliv. Rev*. **140**: 12–32 (2019).

Ning R.Z., Wang F., Lin L., Biomaterial-based microfluidics for cell culture and analysis. *Tredns Anal. Chem*. **80**: 255–265 (2016).

Nugent H.M., Edelman E.R., Tissue engineering therapy for cardiovascular disease. *Circ. Res*. **92**:1068–1078 (2003).

Paloschi V., Sabater-Lleal M., Middelkamp H., Vivas A., Johansson S., van der Meer A., Tenje M., Maegdefessel L., Organ-on-a-chip technology: A novel approach to investigate cardiovascular diseases. *Cardiovasc. Res*. **117**: 2742–2754 (2021).

Park D.Y., Lee J., Chung J.J., Jung Y., Kim S.H., Integrating organs-on-chips: multiplexing, scaling, vascularization, and innervation. *Trends Biotechnol*. **38**: 99–112 (2020).

Park J., Lakes R.S., *Biomaterials: An Introduction* (3rd ed., Springer, New York, 2007).

Peloso A., Katari R., Murphy S.V., Zambon J.P., DeFrancesco A., Farney A.C., Rogers J., Stratta R.J., Manzia T.M., Orlando G., Prospect for kidney bioengineering: Shortcomings of the status quo. *Expert Opin. Biol. Ther*. **15**:547–58 (2015).

Piazza R., *Soft Matter* (Springer, Dordrecht, 2011).

Piluso S., Li Y., Abinzano F., Levato R., Teixeira L.M., Karperien M., Leijten J., van Weeren R., Malda J., Mimicking the articular joint with in vitro models. *Trends Biotechnol*. **37**: 1063–1077 (2019).

Prabhakarpandian B., Shen M.-C., Pant K., Kiani M.F., Microfluidic devices for modeling cell-cell and particle-cell interactions in the microvasculature. *Microvascul. Res*. **82**: 210–220 (2011).

Roveimiab Z., Lin F., Anderson J.E., Emerging development of microfluidic-based approaches to improve studies of muscle cell migration. *Tissue Eng. Part B Rev*. **25**: 30–45 (2019).

Sakthivel K., O'Brien A., Kim K., Hoorfar M., Microfluidic analysis of heterotypic cellular interactions: A review of techniques and applications. *Trends Anal. Chem*. **117**: 166–185 (2019).

Schilders K.A.A., Eenjes E., van Riet S., Poot A.A., Stamatialis D., Truckenmüller R., Hiemstra P.S., Rottier R.J., Regeneration of the lung: Lung stem cells and the development of lung mimicking devices. *Respir. Res*. **17**: 44 (2016).

Shao Y., Fu J., Integrated micro/nanoengineered functional biomaterials for cell mechanics and mechanobiology: A materials perspective. *Adv. Mater*. **26**: 1494–1533 (2014).

Sierra-Sánchez Á., Kim K.H., Blasco-Morente G., Arias-Santiago S., Cellular human tissue-engineered skin substitutes investigated for deep and difficult to heal injuries. *NPJ Regen. Med*. **6**: 35 (2021).

Simon L.R., Masters K.S., Disease-inspired tissue engineering: Investigation of cardiovascular pathologies. *ACS Biomater. Sci. Eng*. **6**: 2518–2532 (2020).

Smith I.O., Ma P.X., Biomimetic scaffolds in tissue engineering. In: Pallua N., Suschek C.V. (eds.), *Tissue Engineering* (Springer, Berlin, 2011).

Solanki S., Pandey C.M., Biological applications of microfluidics system. In: Dixit C.K., Kaushik A. (eds.), *Microfluidics for Biologists* (Springer, Basel, 2016).

Sung B., Kim M.-H., Cell-encapsulating polymeric microgels for tissue repair. In: Khang G. (ed.), *Handbook of Intelligent Scaffolds for Tissue Engineering and Regenerative Medicine* (2nd ed.; Pan Stanford Publishing, Singapore, 2017).

Sung B., Kim M.-H., Liquid-crystalline nanoarchitectures for tissue engineering. *Beilstein J. Nanotechnol.* **9**: 205–215 (2018).

Sung B., Kim M.-H., Abelmann L., Magnetic microgels and nanogels: Physical mechanisms and biomedical applications. *Bioeng. Transl. Med.* **6**: e10190 (2021).

Sung B., In silico modeling of endocrine organ-on-a-chip systems. *Math. Biosci.* **352**: 108900 (2022).

Tan H.-Y., Toh Y.-C., What can microfluidics do for human microbiome research? *Biomicrofluidics* **14**: 051303 (2020).

Tavana H., Chung Y.-K., Kuo C.-H., Takayama S., Microfluidic systems for cellular applications. In: Tian W.-C., Finehout E. (eds.), *Microfluidics for Biological Applications* (Springer, New York, 2008).

Tian C., Tu Q., Liu W., Wang J., Recent advances in microfluidic technologies for organ-on-a-chip. *Trends Anal. Chem.* **117**: 146–156 (2019).

Tonti O.R., Larson H., Lipp S.N., Luetkemeyer C.M., Makam M., Vargas D., Wilcox S.M., Calve S., Tissue-specific parameters for the design of ECM-mimetic biomaterials. *Acta Biomaterialia* **132**: 83–102 (2021).

Tutar R., Çelebi-Saltik B., Modeling of artificial 3D human placenta. *Cells Tissues Organs* **211**: 36–45 (2022).

Whelan I.T., Moeendarbary E., Hoey D.A., Kelly D.J., Biofabrication of vasculature in microphysiological models of bone. *Biofabrication* **13**: 032004 (2021).

Wittmann K., Fischbach C., Contextual control of adipose-derived stem cell function: Implications for engineered tumor models. *ACS Biomater. Sci. Eng.* **3**: 1483–1493 (2017).

Wolfram C.J., Rubloff G.W., Luo X., Perspectives in flow-based microfluidic gradient generators for characterizing bacterial chemotaxis. *Biomicrofluidics* **10**: 061301 (2016).

Van Duinen V., Trietsch S.J., Joore J., Vulto P., Hankemeier T., Microfluidic 3D cell culture: From tools to tissue models. *Curr. Opin. Biotechnol.* **35**: 118–126 (2015).

Xie R., Zheng W., Guan L., Ai Y., Liang Q., Engineering of hydrogel materials with perfusable microchannels for building vascularized tissues. *Small* **16**: 1902838 (2020).

Yesil-Celiktas O., Hassan S., Miri A.K., Maharjan S., Al-kharboosh R., Quiñones-Hinojosa A., Zhang Y.S., Mimicking human pathophysiology in organ-on-chip devices. *Adv. Biosys.* **2**: 1800109 (2018).

Yu F., Choudhury D., Microfluidic bioprinting for organ-on-a-chip models. *Drug Discov. Today* **24**: 1248–1257 (2019).

Zhang B., Korolj A., Lai B.F.L., Radisic M., Advances in organ-on-a-chip engineering. *Nat. Rev. Mater.* **3**: 257–278 (2018).

Index

3D bioprinting 24, 30, 61, 99, 222

acellular hydrogels 112
acute wounds 91
adipose tissue engineering 255
Agrawal, G. 151
Ajay Rakkesh, R. 255
alginate-based composite hydrogels 260
antigen/antibody-responsive hydrogels 8
axonal degeneration 41
Ayan, S. 99

Baino, F. 175
Basnal, Y. 77
Bedir, T. 37
Behere, I. 213
Blessy Rebecca, P. N. 255
bioactive cement 282
bioactive ceramics 276
bioactive glasses 175
biogenic materials 77, 79, 80
bioprinting techniques 24, 108, 250, 298
biosensors 204
bone organoids 219
bone-repairing composites 277
bone tissue regeneration 114, 237
bovine serum albumin 157, 181, 204

cartilage tissue regeneration 29, 213
cell-free approach 220
cell-laden hydrogels 30, 108, 109, 110
cellulose acetate 244
ceramic-polymer nanocomposites 281
ceramics-metal composites 277
ceramics-polymer composites 278
Cesur, S. 37
chitin 24, 48, 83, 104, 133, 281
chondro-inductive molecules 228
chondrogenesis 24, 31, 229
chronic wounds 91, 200
collagen-based composites 239
composite cryogels 195, 228
composite hydrogels 106, 113, 259
conductive polymers 51
copolymeric hydrogels 106
cryogelation 195
cryogels 193, 228

decellularized hydrogel 102
dextran 137, 138, 162, 200
Dhiman, A. 151
Dipin Das, A. K. 131
Dogan. E. 19
Durgalakshmi, D. 255

Ekren, N. 19, 37, 99
electric/magnetic-responsive hydrogels 3
enzyme-responsive hydrogels 7
extrusion-based bioprinting 25, 223

fibrin-based composite hydrogels 262

Ghosh, S. 237
glucose-responsive hydrogels 5
glycosaminoglycans 20, 52, 238
Gorgani, S. 175
Gunduz, O. 19, 37, 99
Gupta, A. 151

Haniu, H. 237
Holkar, K. 213
hyaluronic acid-based composite hydrogels 261
hydrogel scaffold 29, 110, 116, 221, 239, 295
hydroxyapatite 110, 224, 240, 276
hydroxycarbonate apatite 177

icariin 114
induced pluripotent stem cells 30, 91, 304
Ingavle, G. 213
inkjet bioprinting 26

Kargozar, S. 175
Kepekçi, R.-A. 1
Kermani, F. 175

laser-assisted bioprinting 27
light/photo-responsive hydrogels 2

macroporous hydrogels 193
macroporous scaffold 195
magnetic nanoparticles 4, 162, 164, 185, 248
matrigel-based composite hydrogels 262
mesenchymal stem cells 20, 90, 108, 181, 198, 225, 240
methacrylate-based hydrogels 50
methylcellulose 48, 86, 109, 199, 265
methylprednisolone 41
microcontact printing 292
microelectronic chip 292, 304
microfluidics system 289
micromixing 293
Miyazaki, T. 275

Mollazadeh, S. 175
Mostafavi, E. 237

nacre teeth 80
nanofibers 52, 153, 228, 242, 263
natural polymers 87, 133, 215, 223, 244, 258
naturally derived hydrogels 264
nerve regeneration 42, 198
neural tissue engineering 42, 83

open-pore microgel 264
osteoinductive effect 242

pathological modeling 298
pH-responsive hydrogels 5
photopolymerization 24, 44, 104, 166
poly(2-hydroxyethyl methacrylate) 105
poly(amidoamine) 139
poly(ethylene glycol) 22, 50, 104, 263
poly(ethylene glycol)-diacrylate hydrogels 263
poly(lactic-co-glycolic acid) 49, 197, 242, 263
poly(vinyl alcohol) 105, 279, 281
poly(ε-caprolactone) 279, 281
polyacrylamides 105
polydimethylsiloxane 281, 294
polyhydroxyvalerate 250
polysaccharide-based hydrogels 103
pressure/strain-responsive hydrogels 4
protein-based hydrogels 102
pullulan 139, 140

redox-responsive hydrogels 6
Rekha, M. R. 131

Sajeesh, S. 131
Samal, S. K. 151
Savina, I. N. 193
secretome 217, 229
segmental demyelination 41
self-assembly peptides 50
silicone ball 81
stimuli-responsive hydrogels 1
stimuli-responsive microgels 151, 155, 165
Suhag, D. 77
Sung, B. 289
synthetic hydrogels 11, 49, 104, 219

temperature-responsive hydrogels 2
theranostics 151, 165
Thongmee, S. 237
three-dimensional microenvironment 213
tissue mimicry 296
Torun, S. S. 19

ultrasound-responsive hydrogels 4
Ustundag, C. B. 19, 37, 99

vascular tissue engineering 202

Wallerian degeneration 41

Xyloglucan 49

Yıldırım, R. 99

For Product Safety Concerns and Information please contact our EU representative GPSR@taylorandfrancis.com
Taylor & Francis Verlag GmbH, Kaufingerstraße 24, 80331 München, Germany

www.ingramcontent.com/pod-product-compliance
Lightning Source LLC
Chambersburg PA
CBHW060328220326
41598CB00023B/2646

* 9 7 8 1 0 3 2 1 7 0 9 0 9 *